Psychiatric

NURSING

· EXAMINATION ·

REVIEW

Psychiatric

NURSING

·EXAMINATION·

REVIEW

502 QUESTIONS IN PSYCHIATRIC-MENTAL HEALTH NURSING

INCLUDES REFERENCED EXPLANATORY ANSWERS,
STUDY OUTLINE, AND PHARMACOLOGY GUIDE

· EDITED BY ·

SYLVIA K. FIELDS, Ed.D., R.N.
Formerly Director of Undergraduate Program,
Nell Hodgson Woodruff School of Nursing, Emory
University, Atlanta, Georgia

RUTH YURCHUCK, Ed.D., R.N.
Associate Professor, Nell Hodgson Woodruff School
of Nursing, Emory University, Atlanta, Georgia

 MEDICAL EXAMINATION PUBLISHING CO., INC.
an Excerpta Medica company

Main entry under title:

Psychiatric nursing examination review

    Bibliography: p.
    1. Psychiatric nursing—Examinations, questions, etc. I. Fields, Sylvia Kleiman. II. Yurchuck, Ruth. [DNLM: 1. Psychiatric nursing—Examination questions. 2. Psychiatric nursing—Outlines. WY 18 P9763]
RC440.P743   1984   610.73′68   84-6596
ISBN-0-87488-500-0

notice

The editors, authors, and the publisher of this book have made every effort to ensure that all therapeutic modalities that are recommended are in accordance with accepted standards at the time of publication.

    The drugs specified within this book may not have specific approval from the Food and Drug Administration in regard to the indications and dosages that may be recommended by the authors. The manufacturer's package insert is the best source of current prescribing information.

To our Editor, Esther Gumpert,
who somehow managed to maintain sanity
for all of us.

Contents

PART I
Basic Knowledge Essential to the Care of Clients with Psychiatric Problems

PART II
Nursing Self-Assessment and Review

Contributors

Sharon L. Anderson, M.S., M.Ed., R.N., Assistant Professor, Long Island College Hospital, School of Nursing, Brooklyn, New York

Donald G. Barstow, B.A., B.S., M.A., M.S., Faculty, Central State University, Edmond, Oklahoma

Loretta M. Birckhead, M.S., Ed.D., R.N., Psychotherapist and Associate Professor, San Diego State University, San Diego, California

Judy A. Bourrand, M.S.N., R.N., Assistant Professor, Samford University School of Nursing, Birmingham, Alabama

Elizabeth B. Brophy, Ph.D., R.N., Associate Professor, Loyola University of Chicago, Chicago, Illinois

Margery Menges Chisholm, M.S., C.A.G.S., Ed.D., R.N., Associate Professor and Associate Dean for Graduate Study, Boston University, Boston, Massachusetts

Rose Eva Bana Constantino, Ph.D., J.D., R.N., Associate Professor of Psychiatric–Mental Health Nursing, University of Pittsburgh School of Nursing, Pittsburgh, Pennsylvania

Lillian A. Dibner, C.S., Ed.D., R.N., Family Therapist (Private Practice), Associate Professor, Southern Connecticut State University, New Haven, Connecticut

Catherine Dickens, R.Ph., R.N., Staff Nurse and Staff Pharmacist, De Kalb General Hospital, Atlanta, Georgia

Sandra Perrin Gunderson, M.S.N., R.N., Assistant Professor, Psychiatric Mental–Health Nursing, Nazareth College, Kalamazoo, Michigan

Mary Lou Hamilton, M.S., R.N., Assistant Professor, University of Delaware College of Nursing, Newark, Delaware

Jan Heineken, Ph.D., R.N., Associate Professor, San Diego University School of Nursing, San Diego, California

Kathleen T. Heinrich, M.S.N., Certified Mental Health/Psychiatric Adult Clinical Specialist and Assistant Professor of Nursing, University of Hartford, West Hartford, Connecticut

Carolyn C. Hoch, Ph.D., C.S., R.N., Assistant Professor, University of Pittsburgh School of Nursing, Pittsburgh, Pennsylvania

Lynette Wrisley Jack, M.N., R.N., Assistant Professor, Undergraduate Program, University of Pittsburgh School of Nursing, Pittsburgh, Pennsylvania

Jeanette Lancaster, Ph.D., R.N., Professor and Chairman, M.S.N. Degree Program, University of Alabama School of Nursing, Birmingham, Alabama

Donna Gilmore Miller, M.S., R.N., Assistant Professor, FLEX Coordinator, Division of Nursing, Grand View College, Des Moines, Iowa

Joan M. Monchak, M.S.N., R.N., Instructor; Consultant and Therapist, Psychiatric–Mental Health Nursing, Union Memorial Hospital School of Nursing, Baltimore, Maryland

Jane Stacy Mulaik, Ph.D., R.N., Associate Professor, Emory University, Nell Hodgson Woodruff School of Nursing, Atlanta, Georgia

Nancy K. Nally, M.S., R.N., Assistant Professor of Psychiatric–Mental Health Nursing, Hampton Institute School of Nursing, Hampton, Virginia

Rebecca W. Newsome, M.S., R.N., Assistant Professor of Psychiatric–Mental Health Nursing, Hampton Institute School of Nursing, Hampton, Virginia

Beverlyanne Robinson, Ph.D., R.N., Director, Division of Nursing, University of Texas, Austin School of Nursing, Austin, Texas

Carolyn Shinsky Schmidt, Ph.D., C.S., R.N., Assistant Professor, University of Pittsburgh School of Nursing, Pittsburgh, Pennsylvania

Barbara Smith, M.N. Ed., R.N., Assistant Professor, University of Pittsburgh School of Nursing, Pittsburgh, Pennsylvania

Jane Metcalf Smith, M.Ed., M.S.N., R.N., Associate Professor and Coordinator of Nursing Education, Brenau College, Gainesville, Georgia

Hope Titlebaum, M.S., C.S., R.N., Instructor of Psychiatric Nursing, University of Rochester, Rochester, New York; Clinician II, Strong Memorial Hospital, Department of Psychiatry, Rochester, New York

Mary S. Turner, M.S., C.S., R.N., Assistant Professor and Clinician II, University of Rochester School of Nursing, Rochester, New York

Preface

Psychiatric Nursing Examination Review is one of four books in the Medical Examination Publishing Company's Nursing Review Series. The purposes of this book are: (1) to provide the student with a convenient, concise review of the essential content in psychiatric nursing at the conclusion of a course; and (2) to assist the student and graduate nurse in preparing for the National Council Licensure Examination for Registered Nurses (NCLEX-RN).

The book consists of two parts. In Part I, a series of concise outlines identify knowledge essential to the care of clients with psychiatric problems and selected representative health deviations. The health problems are conveniently arranged by body system for easy identification. Part II contains a series of review questions to test one's knowledge of content essential to providing safe care to clients with psychiatric problems and selected health deviations. These questions are similar in focus and content to those included in the NCLEX-RN. The combination of outlined nursing content and review questions should facilitate your self-assessment and the application of pertinent knowledge to the care of clients with psychiatric problems.

Every attempt has been made to ensure the accuracy of content in the outlines and review questions; however, as nursing and medical treatment modalities are constantly changing, some of the information may be superseded by new diagnostic and treatment approaches. Since practices may vary across the country, general principles should be considered rather than specific directives.

The content outlines have been developed by an experienced nursing faculty. Review questions were solicited from experienced clinicians and nursing faculties from across the country. Faculty contributors represent a variety of nursing programs preparing students for licensure as registered nurses. Selection of content for study and correct responses to test items, including identification of nursing behaviors and laws of decision making, represent the contributor's best opinions. The editors can only suggest these areas for review and consideration, since no assurances can be made regarding the actual content on the national examinations.

Acknowledgments

We would like to express our appreciation to the many contributors who assisted us in the preparation of this book. Preparing examination questions according to our stringent guidelines was by no means an easy task. Outline writing is really a challenge given the strict limitations on words and time. We are truly indebted to our secretaries, Kathy Fortune in Atlanta and Mary Ellen D'Orazio in Philadelphia, who kept the Federal Express lines on track. Special thanks are offered to Alan and Steven Yurchuck, whose contributions of patience, encouragement, and understanding have made it possible. Special thanks also to Esther Gumpert, our Editor, who gave us the support and encouragement to achieve our goals. Thank you, thank you.

Introduction

In July 1982, a new test plan format was adopted for the NCLEX-RN. The examination still tests ability to apply nursing knowledge in specific health care situations. However, the test plan that determines selection of items included in the examination now consists of three components: (1) nursing behaviors (i.e., steps of the nursing process), (2) systems of client health requirements (i.e., designated in relation to locus of decision making), and (3) scope of care to be provided and levels of cognitive ability. Brief definitions of these terms, as used by the National Council of State Boards of Nursing, are as follows:

Nursing behavior:

1. Assessing: establishing a data base about a client
2. Analyzing: identifying the client's health care needs and selecting goals of care
3. Planning: designing a strategy to achieve the goals established for client care
4. Implementing: initiating and completing actions necessary to accomplish the defined goals
5. Evaluating: determining the extent to which the goals of care have been achieved

Systems of client health requirements:

Locus of decision making:

1. Centered in nurse when clients are unable to make decisions regarding their physical and/or psychologic status

2. Shared by nurse and client when client is able to exercise partial control in meeting health requirements and to perform selected activities of daily living
3. Centered in clients when they are able to manage their health care needs independently

Levels of cognitive ability:

1. Knowledge: remembering previously learned material
2. Comprehension: ability to grasp the meaning of material, which may be shown by translating material from one form to another, interpreting material, and estimating future trends
3. Application: ability to use learned material in new and concrete situations
4. Analysis: ability to break down material into its component parts so that its organizational structure may be understood

Having completed a course in psychiatric nursing*, and to prepare for the NCLEX-RN, you will find it useful to use this review book as an adjunct to your class notes and nursing texts. The outlines in Part I of the book may be used as a concise review of knowledge essential to providing care to clients with psychiatric problems and common recurring health problems. The content outlines cannot replace a standard nursing textbook or your own class notes, but they may assist you in highlighting significant aspects in the care of clients with psychiatric problems.

In Part II of this book, you will have the opportunity to test your knowledge of the care of clients with psychiatric problems through the multiple-choice questions. The review questions are organized by body system and include aspects of pharmacology, medical management, nutrition, social, and biologic sciences, as well as nursing management of clients with specific health deviations. While it is important to recognize that these questions can only sample the knowledge

---

*Course titles may vary, i.e., Mental and Physical Illness of Adults, Psychiatric Nursing, etc.

base required for safe nursing practice for clients with psychiatric problems, they should nevertheless build confidence both in your grasp of the information and in taking multiple-choice tests. They should also prepare you for the type of questions you will find on the NCLEX-RN examination in that they reflect the structure of the exam in terms of nursing behaviors, locus of decision making, and levels of cognitive ability. As you use these questions to assess your knowledge of the nursing care of clients with representative health deviations, you will find the classification of each item in the section which describes the rationale for the correct answers. Since each answer is keyed to a major nursing textbook, you will also have easy access to additional information about a particular topic.

Some questions may refer to terms considered "nursing diagnoses." These terms may be used in course content both in the classroom and in the clinical areas. To assist you with review a listing of such terms follows this Introduction. We recommend that you attempt to define each of these terms for clarification and understanding before approaching the review process. Try to think of an example for each before or after you review the outline. We believe you will find this helpful as you attempt to answer the assessment questions.

Selected Nursing Diagnoses*

Airway clearance, ineffective.
Bowel elimination, alteration in, constipation.
Bowel elimination, alteration in, diarrhea.
Bowel elimination, alteration in, incontinence.
Breathing pattern, ineffective.
Cardiac output, alteration in, decreased.
Comfort, alteration in, pain.
Communication, impaired verbal.
Coping, family, potential for growth.
Coping, ineffective, family, compromised.
Coping, ineffective, family, disabling.
Coping, ineffective, individual.
Diversional activity, deficit.
Fear.
Fluid volume deficit, actual.
Fluid volume deficit, potential.
Gas exchange, impaired.
Grieving, anticipatory.
Grieving, dysfunctional.
Home maintenance management, impaired.
Injury, potential for (specify). E.g., potential for, poisoning;
    potential for, suffocation; potential for, trauma.

---

*Diagnoses accepted at the fourth and fifth national conferences or recommended
for acceptance.

Knowledge deficit (specify).

Mobility, impaired physical.

Noncompliance (specify).

Nutrition, alteration in, less than body requirements.

Nutrition, alteration in, more than body requirements.

Nutrition, alteration in, potential for more than body requirements.

Parenting, alteration in, actual.

Parenting, alteration in, potential.

Rape-trauma syndrome, rape trauma; compound reaction; silent reaction.

Self-care deficit (specify level): feeding; bathing/hygiene; dressing/grooming; toileting.

Self-concept, disturbance in, body image; self-esteem; role performance; personal identity.

Sensory perceptual alteration, visual; auditory; kinesthetic; gustatory; tactile, olfactory perceptions.

Sexual dysfunction.

Skin integrity, impairment of, actual.

Skin integrity, impairment of, potential.

Sleep pattern disturbance.

Spiritual distress (distress of the human spirit).

Thought processes, alteration in.

Tissue perfusion, alteration in, cerebral; cardiopulmonary; renal; gastrointestinal; peripheral.

Urinary elimination, alteration in patterns.

Violence, potential for.

Cognitive dissonance.

Decision-making, impaired/ineffective (decision made by client produces results other than or less than desired).

Family dynamics, alteration in, family role changes/shifts; dysfunctional coping; stress management patterns; developmental transition; situational transition.

Fluid volume, alteration in, excess, potential for.

Memory deficit.

Rest-activity pattern, ineffective.

Role disturbance.

Social isolation.

[From Kim, M. and Moritz, D. (eds.): *Classification of Nursing Diagnoses,* McGraw-Hill, New York, 1982.]

Activity intolerance.
Anxiety.
Family processes, alteration in.
Fluid volume, alteration in, excess.
Health maintenance alteration.
Oral mucous membrane, alteration in.
Powerlessness.
Social isolation.

Test–Taking Guidelines

In taking examinations, particularly those in a multiple-choice format, there are some helpful hints or guidelines that should be used to improve your test performance. While no special guidelines or techniques can substitute for actually knowing the content to be tested, they can improve your performance on a test. Here are some basic guidelines related to test taking.

Read directions and questions carefully

A special answer sheet is used to record your answers to the questions on the NCLEX-RN examination. It is important to read carefully the directions for selecting the answers to the questions posed, and to record these answers correctly.

Since there is only one best answer to each multiple-choice question, you need to determine what the question is really asking. It is also helpful to make note of any key words and information relevant to answering the question as you read it. After reading a question, formulate an answer to it in your own words. While it is tempting to reframe questions and make them into the questions you would prefer to answer, it is very important to answer the questions as they are actually stated.

SOURCE: Adapted, with permission, from Yurchuck, R. (ed.): *Commission on Graduates of Foreign Nursing Schools Examination Review.* Garden City, NY: Medical Examination Publishing Co., 1983, pp. 10–12.

Select the best answer for each question

Having read a question carefully and formulated an answer in your own words, examine the various options. On the basis of your knowledge, you should be able to eliminate options that are obviously incorrect. This will give you more time to concentrate on selecting the correct option from those that remain and appear plausible.

When several options appear to be correct, try to determine the differences among the options and ask yourself which one best answers the question as posed. Remember that a correct answer is never partially wrong. The broader or more general option is often correct because it may encompass information provided in other option choices unless a very specific answer to the question is called for. Options that reflect specific hospital policies, rules, or regulations are inappropriate for broad-based examinations such as the NCLEX-RN.

Words such as "all," "never," "only," "no," "always," "except," and "every" appearing in either the stem or the options place special limitations on potentially correct answers; use caution in selecting answers to questions in which these words appear in the stem or in the options. Remember that when a question asks you to choose which option is incorrect or an exception to the information in the stem, an incorrect statement or exception is the correct answer.

Another way to eliminate incorrect answers to a question is to determine any grammatic inconsistency between an option and the stem. Each option should complete the question posed in the stem in a grammatically consistent way. Just test each option against the actual question. If one or more options do not meet this basic criterion it (or they) can be eliminated from consideration as correct options.

In questions relating to nurse-patient communication, focus on the patient's feelings and concerns

If the patient's feelings or concerns are overlooked, a potentially correct answer can be eliminated as incorrect. A response that focuses on the patient's feelings, accepts the patient as she/he is, or attempts to establish good rapport with the patient is likely to be correct.

Use the testing time wisely

The NCLEX-RN examination has a specific time limit, thus it is important to pace yourself during the testing period. Allow about 1 minute to answer each question, mark the correct answer, and move on to the next question. If you are uncertain about the best answer, place a light mark beside that number on the answer sheet so that you can return to it later. It is important to attempt answering every question but do not spend too much time on any one. By moving on you will be able to answer more questions during the testing time. If time permits you can return to the questions about which you were uncertain.

If you do not know the correct answer to a question, it is better to make an educated guess as to the answer rather than leave an answer blank. By using some of the test-taking guidelines just outlined, you should be able to eliminate some of the options as incorrect; the more options you can eliminate the greater the probability of correctly answering the question. Remember you have a 25% chance of guessing the correct answer to a four-option, multiple-choice question.

If you complete the examination before the end of the testing period, use this time to answer questions about which you were uncertain and to review your answers to all questions. Generally it is best *not* to change your answer to a question unless you are sure your original answer is incorrect.

disclaimer

The authors have made every effort to thoroughly verify the answers to the questions which appear in Part II. However, as in any text, some inaccuracies and ambiguities may occur; therefore, if in doubt, please consult your references.

The Publisher

PART I

Basic Knowledge Essential to the Care of Clients with Psychiatric Problems

PART 1

1

Study Outline

Jane Mulaik and Catherine Dickens

CONTENTS

1

OUTLINE

I. Overview

A. *Introduction*

A historical perspective of the treatment of mental illness and knowledge about the theories of personality are necessary for understanding the nurses' role and the treatment approaches used for patient/clients with mental illness or emotional disturbance. The nursing process of assessment, planning, intervention, and evaluation is described as are personality theories, treatment approaches, behaviors manifested by patients (clients) with various mental conditions, and nursing interventions used to treat these conditions. The psychiatric-mental health nurse's role and the legal and ethical issues in psychiatry are also outlined.

B. *History of treatment of mental illness*

Historically psychiatry, the care and treatment of the mentally ill, has undergone three "revolutions" related to the care of psychiatric patients (Clunn and Payne, 1982). Before the eighteenth century individuals who were mentally disturbed were called "hopelessly insane," "dangerous people," or "possessed by demons." They were isolated, beaten, chained, frightened by bizarre methods to "bring them to their senses," or even killed. In late eighteenth-century France Phillipe Pinel, a chief physician for Napolean, unlocked the chains of patients in a large hospital for the insane and instituted more humane treatment. Pinel's act changed from monstrous to human the way the mentally ill were viewed. This was the first psychiatric revolution.

During the next 100 years the mentally ill were gathered together in large institutions or "insane asylums" which were often built in isolated areas to separate the "insane" from other members of society. The approach was to treat the patient by providing for his physical needs and by punishing "bad" behavior. Mental illness was often viewed as a failure of will. In general, the treatment was more humane, although not very effective. Few physicians and fewer nurses treated these patients. Instead a large number of untrained attendants and some of the less disturbed patients cared for those who needed more help.

The second psychiatric revolution occurred when Freud developed his theory of the unconscious in the 1890s. If behavior was unconsciously motivated, patients could not be held responsible for behavior they could not control. After Freud many theorists developed psychoanalytic theories. Some based their theories on Freudian concepts of unconscious conflict, and others such as Jung and Adler, based their theories on very different concepts. Neofreudians and ego psychologists, such as Karen Horney, Harry Stack Sullivan, Anna Freud, Leopold Bellak, Erik Erikson, and others, further developed psychoanalytic theory based on Freud's teachings. Although psychoanalytic theory was helpful in the treatment of neurotics rather than psychotics, it nevertheless influenced the development of psychiatric treatment approaches for all patients and increased the interest of physicians, nurses, and the general public in the study of the mind and of mental processes.

Two psychiatrists who worked with schizophrenic patients in the early 1900s were Emile Kraepelin, who classified schizophrenic subtypes, and Eugene Bleuler who described the four "A"s, symptoms of schizophrenia—autism, apathy, ambivalence, and associative looseness. Treatment of many psychotic patients during the period 1900–1940 was custodial rather than therapeutic except for the select few who could afford psychoanalytic treatment. More nurses were involved in the care of hospitalized patients with the advent of somatic therapies in the 1930s. When electro-convulsive therapy, insulin therapy, pentylene-tetrazol (metrazol) therapy, or psychosurgery was used, nurses were more active in providing supportive care to patients and also directed the care provided by attendants.

Major changes occurred in psychiatric care during and shortly after World War II. Nurses were involved with the care of servicemen who had mental breakdowns. Treatment of men in crisis from combat was found to be more successful if it was short and intense, and men were returned to duty as quickly as possible. In 1946 the National Mental Health Act authorized the establishment of the National Institute of Mental Health whose mission was to support training of personnel (nurses, doctors, social workers, psychologists), promote research, provide new treatment facilities, and develop pilot projects for new treatment modalities. The Mental Health Act eventually resulted in 8000 psychiatric nurses prepared with master's degrees and also helped to increase the total number of nurses in mental health facilities from 21,000 to 39,000 in 11 years (Clune and Payne, 1982). Treatment facilities increased, and treatment was provided for many more patients.

In the 1950s three important events occurred that were precursors to the third psychiatric revolution. Psychotropic drugs, e.g., thorazine and other phenothiazine tranquilizers were discovered as were the antidepressant drugs, e.g., isoniazid (an antituberculosis drug), other MAO inhibitors, and the tricyclics, such as imipramine. These drugs enabled nurses, physicians, and others to communicate more effectively with patients because patients on psychotropic drugs were able to perceive reality and control their own behavior. The second event was the development by Maxwell

Jones, a British psychiatrist of the "therapeutic community" concept. In Jones' view the patient was expected to take an active part in his treatment and to participate as a responsible person in the group or community. This was seen as a "therapeutic milieu" in which all aspects of the environment—the staff, the patients, the physical setting, and the program—were geared toward treatment of patients. Nurses were actively involved in helping to maintain and promote a therapeutic milieu.

During the 1950s a third event or series of events occurred. New, brief treatment modalities were developed by psychologists and psychiatrists. Psychoanalytic approaches that were originally espoused by Freud, Jung, Adler, and other theorists who followed them assumed less importance. Brief therapies, some based on Pavolvian classical conditioning (e.g., desensitization to phobias developed by Wolpe and others) and operant conditioning based on Skinner's approach (e.g., the "token economy" described by Allyn and Azrin) were developed. Family therapy approaches were developed by Nathan Ackerman, Jay Haley, and others. These therapies were all based on learning theory. Bateson, Satir, and others developed the communication approaches that became the human potential movement, which was less a treatment approach than it was a way for the normal or mentally healthy individual to grow emotionally. A number of psychologists developed theories of behavior such as Abraham Maslow's theory that human motivation changes and growth occurs when needs are met, or Gordon Allport's theory that personality is the result of basic human traits. Existential philosophy was the basis for phenomenological personality theory that influenced Carl Rogers and Viktor Frankl who emphasized experiencing the self and "being in the world." Rogers and Frankl were theorists who also were therapists and treated people with mental problems. Other theorists who studied personality both during and after the 1950s were: Jean Piaget, who described cognitive development in the child; Albert Bandura, who developed a theory of social learning; and field theorists such as Kurt Lewin who noted the influence of the social group on behavior.

A greatly increased interest and understanding of personality and behavior, new brief treatment approaches that included both somatic treatment and learning approaches, and increased numbers of personnel set the stage for the third revolution in psychiatry—the community mental health movement. The Community Mental Health Act brought about a marked change in the treatment of mental patients. Treatment was shifted from large hospitals to community mental health centers. There was a mass exodus of patients (deinstitutionalization) from hospitals back to families, or to community foster homes, or to apartments or nursing homes, or in some cases to no homes at all. Psychotropic drugs made outpatient treatment possible. Larger numbers of prepared personnel, including psychiatric nurse clinicians using short therapies and learning approaches, made outpatient psychotherapy feasible. Currently outpatient treatment is still the norm with inpatient treatment used for crisis stabilization.

C. *Changes in the psychiatric-mental health nurse role during the twentieth century*

   1. The nurse's role has changed from custodial to technical to professional. The professional nurse:
     a. Maintains a therapeutic milieu to provide structure for patients
     b. Provides somatic treatments, i.e., medications
     c. Functions as an expert communicator with individuals and groups to assist patients with problem-solving and development of life skills

d. Teaches patients about health maintenance
e. Collaborates with the interprofessional team to plan patient care and work with families
f. Manages the psychiatric unit
g. Directs the work of nursing aides or technicians
h. Acts as liaison with other professionals to provide follow-up care for discharged patients

2. The majority of professional nurses with psychiatric experience function in psychiatric hospitals or in general hospital psychiatric units.

3. Some also function in clinics or in patient units that provide detoxification for alcohol and drug-abuse patients.

4. The Mental Health Act provided for advanced preparation of psychiatric clinical nurse specialists. The psychiatric clinical nurse specialist:
   a. Has a master's or doctoral degree
   b. May function in a wide variety of settings and provides a different level of service
   c. Functions as a psychotherapist in private or group practice similar to other disciplines, i.e., psychiatry and psychology
   d. Is a specialist in individual, group, or family therapy
   e. Practices in community mental health settings as a primary therapist for selected clients and as a case manager for other clients
   f. Provides direct care, teaching, and consultation to other professionals, such as teachers
   g. Involved in the promotion of positive mental health in schools, etc.
   h. Acts as a consultant-liaison nurse in a general hospital assisting nonpsychiatric nurses to deal with emotional crises in their medical-surgical patients
      1) May function as an educator in a school of nursing, in hospital inservice programs, and in research

5. Psychiatric nurses developed theories of nursing: i.e., Hildegard Peplau, Ida Orlando, and June Mellow.
   a. Defined nursing as a deliberate process, not intuition
   b. Peplau's theory based on Sullivan's theory of interpersonal development: nursing is an interpersonal process through which nurse and patient develop.
   c. Orlando defined nursing as a process of inquiry in which the nurse helps the patient define his need and discover his own solution.
   d. Mellow emphasized corrective emotional experiences for schizophrenic patients to alter their view of themselves and their world.

6. Summary of the psychiatric-mental health nurses role today
   a. Emphasizes communication and caring to help the patient move toward improved mental health
   b. Expanded interprofessional responsibility

D. *Mental health and mental disorders (Conceptual models):*

1. Definitions of mental health
   a. Psychological well-being or
   b. Adequate adjustment which conforms to community based norms

2. Descriptions of wellness behaviors
   a. Reasonable independence
   b. Ability to work and be productive
   c. Ability to form and keep satisfying interpersonal relationships
   d. Ability to cooperate
   e. Ability to deal with frustration
   f. Ability to accept oneself

3. Mental health is a relative state and a dynamic one

4. Mental health: mental disorder is conceptualized as a health-illness continuum with the population scattered along this continuum
   a. Individuals move up and down the continuum
   b. The move is not far in either direction except over time
   c. The individual person's abilities and strengths and the stresses of the environment interact to affect the person's mental health or lack of it

5. The "medical model" of mental disorders. The discussion in the preceding paragraph describes a view of mental disorder that is classed as the "medical model." The underlying assumption is that mental disorder is an illness, has symptoms, can be treated, and is analogous to a physical illness. Although causes are not known for most mental disorders such as schizophrenia, it is presumed that there is likely to be some underlying disease process, e.g., a genetic problem, a biochemical disorder, or some other malfunctioning body process. Many individuals working with persons manifesting mental disturbance subscribe to this theory.
   a. *Diagnostic and Statistical Manual,* 1980 *(DSM III)* describes mental disorders in relation to five axes or categories
      1) Axis I includes severe mental disorders: neurotic disorders, e.g., anxiety disorders, phobias, and psychotic disorders, e.g., schizophrenia, manic depression, organic brain syndromes

 2) Axis II: developmental disorders and personality disorders
 3) Axis III: physical disease relevant to mental disorders
 4) Axis IV: measure of severity of psychologic stressors
 5) Axis V: measure of level of function in the past year
   b. Psychotic disorders: most severely ill
 1) Primary symptom: not being in touch with reality
 2) Other symptoms, i.e., poor communication, inability to relate adequately to others, very poor self-concept, etc.
   c. Neurotic disorders: mild to moderately ill
 1) Maintain contact with reality
 2) Have behaviors that disrupt life and limit relationships, i.e.,
   a) High anxiety levels
   b) Depression
   c) Difficulty in maintaining satisfying interpersonal relationships, etc.
   d. Personality disorders
 1) Manifest behaviors that are often lifelong
 2) Which do not greatly interfere with the person's chosen life-style, but which may be disturbing to others, e.g., behaviors such as antisocial behavior and indifference to concerns of others as seen in the antisocial personality
 3) Very self-centered behavior as observed in the narcissistic personality, etc.

6. The "psychodynamic model" of mental disorder
   a. Mental disorder viewed not so much as an illness but rather as a disturbance in psychological forces

      b. Schizophrenia may be seen as a psychological condition in which the forces of the id (drive) overwhelm the ego (part of the personality in touch with reality which controls overt behavior)

      c. Results in the failure of repression (an ego defense mechanism) so that unconscious thoughts rise to the level of consciousness and the person loses contact with reality

7. "Social" model of mental disorders*

      a. Source of person's inability to deal with his life satisfactorily results from a problem in the environment and not from the person

      b. Society and social forces are often so severe or disruptive to an individual that he cannot deal effectively with them

      c. A marked change in the environment needed

      d. Family, the person's social group, and the community are important influences

      e. The person should not be considered as ill, nor seek to be treated that way, but rather he should be treated with understanding as a responsible person, able to deal with his problem with help, and worthy of love

      f. Person may need to get out of situation causing the stress until he can be helped to deal with it or alter it

      g. The interaction of the person with environment is an important aspect of this model, but the source of the problem is often seen to be the environment not the individual*

8. Treatment approaches

      a. Vary in each of these models. May be eclectic: a variety of treatment approaches, some "borrowed" from a different model are used in working with patients or clients

---

*This is the view of Thomas Sasz, R. D. Laing, and others who have developed different approaches to treatment of mental disorder and see the disorder as an opportunity for the person to grow and to change.

b. Medical model emphasizes somatic treatments (drugs) with psychotherapy, milieu therapy, and occasionally brief conditioning therapies
c. Psychoanalytic approach emphasizes psychoanalytic psychotherapy, but may use somatic treatment, milieu, and rarely brief therapies
d. Social model emphasizes relationship therapy and environmental change
e. In practice, different practitioners, regardless of discipline, may use different therapies

It is apparent in all of the models of mental disorder that there is an interaction of the individual and his environment. Stress may arise from the interplay of forces to which the individual may respond with any of a wide variety of behaviors.

13. Cultural and social differences can strongly affect the way the individual responds to his environment
a. Cultural differences in response patterns may be misinterpreted if the nurse is not so attuned.
b. Awareness of the conflict such differences may produce either within an individual or between individuals is important for the nurse and other health workers to understand and to deal with effectively.

E. *Nursing Process*

1. Overview of nursing process applied to psychiatric-mental health nursing
a. Communication
1) The nurse, to be effective in working with any patient, must be aware of her/his own attitudes, self-concept, and feelings
2) Must be able to communicate effectively with others
3) Must be aware of her/his communication approaches

4) Must be skilled in facilitating communication through both verbal and nonverbal means

5) Must recognize and avoid the use of inappropriate communication approaches, e.g., being overly reassuring or directing

b. Phases of the nurse-patient realtionship

1) An initial, getting-acquainted phase during which the relationship is structured and assessment is carried out

2) A working phase during which problems are discussed, goals set, and problems resolved

3) A terminating phase during which separation is dealt with

c. The nursing process with the psychiatric patient

1) Assessment

a) Psychological

(i) The precipitating problem

(ii) The dynamic issue

(iii) The patient's strengths and coping (defense mechanisms)

(iv) The mental status examination

b) Social

(i) Social workers assume responsibility

(ii) Nurse contributes data regarding family

c) Behavioral

(i) Patient's ability to relate to others

(ii) Maladaptive behaviors are noted

d) Physical

(i) General appearance

(ii) Gait

(iii) Posture and stature

(iv) Neurologic examination

2) Nursing diagnosis and goal setting
   a) May use *DSM–III* (clinical specialist)
   b) May list problems, i.e., depressed, anxiety, etc.
   c) Set collaboration by nurse and patient
   d) Determine long-term goals and break down into attainable short-term goals

2. Planning and specific interventions
   a. Interactional, or validating concerns
      1) Allowing ventilation of feelings
      2) Problem solving with client, with family
      3) Providing information
      4) Teaching
   b. Administering medications ordered
   c. Providing for basic physical needs, for touch, and for a pleasant appropriate environment
   d. Restraints or seclusion if needed
   e. Social: encouraging appropriate activities and providing structure, i.e., music, art, exercise, play therapies
   f. Making referrals
   g. See patient as an individual with a family and a community to which he/she will return as soon as feasible

3. Evaluation
   a. Informal by nurse; carried out continuously
   b. Plans or interventions may be altered if needed
   c. Formal evaluation of care plans and progress done on a regular basis by interprofessional team

II. **Social, legal, ethical and professional concerns of psychiatry-mental health**

A. *Community mental health movement*

1. Federal legislation, 1963, established centers
   a. Medicare
   b. Medicaid

   2. Mental health professional team
      a. Psychiatrist (M.D.)
      b. Psychologist (Ph.D.)
      c. Psychiatric social worker (A.C.S.W.)
      d. Psychiatric nurse clinical specialist (M.N., M.S.N.)

   3. Concepts of intervention: primary (promotion of health), secondary (prevention of illness when at risk), tertiary (prevention of complications or long-term/chronic illness when acute illness occurs)

   4. Civil rights movement

   5. Women's rights

   6. Gay rights

   7. Consumer movement
      a. Standards for patient care
      b. Accountability
      c. Care of underserved populations: minorities, women, children, elderly, mentally ill

B. *Mental health problems with social significance*

   1. Alcohol and drug abuse

   2. Child abuse

   3. Mental retardation

   4. Physically handicapped

   5. Learning disabilities

   6. Prison populations

C. *Legal issues in mental health care*

   1. Competency vs commitment

   2. Types of admission
      a. Voluntary (most patients in psychiatric care settings)

b. Emergency involuntary: dangerous to self or others (complaint of two witnesses, i.e., family, police, physician); time-limited (usually 1–2 weeks, varies state by state)

c. Judicial: indefinite involuntary commitment requiring a court decision; primarily criminal cases

3. Legal rights; vary by state
   a. Right to vote
   b. Right to manage financial affairs (if unable, legal guardianship established)
   c. Right to execute legal documents

4. Informed consent and patients' rights
   a. Right to confidential treatment
   b. Right to informed consent
   c. Right to refuse treatment
   d. Right to least restrictive alternative environment
   e. Permission must be obtained for aversive treatments: electroconvulsive therapy, etc.
   f. Right to aftercare

5. Malpractice: negligence (civil suit)
   a. Nurse is accountable for all actions
   b. Must provide care in accordance with what is professionally defined as appropriate treatment according to diagnosis and unique factors of each patient's needs, the setting, and the given circumstances
   c. Nurse must recognize "rights" of each patient

6. Confidentiality and privilege
   a. The nurse must recognize the patient's right to confidentiality
   b. Information in the patient's record should not be discussed outside the treatment team conference or with those not directly involved in the treatment plan

      c. Information gained from the patient belongs only to the team and in the record and should not be shared with those outside the treatment team

      d. In the event of law such as pending legal action the nurse should seek legal counsel

III. Theoretical foundations from the behavioral sciences

A. *Personality theories*

    1. Psychoanalytic theories
      a. Freud
        1) Structure of personality
          a) Unconscious, preconscious, conscious mind
          b) Id, ego, superego
        2) Sources of energy and motivation: unconscious, conflicting drive toward love and death
        3) Source of illness/maladaptation: unconscious conflict produces anxiety which produces symptoms
        4) Development: psychosexual periods: oral, anal, oedipal, latent, adolescent, adult
      b. Jung
        1) Structure of personality
          a) Personal unconscious: life experience of individual
          b) Collective unconscious: total experience of the race
        2) Motivation: collective unconscious of fears, need, desires as motivating force
        3) Source of illness: interactions of unconscious with social experience and personality type (introvert, extrovert)
      c. Ego psychologists
        1) Anna Freud

a) Ego defense mechanisms: repression, regression, denial, displacement, projection, undoing, isolation, identification, reaction formation, sublimination, suppression

2) Leopold Bellak
   a) Ego functions: reality testing, judgments, controlled impulse, object relations, thought processes, adaptive regression, defensive functioning, stimulus barrier, autonomous functioning, synthesis integration, mastery competence

3) Erik Erikson
   a) Eight developmental stages of man: trust, autonomy, initiative, industry, identity, intimacy, generativity, integrity

d. Neofreudian psychologists
   1) Harry Stack Sullivan
      a) Structure of personality: interaction results in three aspects of ego—"good me," "bad me," "not me"
      b) Source of energy/motivation: need for physical security and satisfaction in relationships
      c) Source of illness/maladaptation: breakdown of communication process between individual and significant other; intrapsychic conflict resulting from interpersonal conflict
      d) Development: biologic drives interacting with social environment

   2) Karen Horney
      a) Structure of personality: real vs idealized self
      b) Developmental goal: self-actualization, self-realization
      c) Motivation: to reach self-actualization

d) Source of illness/maladaptation: conflict with significant others produces
   hostility which produces neurotic
   trends

2. Psychological theories
   a. Humanistic theory: unique to human be-
      havior
      1) Abraham Maslow
         a) Personality structure: healthy psyche
            in all
         b) Motivation: Hierarchy of inherent
            needs from basic survival to self-
            actualization
         c) Source of maladaptation: unmet needs
            resulting from a limiting environment
         d) Change: increase self-knowledge and
            mobilize resources toward self-actual-
            ization
   b. Trait theory
      1) Gordon Allport
         a) Personality structure based on indi-
            vidual and common traits
         b) Motivation: unique to person; situa-
            tional and moves person toward
            autonomy
      2) Raymond B. Cattell
         a) Personality structure: Basic 16 per-
            sonality factors determined by factor
            analysis
   c. Field theory
      1) Gestalt psychology: viewing the parts
         and giving structure to the whole
      2) Kurt Lewin
         a) Personality structure: a set of vectors
            in a field of forces
         b) Primary concept: life space which
            consists of psychological environment
            and the person

d. Phenomenological theory
  1) Carl Rogers
    a) Personality structure: "self" results from interaction of the individual with his environment
    b) Motivation: self-actualization to become a fully functioning person
    c) Source of maladaptation: lack of experiencing unconditional positive regard from others
    d) Change: experience self-worth through unconditional positive regard of another person
  2) Existential philosophy—"being in the world"
    a) Viktor Frankl's logotherapy
      (i) Man has three dimensions: physical, psychological, and spiritual, which is the most human aspect
      (ii) Motivation: to find meaning for life
      (iii) Source of maladaptation: anxiety resulting in the inability to take responsibility for overcoming existential frustration (lack of meaning) in one's life
      (iv) Change: take responsibility for one's life and for the search for meaning

B. *Learning theories*

  1. Cognitive theory
    a. Piaget
      1) Cognition: occurs through accommodation and assimilation
      2) Stages of intellectual development: sensori-motor, preoperational, concrete operations, formal operations

2. Stimulus-response theory
   a. B. F. Skinner: operant conditioning
      1) Basis for behavior: reinforcement
      2) Personality structure: mental capacity, thoughts, etc., do not exist in this theory. Man and animal respond similarly to environmental stimuli.
      3) Maladaptation: occurs because unwanted or undesirable behaviors are reinforced
   b. Pavlov: classical conditioning
      1) Behaviors paired in time and connected as cue and response
      2) Extinction: when conditioned stimulus is presented repeatedly without unconditioned stimulus, extinction of response occurs.
      3) Stimulus generalization: a second stimulus similar to a first stimulus will produce some response.

3. Modeling or social learning theory
   a. Albert Bandura
      1) Basic premise: behavior is learned by observing others as well as by reinforcement.
      2) Personality: a product of past learning experiences and childhood models
      3) Motivation: stimuli are selectively attended and are self-activated in accordance with learned anticipation.
      4) Change: occurs by attending to different models of behavior

C. *Psychological equilibrium theory*

1. Definition of psychological equilibrium: balance process of interaction between the person and his environment

2. Definition of mental health: mind-body well-being

3. Concept of mental distress
    a. Expression of distress occurs through feelings, thoughts, and behaviors
    b. Use of ego defense mechanisms increases
    c. Symptoms of mental disorder occur when defense mechanisms are insufficient and are also a defense

4. Concept of abnormality
    a. Behaviors that cause pain
    b. Behaviors that are unusual in society
    c. Behaviors that deviate from the norm

D. *Social science theories*

1. Group dynamics
    a. Types of groups: task, social, encounter, therapy (see Table 1)
    b. Membership: selection, roles
    c. Leadership roles
    d. Group goals, norms, consensus
    e. Phases of group development
    f. Characteristics of successful groups

2. Systems theory—von Bertalanffy
    a. Definition of a system: set of interacting units within a boundary, which filters inputs and outputs
    b. Living or open systems vs nonliving or closed ones
    c. Crucial mechanisms: feedback loop
    d. Subsystem of general systems theory: communication, a social interchange (J. Reusch)

E. *Psychiatric nursing theory and role*

1. History of psychiatric nursing
    a. Custodial care: 1850–1950
    b. Therapeutic milieu: 1950–present
    c. Nurse-therapist: 1950–present

TABLE 1 Types of Groups

TYPE OF GROUP	LEADER	TYPE AND NUMBER OF MEMBERS	PURPOSE	TIME PERIOD
Task	Chairman	No specific number but 10 or 12 is comfortable. Individuals are members of a work group, e.g., nurses, salesmen, etc.	To complete a task, e.g., develop a program, plan, a campaign, etc.	Indefinite; continues until job is done; usually disbanded then. A new group may be formed for a new task.
Social	None	No specific number. May vary greatly from day to day. Members have mutual friendships and interests.	To enjoy each other's company, support, enjoy an activity	Indefinite; often continues for years. Members may come and go.
Encounter	Trainer or Facilitator	9–12 members who are self-selected. Individuals are "normal," i.e., have no mental problems.	To grow emotionally, experience greater self-understanding	Brief, often intensive meetings 2 or 3 daily for 4–5 days or less

Psychotherapy	Therapist	9-12 members, occasionally more, members are selected by therapist and have some type of mental/emotional problem or a crisis. Members usually are strangers.	To treat the disorder, to improve the functioning of individual members, to assist members to deal with crisis	Usually limited to several meetings weekly for a period of weeks (e.g., 10-12). Some group therapies are ongoing, but most are time limited.
Self-help	None	No specific number, may be small group of 10-12 or larger one of 20. Individuals have a life problem in common, e.g., alcoholism (AA or Al-Anon), overweight, a specific disease.	To assist each other with ways of handling the specific problem to give support	Ongoing; members come and go

2. Mental Health Act, 1946
   a. Nurse Training Act for preparation of psychiatric nurse specialists

3. General nursing theory
   a. Martha Rogers' theory of unitary man states that mind and body are one, that man constantly grows and develops, reaching higher planes until death.
   b. Sister Callista Roy's adaptation model states that man is a system, that the nurse provides appropriate input to help alter the system.

4. Psychiatric nursing theory
   a. Hildegarde Peplau's theory of interpersonal relations demonstrates that through nurse-patient interaction the patient improves and grows and so does the nurse.
   b. June Mellow described nursing therapy with schizophrenic patients. The nurse provided "corrective emotional experiences" to change the patient's behavior.
   c. Ida Orlando's process of inquiry states that nurses interact to assist the patient to identify the problem he suffers from and the solution(s) he seeks.

5. Roles of the psychiatric nurse
   a. Traditional caretaker role: supportive services
   b. Clinical nurse specialist
      1) Case management with patients
      2) Therapy with patients
      3) Educator with patients, nurses, others
   c. Collaborator with other disciplines
   d. Researcher role

6. Functions of the psychiatric nurse (ANA Standards)
   a. Provide therapeutic milieu
   b. Address here-and-now issues
   c. Surrogate parent

d. Care of physical health
e. Increase patients' social competency
f. Conduct psychotherapy
g. Function as a leader
h. Participate in community
i. Teach

IV. Theoretical foundations from the biophysical sciences

A. *Brain and nerve function in relation to body processes*

1. Feelings
   a. Source: hypothalamus, reticular activating system
   b. Consciousness

2. Thought processes
   a. Memory
   b. Attention
   c. Sensory perception

3. Regulation of body processes
   a. Sleep
   b. Appetite
   c. Activity

4. Cranial nerve function

5. Autonomic nervous system function
   a. Sympathetic: fight-flight
   b. Parasympathetic

6. Sensory and motor nerves, spinal chord reflex responses

B. *Biochemical factors within cells*

1. Brain amine changes
   a. Dopamine, serotinin levels in schizophrenia
   b. Norepinephrine levels in depression

2. Endorphins and receptor sites in addiction

3. Metabolism of toxic substances: drugs, poisons, and withdrawal

C. *Historic medical theory of mental illness*

1. Emile Kraepelin
   a. Developed a system of classification of mental illness based on description of behaviors. This is basis of modern classification.
   b. Saw mental illnesses as a biomedical problem. His concepts form basis of today's medical model of mental disease.
   c. Described the subtype of dementia praecox (schizophrenia): simple, catatonic, paranoid

2. Eugene Bleuler: theory of four As of schizophrenia
   a. Developed the term schizophrenia or split mind
   b. Described four principal symptoms of schizophrenia (four As)
      1) Autism: behavior whose meaning is unique to the individual
      2) Ambivalence: experiencing contradictory feelings at the same time toward an object
      3) Apathy: indifference, lack of feeling of pleasure or pain
      4) Associative looseness: having little or no connection between thoughts

D. *Genetic factors in mental illness*

1. Twin studies: schizophrenia, manic-depressive illness

2. Studies of multigenerational families and adoptive families of persons with mental illness and/or alcoholism

E. *Neurophysical changes in brain and nervous tissue secondary to mental distress*

1. Focal lesions: tumor, trauma

2. Nonfocal lesions: epilepsy

3. Structural brain changes in Alzheimer's disease, other dementias, and schizophrenia

4. Behavioral changes resulting from neurologic disease, metabolic disease, or environmental deficit (e.g., multiple sclerosis, diabetic acidosis, hypoglycemia, hyper- or hypothyroidism, oxygenation, increased or decreased temperature)

F. *Physiologic responses secondary to mental distress*

1. Psychophysiologic disorders
   a. Cardiorespiratory disorders: arrhythmias, asthma
   b. Gastrointestinal disorders: ulcers, colitis
   c. Sexual dysfunction
   d. Neuromuscular/joint disorders: arthritis

2. Medical complications of addiction: hepatitis, cirrhosis

3. Selye's stress adaptation model: alarm, resistance, adaptation

G. *Genetic defects/birth trauma/metabolic disorders associated with mental retardation*

V. **Therapeutic processes: conceptual models for nursing intervention**

A. *Psychological model*

1. Theorists: Freud, Sullivan, Erikson, ego psychologists; existential and humanistic psychologists; Peplau, Mellow, Orlando, others

2. Nurse-patient relationship
   a. Working with the here and now
      1) Managing feeling states
      2) Managing defensive thinking
   b. Accepting and using the parent surrogate role
      1) Encouraging talking

2) Listening
3) Bearing painful feelings
4) Empathy
5) Setting limits
6) Support
7) Providing a corrective experience

c. Conducting psychotherapy
1) Focus on individual patient, family, or group
2) Nurse's personal responsibility for outcome

B. *Social interactive model*

1. Theorists: Sullivan, Meyer, systems theorists

2. Nursing activities in the social model
a. Providing a therapeutic milieu
1) Developing unit climate
2) Providing structure for patient's day
3) Providing for activities of daily living
b. Assuming the role of social agent
1) Providing for occupational, recreational, art, and other therapy
2) Developing social skills
3) Setting goals for interaction, activities
4) Evaluating activities
c. Providing leadership to nurses, collaborating with other disciplines
d. Engaging in social and community action roles

C. *Behavioral model*

1. Theorists: Pavlov, Watson, Guthrie, Skinner, Wolpe, Ayllon, Bandura

2. Use of conditioned learning theory
a. Reinforcement of appropriate behavior; "token economy"
b. Nonreinforcement of inappropriate behavior, "time out"

3. Behavior therapy or modification
   a. Relaxation therapy, desensitization
   b. Aversive therapy
   c. Modeling

4. Patient teaching
   a. Teaching with reference to emotional health, e.g., smoking, obesity
   b. Teaching specific responses to anger and other feelings
   c. Teaching social skills, how to interview for job

D. *Biologic model*

1. Theorists: Kraepelin, Bleuler
   a. Psychiatric illness as disease

2. Treatment with antipsychotic, antidepressant, and other psychotropic drugs

3. Assessing and caring for somatic health problems including response to various treatments

4. Treatment with electroconvulsive therapy; insulin therapy
   a. Purposes, procedure, contraindications, outcome, and complications of treatment
   b. Providing patient support and teaching about a treatment

5. Other treatments: psychosurgery, hydrotherapy

E. *Selection of model*

1. Immediacy of social situation

2. Use of eclectic model

3. Need to change models

VI. Communication and nurse-patient interaction

A. *Attitudes, feelings, behaviors of the nurse*

1. Self-assessment by nurse

a. Assessing problems, feelings, concerns at present
b. Assessing personality, values, strengths overall

2. Developing positive responses
   a. Developing comfort in professional role
   b. Communicating respect
   c. Maintaining hope, optimism
   d. Developing sensitivity and caring
   e. Maintaining appropriate involvement
   f. Developing patience, persistence

3. Recognizing and dealing with nurses' negative feelings
   a. Being judgmental
   b. Feelings of pessimism
   c. Feelings of omnipotence
   d. Needing to reassure

4. Recognizing and dealing with nontherapeutic approaches
   a. Being overly reassuring
   b. Being overly directive
   c. Being psychoanalytic
   d. Labeling
   e. Having difficulty listening to or bearing painful feelings
   f. Being overinvolved with patient
   g. Being overidentified with problem
   h. Need to have patient more independent or dependent than he is

B. *Phases in the nurse-patient relationship*

1. Initial phase
   a. Getting acquainted
   b. Assessment
   c. Structuring relationship
   d. Developing comfort

2. Working phase
   a. Discussing and prioritizing problems

    b. Setting goals

    c. Focusing

    d. Encouraging expression of thoughts and feelings

    e. Observing and assessing behavior during interaction

3. Termination
   a. Assessing nurse's and patient's feelings about separation
   b. Preparing for termination: begins with first interview
   c. Reviewing and summarizing progress and changes
   d. Sharing feelings about relationship

C. *Types of interaction*

1. Social interaction
   a. Exchange of nurse's and patient's thoughts and feelings about a topic
   b. Purposes: encourage socialization and develop patient's social skills; increase comfort

2. Therapeutic interaction
   a. Focus: on patient and his concerns
   b. Expression of thoughts and feelings by patient, not by nurse
   c. Structure: goal-directed; time-limited
   d. Type of therapeutic interview
      1) Fact-finding
      2) Patient-oriented problem solving
   e. Phases of interview
      1) Initial
      2) Working
      3) Terminating
   f. Helpful verbal responses
      1) Useful questions (exploring): who, what, where, when, e.g., "Tell me more about . . . ."

2) Restatement, reflection, focusing, e.g., "You say you were confused and angry. What were you thinking?"

3. Clarifying, validating, e.g., "you finished the course work and graduated?"

4) Linking, confronting, e.g., "You left right after the accident."

5) Summarizing

g. Helpful nonverbal responses

   1) Observation of patient's nonverbal responses

   2) Awareness of nurse's nonverbal response

   3) Use of nonverbal to convey closeness, allow distance

   4) Silence: time to reflect

h. Nonhelpful responses

   1) Reassuring, agreeing, e.g., "This is only a minor setback, you'll be out of here soon."

   2) Probing, e.g., "Why were you so angry with her?"

   3) Rejecting, e.g., "Why are you carrying on? That really didn't hurt."

   4) Defensive, e.g., "What do you mean the food is terrible!"

   5) Advising, e.g., "You really shouldn't be so frightened."

   6) Belittling, e.g., "That's a ridiculous idea."

   7) Cliche, e.g., "Nothing can be that bad."

   8) Judgmental, e.g., "Why don't you stop complaining?"

i. Silence

   1) Reflection: helpful

   2) Nonhelpful: confused, disturbed, resistive

VII. Nursing process

   A. Assessment and data collection

     1. Entry into the health system

2. Involving the patient and setting goals

3. Psychological assessment
   a. Dynamic issue: what is underlying intra- or interpersonal problem?
   b. Precipitating cause or event
   c. Defense mechanisms, what are principal mechanisms the patient uses to defend himself against anxiety? (see Table 2)
   d. Patient strengths, e.g., youth, health, strength, intelligence; family support system, job, etc.
   e. Mental status examination
      1) Appearance: e.g., appropriate dress, grooming, physical appearance, expression, gestures
      2) Mood: depressed, anxious, happy, apathetic, euphoric
      3) Speech: clear, understandable, self-initiated; note blocking, inappropriate, looseness or tightness of associations
      4) Affect: feeling at the moment e.g., happy, sad
      5) Thought: appropriateness of content, to the point, rapid or slow in flow of ideas, ability to abstract (understand proverbs)
      6) Perception: does person perceive reality; hallucinations or delusions
      7) Intellect: normal, dull, highly intelligent
      8) Memory: note long-term memory (names, history) and short-term memory (list words or numbers and ask to recall them)
      9) Orientation x4: oriented to time, place, person, situation
      10) Judgment: good or poor

4. Social assessment
   a. Family's communication style: Which members talk and form alliances?

TABLE 2   Definitions of Defense Mechanisms

Types of defense mechanisms: Defense mechanisms are used to reduce anxiety. There are many types of defense mechanisms. Those more commonly used are listed here and briefly defined.

1. Displacement: feelings are distorted, separated from the original object, and discharged toward a substitute object. Example: A father, embarrassed in a public meeting by his boss, comes home and ridicules his son in front of the son's friends.
2. Denial: painful or anxiety-inducing aspects of reality are blocked out. Example: Mother has been told her child is severely retarded; she still plans ahead for college since Uncle Joe was a slow child and he earned a Ph.D.
3. Compensation: a real or imagined inadequacy is alleviated by substituting another goal to maintain one's own self-respect and gain others' approval. Example: The frightened boy becomes a daredevil auto racer.
4. Regression: behavior patterns characteristic of an earlier period are displayed. Example: A 5-year-old boy is hospitalized and begins to suck his thumb.
5. Conversion: feelings become unbearable and are rechanneled somatically. Example: A man wants to beat up a friend but can't close his hand into a fist, because his fingers won't curve.
6. Projection: undesirable feelings are attributed to others. Example: Archie Bunker calls Edith a "dingbat."
7. Rationalization: unacceptable feeling responses are justified or excused with logical reasons. Example: A girl cannot afford a dress she likes, so she says, "It made me look too fat anyway."
8. Sublimation: unacceptable impulses are discharged indirectly in constructive activities. Example: Children make mud pies or fingerpaint instead of smearing.
9. Reaction formation: unresolved conflicts between feelings or impulses are alleviated by reinforcing one, repressing the other. Example: Hostile woman gushes sweetness and "loves" everyone.
10. Identification: feelings, qualities, attributes of someone admired are imitated until they become an actual part of the individual. Example: Boy who imitates father becomes very much like his father.
11. Isolation: certain feelings, ideas, are set apart from others; the emotional and the intellectual content are separated. Example: Nurse stresses "humanistic" hospital care, but refuses to let parents stay with their sick children.

TABLE 2   (cont'd)

12. Introjection: feelings, values, attitudes of another assimilated into his own ego or supergeo. Example: Small child whose parents literally become a part of him.
13. Undoing: actions are negated by other actions. Example: Man proposes on a romantic night, does not again mention marriage to the girl and introduces her to his best friend.
14. Condensation: a group of ideas is expressed by a single word and the single word is reacted to with all the emotions associated with the group of ideas. Example: Any four letter word associated with sex.
15. Repression: unwanted feelings are kept from awareness. Example: Girl is jealous of her brother but has never been aware of it.
16. Suppression: unwanted feelings are consciously kept out of awareness. Example: Scarlet O'Hara's "I'll think about that tomorrow."
17. Transference: The projection of feelings, thoughts and wishes onto others, and the person is reacted to as if he were someone from the past. Behaviors appropriate in that part, earlier interaction are activated.
    a. Transference is basic to the psychoanalytic process, skillfully cultivated by the therapist to reenact, reexperience, and work through past traumas. Transference may be either positive or negative.
    b. Countertransference is the reaction of the therapist to the patient and can also be a positive or negative factor in the therapeutic process.

SOURCE: Reprinted, with permission, from Clunn, P.A. and Payne, D.B., *Psychiatric Mental Health Nursing: Nursing Outline Series*, 3rd Ed., Garden City, N.Y.: Medical Examination Publishing Co., 1982, pp. 38-40.

    b. Family's perception of illness and goals, same as patient's or not; desire for patient recovery
    c. Genogram: assessment tool to "map" family members and show generations. (see Figure 1)

  5. Behavioral assessment
    a. Types of relationships
    b. Assessment of maladaptive behaviors

  6. Physical assessment

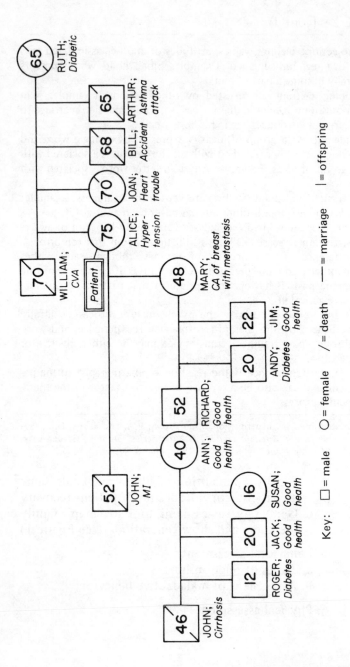

Figure 1 Example of a genogram. (Reprinted, with permission, from Sherman, J.L., Jr., and Fields, S.K.: *Guide to Patient Evaluation*, 4th Ed. Garden City, N.Y.: Medical Examination Publishing Co., 1982, p. 39.)

       a. Assessment by history of patient's physical status and changes in body systems

       b. Physical examination and laboratory study as indicated i.e., blood pressure and CBC for "fatigue"

B. *Diagnostic process*

    1. Medical diagnosis by a physician

       a. *DSM III: Diagnostic and Statistical Manual for Mental Diseases.* 3rd Ed., 1980.

          1) Purpose is to provide a listing and numbering of categories of mental disorders to provide a standard format for diagnosis and to provide a classification for statistical and research purposes

          2) Method of classification is on five axes. Axis I and II encompass all of the mental disorders. Axis III, IV, and V provide additional clinical information that is helpful for treatment and for research

             a) Axis I: includes psychotic disorders, neurotic disorders, specific childhood diseases, e.g., schizophrenia, manic-depressive disorder, anxiety disorders, chronic and acute brain syndromes, attention disorder, phobias, etc.

             b) Axis II: includes the personality disorders, e.g., borderline personality, hysterical personality, antisocial personality, etc.; and certain developmental disorders, e.g., adolescent adjustment reaction, learning disabilities, etc.

             c) Axis III: includes physical disorders that are potentially relevant to understanding the individual's mental disorder, e.g., underlying neurologic disease, cirrhosis in case of an alcoholic patient, etc.

        d) Axis IV: measures the severity of the psychologic stressors. Rated on a scale from 0–5 in comparison with an "average person"

        e) Axis V: is the highest level of adaptive functioning for the past year. Rated on a scale from 1 or "superior" functioning to 7 or "grossly impaired in all functional areas"

    2. Nursing diagnosis: psychiatric clinical nurse specialists utilize *DSM III.* Other psychiatric nurses list problems or selected nursing diagnoses.

C. *Planning nursing care*

    1. Determining priorities

    2. Setting long-term and short-term goals
        a. Negotiating changes for any goals on which the patient and nurse disagree

    3. Providing for activities of daily living and safety

    4. Providing structure, i.e., planning and carrying out daily activities

    5. Providing for expression of feeling, problem-solving

    6. Providing for socialization needs

    7. Obtaining other services as needed, e.g., social service, vocational planning

    8. Maintaining family contacts

    9. Planning for future, discharge; plan with patient and family

D. *Maintaining records*

    1. Use of problem-oriented medical record (POMR); subjective objective assessment plans (SOAP) format

2. Importance of record

3. Purpose of nursing note

4. Type of nursing records

E. *Evaluation*

1. Evaluation of nursing service to patient

2. Evaluation of interdisciplinary team

VIII. Pharmacologic therapy

A. *Historic perspectives*

1. Discovery of neurotransmitters: acetylcholine and norepinephrine, 1921

2. Use of rauwolfia for hypertension and noted side effect of calmness in 1940s

3. 1950: rauwolfia used for treatment of schizophrenias

4. 1950s: lithium discovered and used with manic patients

5. 1952: monoamine oxidase (MAO) inhibitors discovered through use of antituberculosis drug which relieved secondary depression

6. After 1950 synthesis of chlorpromazines in France; similar substance haloperidol synthesized in United States 1960

B. *Legal issues*

1. Informed consent

2. Right to refuse medication and other treatment

C. *Neurotransmitters*

1. Receptor sites and drug action
   a. Action occurs at receptor site of neuron cell synapse

   b. Drug acts to increase or inhibit the release of neurotransmitter

2. Primary neurotransmitters
   a. Acetylcholine
      1) Site of action: brain and throughout the body in parasympathetic portion of autonomic nervous system
      2) Type of action: cholinergic
   b. Norepinephrine and epinephrine
      1) Site of action: brain and throughout the body in sympathetic portion of the autonomic nervous system
      2) Type of action: adrenergic

3. Brain amines
   a. Catecholamines
      1) Norepinephrine and epinephrine; decreased availability in depression, increased availability in mania
      2) Dopamine: increased availability in schizophrenia
         a) Location: secreted in basal ganglia
         b) Synthesis: from tyrosine
   b. Serotonin: decreased amounts in Down's syndrome and decreased amounts in insomnia
      1) Location: found in brain and throughout the body
      2) Synthesis: from tryptophan
   c. Gamma-aminobutyric acid (GABA): decreased amount produces dystonia in Huntington's chorea
   d. Presence of brain amines: inferred from presence of metabolic end-products in urine, spinal fluid

D. *Classification of psychotropic drugs* (see Tables 3–5)

1. Antipsychotic drugs

TABLE 3 Equivalent Dosages and Usual Daily Dosage Ranges
of Oral Forms of Antipsychotic Agents

GENERIC NAME	TRADE NAME	APPROXIMATE EQUIVALENT DOSAGE (mg)	USUAL DAILY DOSAGE RANGE (mg/day)	
			ACUTE	MAINTENANCE
Phenothiazines				
Aliphatic				
Chlorpromazine[a]	Thorazine	100	300–1600	100–400
Triflupromazine	Vesprin	25	75–150	25–100
Piperidine				
Mesoridazine	Serentil	50	150–400	50–200
Piperacetazine	Quide	10	40–160	20–50
Thioridazine[a]	Mellaril	100	300–800	100–400
Piperazine				
Acetophenazine	Tindal	20	60–120	40–80
Butaperazine	Repoise	10	30–100	10–40
Carphenazine	Proketazine	25	75–400	25–150
Fluphenazine	Prolixin } Permitil	2	6–60	2–8
Perphenazine	Trilafon	8	16–64	8–24
Prochlorperazine[a]	Compazine	15	50–150	20–60
Trifluoperazine	Stelazine	5	15–60	5–15

TABLE 3 (cont'd)

GENERIC NAME	TRADE NAME	APPROXIMATE EQUIVALENT DOSAGE (mg)	USUAL DAILY DOSAGE RANGE (mg/day)	
			ACUTE	MAINTENANCE
Thioxanthenes				
Chlorprothixene	Taractan	100	300–600	75–400
Thiothixene	Navane	5	15–60	6–30
Butyrophenones				
Haloperidol	Haldol	2	6–100	2–8
Dihydroindolines				
Molindone	Moban } Lidone }	10	40–225	15–60
Dibenzoxazepines				
Loxapine	Loxitane } Daxolin }	15	50–250	20–75

[a] Also available generically.

SOURCE: Reprinted, with permission, from Pirodsky, D.M.: *Primer of Clinical Psychopharmacology: A Practical Guide.* Garden City, N.Y.: Medical Examination Publishing Co., 1981, pp. 8-9.

TABLE 4   Approximate Daily Dosage Ranges of Antidepressant Drugs

GENERIC NAME	TRADE NAME	USUAL DAILY DOSAGE RANGE (mg/day)	
		INPATIENT	OUTPATIENT OR MAINTENANCE
Tricyclic antidepressants			
Tertiary amines			
Amitriptyline[a]	Elavil, Endep	150–300	50–150
Doxepin	Sinequan, Adapin	150–300	50–150
Imipramine[a]	Tofranil, Presamine	150–300	50–150
Trimipramine	Surmontil	150–300	50–150
Secondary amines			
Desipramine	Norpramin, Pertofrane	150–300	50–150
Nortriptyline	Aventyl, Pamelor	75–200	25–100
Protriptyline	Vivactil	30–60	10–30
Amoxapine	Asendin	150–300[b]	100–300[c]
Monoamine oxidase inhibitors			
Phenelzine	Nardil	45–75	15–45
Tranylcypromine	Parnate	20–30	10–20

[a] Amitriptyline and imipramine are also available generically.
[b] May be cautiously raised up to 600 mg/day if no response after 2 weeks.
[c] May be cautiously raised up to 400 mg/day if no response after 2 weeks.

SOURCE: Reprinted, with permission, from Pirodsky, D.M., *Primer of Clinical Psychopharmacology: A Practical Guide*, Garden City, N.Y.: Medical Examination Publishing Co., 1981, pp. 40–41.

TABLE 5   The Benzodiazepines

GENERIC NAME	TRADE NAME	USUAL DAILY DOSAGE RANGE (mg/day)[a]	DURATION OF ACTION
Antianxiety agents			
Chlordiazepoxide[b]	Librium	15–100	Long
Clorazepate dipotassium	Tranxene	15–60	Long
Clorazepate monopotassium	Azene	13–52	Long
Diazepam	Valium	6–40	Long
Lorazepam	Ativan	1–6	Intermediate
Oxazepam	Serax	20–120	Short
Prazepam	Centrax	20–60	Long
Sedative-hypnotics			
Flurazepam	Dalmane	15–30 (at bedtime)	Long
Temazepam	Restoril	15–30 (at bedtime)	Short

[a] Higher doses may be needed for the treatment of alcohol withdrawal.
[b] Chlordiazepoxide is also available generically.

SOURCE: Reprinted, with permission, from Pirodsky, D.M., *Primer of Clinical Psychopharmacology: A Practical Guide*, Garden City, N.Y. Medical Examination Publishing Co., 1981, p. 95.

a. Phenothiazines
b. Thioxanthene
c. Butyrophenone
d. Dosage and monitoring
e. Toxicity and side effects
f. Overdosage
g. Adverse interactions, nursing implications

2. Antidepressant drugs
   a. Tricyclics
   b. Monoamine oxidase inhibitors
   c. Dosage and monitoring
   d. Toxicity and side effects
   e. Overdosage
   f. Interactions, nursing implications

3. Antianxiety drugs and sedatives
   a. Benzodiazepam
   b. Antihistamines
   c. Sedatives
   d. Analgesics
   e. Hypnotics
   f. Dosage and monitoring
   g. Toxicity and side effects
   h. Overdosage
   i. Withdrawal effects
   j. Interactions, nursing implications

4. Antimanic drug
   a. Lithium
   b. Dosage and monitoring
   c. Side effects and toxicity

5. Stimulant drugs
   a. Amphetamines
   b. Dosage and monitoring
   c. Toxicity and side effects
   d. Adverse interactions, nursing implications

6. Antiparkinsonian drugs
   a. Trihexyphenidyl (Artane)

   b. Benztropine (Cogentin)
   c. Dosage
   d. Side effects, toxicity
   e. Adverse interaction, nursing implications

IX. Psychotherapy methods

A. Schools of psychotherapy

1. Psychodynamic
   a. Basic concepts: instinctual conflict; sexual repression
   b. Treatment model: medical
   c. Therapist role: interpreter, reflector
   d. Technique: interpretation

2. Behavioral
   a. Basic concepts: anxiety; learned habits
   b. Treatment model: educational
   c. Therapist role: shaper, advisor
   d. Technique: conditioning, reinforcement

3. Experiential
   a. Basic concepts: alienation, existential despair
   b. Treatment model: existential or adult to adult
   c. Therapist role: interactor, acceptor
   d. Technique: encounter, experiential

B. Psychiatric-mental health nurse as primary psychotherapist

1. Selecting the conceptual model

2. Therapeutic role with the client; transference

3. Therapeutic approaches
   a. Individual
   b. Group
   c. Family

4. Collaboration with colleagues

5. Community responsibilities

C. *Group therapy*

1. Types of therapy groups
   a. Psychodynamic: traditional, insight-oriented group conducted by a therapist who selects 10–12 members. Generally used for non-psychiatric persons. Purpose is to gain insight into problems and insight into self. Usually time-limited, once, or twice weekly for 10–12 weeks.
   b. Gestalt: psychodynamically oriented, use of role playing, dramatization, focused on one member at a time. Purpose to gain insight. Developed by psychotherapists such as Fritz Perls. Group members are selected and screened by therapist. Approach is used for normal or neurotic persons. Time-limited by number in small group and time needed to explore problems.
   c. Training group (T group): Brief, insight-oriented group for well-functioning persons (e.g., students, executives, professionals) to learn how they affect others, gain insight, change behavior. Selected and screened by trainer; 10–12 people; time-limited to four or five sessions.
   d. Crisis group: small group of self-selected individuals with a specific problem, e.g., newly diagnosed cancer patients, parents who lost a child through death. Therapist conducts group of people dealing with a particular life crisis. Time-limited to one or two times week for 6–8 weeks.
   e. Family therapy: all members of a family living together seek help for identified patient (often a child). Therapist meets weekly with all family members for 6–8 weeks. Purpose is to strengthen family ties, develop more effective interrelationships. Family is seen as a system with change in one member producing change in others.

f. Self-help groups: members are self-selected to deal with a particular problem. e.g., alcoholism (AA or Al-Anon) or weight problem, etc. Group is usually ongoing, no lime limit and members come and go.

2. Effectiveness of therapy groups
   a. Learning
   b. Catharsis
   c. Cohesiveness
   d. Hope

3. Leadership functions
   a. Selection of members
   b. Guidelines development
   c. Facilitating interaction, linking behaviors, and understanding
   d. Bringing closure

D. *Family therapy*

1. Types of families

2. Functions

3. Dynamics of family living

4. Family assessment
   a. Structure of family system
   b. Roles and relationships
   c. Ability to perform tasks
   d. Goal achievement processes

5. Nursing role in intervention

6. Referral

E. *Self-help groups*

1. Organization

2. Developing guidelines

3. Group structure

4. Group dynamics

F. *Play therapy*

   1. Purposes: learning vs expressive

   2. Therapist role

X. Nursing Intervention in Selected Crises

A. *Crisis theory and intervention*

   1. Crisis theory
      a. First described by Eric Lindemann and defined by Gerald Caplan
      b. Caplan's definition: ". . . a psychological disequilibrium in a person who confronts a hazardous circumstance that constitutes an important problem which for the time being he can neither escape nor solve with his customary problem solving resources."
      c. Person either functions better or worse as a result of the crisis. There is opportunity for growth.

   2. Typology of crisis
      a. Internal or developmental: predictable changes in one's life that occur with everyone as described in Erik Erikson's "Eight Stages of Man."

Stage	Age
Basic trust vs mistrust	Infancy: 1 year
Autonomy vs shame, doubt	Toddler: 1–3 years
Initiative vs guilt	Preschooler: 3–5 years
Industry vs inferiority	School age: 6–12
Identity vs role confusion	Adolescence
Intimacy vs isolation	Young adult
Generativity vs stagnation	Adult
Ego integrity vs despair	Older adult

3. Assessment
   a. Perception of event
   b. Support systems
   c. Coping mechanisms
   d. Diagnosis

4. Intervention
   a. Goals
   b. Models of intervention
      1) Problem-solving partnership
      2) Crisis counseling
      3) Telephone counseling
      4) Hospitalization

B. *Psychiatric-mental health emergency*

1. Definition: sudden acute onset of disordered, inappropriate behavior requiring immediate intervention

2. Types of emergency situations
   a. Suicidal or homicidal crisis
   b. Drug overdose/drug withdrawal
   c. Sudden onset of psychosis, confusion
   d. Severe grief reaction, dying
   e. Response to severe trauma, e.g., accident, rape

3. Nursing roles in psychiatric-mental health emergency
   a. Consultant to nursing staff
   b. Educator-facilitator as liaison with medical staff
   c. Direct service

4. Nursing process
   a. Assessment
      1) Psychological: behavioral status or mental status examination
      2) Social relationships
      3) Biologic states: physical examination and history by physician or other

          4) Nature of crisis request
      b. Interventions
          1) Interactional
              a) Validate concern; identify strengths
              b) Allow ventilation of feelings
              c) Reassure through information
              d) Facilitate problem solving with client and family
          2) Psychopharmacologic
          3) Physical/environmental
              a) Provide for basic needs
              b) Use of restraints, seclusion
              c) Use of touch to communicate
              d) Provide a pleasant physical environment
          4) Social
              a) Encourage appropriate activities and provide structure
          5) Initiate and facilitate referrals
      c. Legal aspects of care for psychiatric emergencies
          1) Patient's rights
          2) Care provider's rights and responsibilities for protection of self and others

XI. Situational crises and behavioral response

  A. Suicidal crisis

    1. Pathogenesis
      a. Suicide is destructive aggression turned inward
      b. Eleventh major cause of death: 25,000 +/yr; 250,000+ attempts
      c. High rates: societies with social unrest, cold climates, and social atmosphere where independence and individual performance valued, e.g., United States, Japan, Germany. Lower in Jewish and Catholic communities

where act is disapproved. The rate is rising in single persons and married persons without children; men in general (especially older); whites; older persons; adolescents; and 20 to 30-year-old urban blacks.

d. Risk factors
   1) Prior suicide attempt
   2) Loss of significant realtionship especially parents early in life, spouse, lover
   3) Loss of job, money or social position
   4) Depression or recovery from depression or disrupted life situation
   5) Drug and alcohol abuse
   6) Severe physical illness leading to change in body image or life situation

2. Assessment
   a. Demographic and social variables as related to risk
   b. Clinical variables of individuals at high risk: depression, unemployment, schizophrenia, alcholism, malignancy, delinquency, divorce, family discord
   c. Assessment of lethality: plan, method, prior attempts, resources, and communication with significant others
   d. Psychodynamics of suicide: alienation, isolation, rejection, unexplained change in behavior, careful to careless—impulsive

3. Nursing management
   a. Outpatient
      1) Telephone hot-line
      2) Crisis counseling: family, individual
   b. Inpatient
      1) Agitated vs retarded behavior
      2) Providing a therapeutic environment
         a) Physical safety
         b) Establishing a nurse-patient relationship

       c) Maintaining family and community
          ties
       d) Increasing patient self-esteem
    c. Postintervention: support for bereaved sur-
      vivors of a suicide

B. *Crisis of unresolved grief*

  1. Normal grief
    a. Characteristic behaviors/stages: denial, accep-
      tance, restitution
    b. Time for resolution
      1) Meaning of loss
      2) Previous losses
      3) Individual strengths and external support
    c. Grief as a social process

  2. Unresolved grief
    a. Reasons for failure to grieve
      1) Social factors: negation of loss, unspeak-
         able loss, role of strong one, uncertainty,
         inadequate social support
      2) Psychological factors: guilt, narcissistic
         loss, resistance to mourning, multiple
         losses, reawakening an old loss

  3. Diagnosis of unresolved grief: behavior

  4. Nurses reactions to grief

  5. Intervention
    a. Assessment of level of depression
    b. Establishing a relationship and working
      through
    c. Referrals

C. *Rape crisis*

  1. Assessment
    a. Determining crisis request of the victim and
      type of help needed: medical, psychological,
      police
    b. Assessing coping behavior of the victim

2. Intervention
   a. Establishing a relationship with victim
   b. Working phase: dealing with details of assault
   c. Follow-up care
   d. Accountability

D. *Child abuse/neglect*

1. Pathogenesis
   a. Scope of the problem: 200,000 cases reported in 1 year
   b. Risk factors: family discord, family financial crisis, poor coping methods, lack of community resources

2. Assessment
   a. Physical signs: fractures, burns, bruises
   b. Behavioral signs: inappropriate and ineffective responses socially
   c. Signs of neglect: malnutrition, delayed growth and development

3. Plan and intervention
   a. Interview of family
      1) Family composition, economic and social situation, problem-solving methods
      2) History of child growth and development
      3) Present history
      4) Development of plan for care of child, treatment of parents
   b. Parental treatment
      1) Crisis groups
      2) Self-help: parents anonymous
   c. Need for interagency collaboration
   d. Legislation regarding child abuse
   e. Prevention

4. Evaluation
   a. Consistency in attending crisis and self-help groups
   b. Progress towards treatment goals

E. *Substance abuse*

1. Epidemiology of alcohol abuse
   a. Theories of causation—genetic, biochemical, psychosocial
   b. Family history of psycho-social-economic stress
   c. Legal definition of inebriation when blood levels of alcohol over 0.15% (varies by state)

2. Physiologic action of alcohol
   a. Primarily metabolized in liver
   b. Central nervous system depressant
   c. Initial stimulating response due to relaxation of inhibition
   d. In large amounts depresses respiratory center

3. Social effects
   a. Almost 10 million alcohol abusers in United States
   b. Affects spouses and children
   c. Causes significant number of automobile accidents, homicides and suicides

4. Medical complications
   a. Acute and chronic gastritis and pancreatitis
   b. Alcoholic hepatitis
   c. Anemia
   d. Peripheral neuropathy
   e. Laennec cirrhosis
   f. Cerebellar degeneration
   g. Wernicke-Korsakoff syndrome (amnesia, confabulation, disorientation, coma)

5. Assessment of the alcohol abuser
   a. Medical biologic assessment: evidence of delirium tremens, hepatitis, cirrhosis, organic brain dysfunction, other medical disorders and/or multiple drug abuse
   b. Behavioral assessment: drinking patterns, amount of alcohol intake, change in job to allow for drinking, etc.

      c. Social assessment: family history of alcoholism, changes in patterns of socializing, family problems

      d. Psychologic assessment: feelings of depression, loneliness and low-self-esteem, increased denial, rationalization and guilt

  6. Treatment of the alcoholic client

      a. Detoxification

        1) Selection of inpatient or outpatient site

        2) Medications

        3) Referral to Alcoholics Anonymous (AA)

      b. Rehabilitation treatment

        1) Selection of inpatient or outpatient site

        2) Setting treatment goals collaboratively with client

        3) Therapeutic milieu: increased and varied activity, structure, socialization

        4) Adequate nutritional program

        5) Group therapy (treatment triad)

        6) Educational program

        7) Involvement of family in family therapy, Al-Anon or both

        8) Involvement of client in AA

        9) Medication: evaluation of maintenance

      c. Nurse/staff attitudes toward alcoholic critical

        1) Self awareness preparation through group process prior and during employment

        2) Continuing education essential

      d. Nurses role in prevention of alcoholism

        1) Group at risk, risk factors

        2) Educational programs

  7. Pathogenesis of drug abuse

      a. Definition of drug abuse, drug addiction, drug habituation, drug intoxification (see Table 6).

      b. History of drug abuse

      c. Types and effects of drugs commonly abused

        1) Narcotics

        2) Sedatives, hypnotics

TABLE 6   Definitions Related to Drug Abuse

TERM	DEFINITION
Drug abuse	Excessive, harmful use of drugs. An increasing ingestion of drugs that can lead to myriad problems: medical, social, and legal.
Drug addiction	A state of having yielded to a practice that is habit forming to such an extent that its cessation causes severe physical trauma. Drugs commonly causing addiction are opiates, alcohol, and barbiturates. Both physical and psychic dependence are present, but the physical dependence is what defines addiction.
Drug habituation	A state of being psychically dependent on something. Drugs commonly causing habituation are marijuana, hallucinogens, and stimulants such as cocaine and amphetamines.
Drug intoxication	A state of being affected temporarily with diminished control over the physical and mental powers, usually because of drug use.

SOURCE: Adapted from Reichert, K.E.: *Primary Care of Young Adults*, 2nd Ed. Garden City, N.Y.: Medical Examination Publishing Co., 1983, p. 91.

3) Stimulants
4) Hallucinogens
d. Types of drug users: experimenters, social users, chronic abusers

8. Assessment of drug abusers
   a. Establishing a relationship
   b. Evaluating drug use through interviewing client, his family and associates, physical examination and laboratory tests

9. Plan and intervention
   a. Emergency treatment programs
      1) Overdosage
      2) Determining type of drug used from persons on scene

3) Emergency treatment: CPR or maintain airway, intravenous therapy
4) Administer antidote
5) Provide for other medical treatment and referral

b. Hallucinogenic crisis
1) Symptoms and type of drug
2) Quiet environment
3) Need for presence of close friends
4) Medication: rare
5) Approach: "talking down" (except PCP intoxication)
6) Referral as needed

10. Rehabilitation treatment program
a. Selection of type of program, usually out-patient
1) Drug counseling programs
2) Day-care program
3) Methadone maintenance program for narcotic abusers
4) Self-help groups: Narcotics Anonymous (NA) and residential programs (Synanon)
b. Types of therapy: group more beneficial
c. Treatment triad: professional, recovered addict, and client essential in drug treatment programs

11. Nurse's role in prevention
a. Educational programs: parents and youth
b. Counseling for teens and preteens

F. *Sexual dysfunction*

1. Pathogenesis: impotence, frigidity, dyspareunia
a. Causes: physical, emotional, social

2. Assessment
a. Sexual history
b. Physical assessment
c. Interprofessional evaluation

3. Plan and intervention
    a. Individualized
    b. Surgery, hormone administration
    c. Psychological

4. Transexualism, gender identity crisis
    a. Etiology: varied theories
    b. Treatment: may or may not be indicated
    c. Psychological counseling

XII. Clinical syndromes

A. Psychophysiologic disorders (psychosomatic)

1. Stress and adaptation theories (Selye, Dubos)
    a. Homeostasis
    b. General adaptation syndrome
    c. Levels of anxiety and autonomic response

2. Effects of stress result from
    a. Prior stressors affecting individual
    b. Individual perception of the stress
    c. Genetic predisposition

3. Types of psychophysiologic disorders
    a. Cardiovascular
        1) Type A (competitive, hard driving) vs type B personality
        2) Dynamic issue: frustration, anger, competition
        3) Disorders: coronary artery disease, hypertension
    b. Gastrointestinal disorder
        1) Gastric ulcer
            a) Incidence and prevalence: ulcer is the most frequently encountered psychosomatic condition; now more common in men compared with late nineteenth century when it was prevalent in women; occurrence is more

frequent in those subject to depression and alcoholism but infrequent in schizophrenia; occurs in children

b) Causative factors: a high level of emotional stress and a high level of plasma pepsinogen

c) Dynamic issue: repressed anger over dependency needs

2) Anorexia nervosa

a) Incidence and prevalence: formerly thought to be uncommon, it is being seen in increasing numbers. Adolescents, especially young women, are most common groups affected. Self-concept is that of someone overweight even though person is actually starved. Estimated cases 5–75 per 100,000 population. Mortality is 5–15%.

b) Symptoms: refusal to eat is common. Occasional overeating followed by self-induced vomiting occurs. Bulimia: excessive overeating ("gorging"), followed by self-induced vomiting. Marked weight loss, amenorrhea are common.

c) Dynamic issue: conflict over dependency and a struggle for control with parents especially the mother. Conflict over sexual development. Thus separation, identity, and control are issues.

3) Ulcerative colitis

a) Incidence and prevalence: increasing numbers of individuals are being diagnosed with this disorder. Occurrence is principally in late adolescence or young adulthood in both males and females. The diagnosis is also being made in children.

b) Causative factors: external stress, especially grief over loss, either death of a close family member or friend or severe loss of self-esteem secondary to job loss, school failure, leaving home, marriage failure. Attack often occurs several weeks after loss. Recently the interaction of possible physical factors, such as immune reaction, latent virus infection are being investigated as possible associated factors.

c) Dynamic issue: grief over loss, especially loss of having dependency needs met. Separation is an issue.

4) Respiratory

a) Disorders: hyperventilation, asthma

b) Incidence and prevalence: hyperventilation occurs as a rapid response to anxiety. No particular age or sex is noted as having this problem more often than others. Symptoms of rapid, shallow breathing produce faintness, rapid pulse, and air hunger. Alteration in acid-base balance may occur.

c) Dynamic issue in hyperventilation: anxiety or fear

d) Incidence and prevalence of asthma: occurs more commonly in children of either sex but also occurs and persists with adults. Emotional stress brings on attacks; however some attacks may be due to a conditioned response.

e) Causative factors: emotional stress due to situation involving separation. Other factors appear to be related to severe allergy in some individuals or to interaction between allergic factors and emotional factors.

          f) Dynamic issue in asthma: separation

      5) Musculoskeletal: arthritis

4. Assessment of psychophysiologic condition
   a. Careful assessment of psychological and environmental factors

5. Coordination of medical and psychological treatment

B. *Anxiety disorders (neurotic behavior)*

1. Characteristics of neurotic behavior
   a. Biologic: symptoms of physical illness
   b. Psychological: problems with interpersonal relationships, anxiety
   c. Sociocultural: changes in social roles, feelings of guilt
   d. Difference in neurotic vs psychotic behavior

2. Differences between psychotic and neurotic disorders (see Table 7 for criteria of each). Psychosis implies wider, more severe personality disturbance with more extreme defenses and poorer contact with reality compared with neurotic disorders. (*DSM III* uses the term "anxiety disorders" rather than "neurotic".)

3. Theories of neurotic behavior
   a. Psychodynamic (Freud): conflict between impulses (id) and reality (ego) producing anxiety
   b. Interpersonal (Sullivan): anxiety arising out of disturbed interpersonal relationships
      1) Peplau: levels of anxiety

4. Clinical types
   a. Anxiety reaction
      1) Characteristic behaviors: varies from fatigue to panic, includes somatic symptoms (dry mouth, dizziness, rapid heart rate), feelings of sadness, irritability
   b. Hysterical behavior

TABLE 7   Criteria Differentiating Psychoses from Neuroses

	PSYCHOSES	NEUROSES
Behavioral syndromes	Overactivity Impulsivity Retardation Suspiciousness Idiosyncratic oddities Withdrawal	Apprehensiveness Anxiety attacks Phobias Obsessions Compulsions Conversion reactions Fugues Amnestic confabulatory states Repetitive
Psychologic defenses	Denial Regression Introjection Projection Identification (pathologic)	Repression Displacement Isolation Reaction-formation Undoing Substitution Conversion
Affect	Elation Depression Apathy Ambivalence Inappropriateness	Responsive
Ego functions	Impaired Reality relation distorted Confused Idiosyncratic	Intact but constricted Reality oriented
Interpersonal relations	Object relations ambivalent or seriously impaired Sexual relations confused	Object relations maintained Emotional lability Dramatization or constriction Impaired heterosexual relations

SOURCE: Reprinted with permission from Kolb, L. and Brodie, H.K., *Modern Clinical Psychiatry*, 10th Ed. Philadelphia, W.B. Saunders Co., 1982, p. 465.

1) Conversion type
   a) Physical response related to psychic conflict
   b) Differentiating hysterical response from a specific physical disorder and from malingering
2) Dissociative type: amnesia, sleepwalking

c. Obsessive: compulsive behavior
   1) Definitions: obsession, compulsion
   2) Purpose: control anxiety through repetitive ritual or thoughts

d. Phobias
   1) Incidence and prevalence: phobias (marked fear of an object or situation) are extremely common in childhood and generally disappear without treatment. Phobias in adults persist for longer periods. While common they are rarely diagnosed because they are often associated with anxiety disorders.
   2) Specific objects feared: animals are common; heights, enclosed places, particular buildings, locations or specific situations; rarely, open areas
   3) Dynamic issue: anxiety, often it is displaced from an unknown source to a known, obvious one that may be symbolically related. Purpose is to avoid a feared situation. Occasionally situational phobias will generalize if the avoidance pattern fails.

5. Nursing care
   a. Nurses response: feelings of anger, frustration, helplessness
   b. Assessment
      1) Determine pattern of client behavior
      2) Set goals: decrease anxiety and fears, verbalize freely, increase self-esteem, increase socialization, decrease manipulation and dependency needs

    c. Nursing intervention
        1) Consistent
        2) Set limits
        3) Permit choices
        4) Behavior modification for selected situations
        5) Evaluate

C. *Affective disorder*

  1. Depression
      a. Definitions: depressed mood vs grief vs clinical depression
      b. Types of depression: bipolar (manic-depressive) vs unipolar endogenous depression; endogenous vs exogenous (reactive)
      c. Behaviors typical of depression
          1) Feelings of sadness, worthlessness, guilt, low self-esteem, helplessness, and hopelessness
          2) Somatic responses: decreased sleep, weight loss, decreased appetite, loss of energy, decreased sexual interest
          3) Slowed thoughts, inability to think, inability to work, slowed speech, slowed movement
      d. Incidence and prevalence of depression: National Institute of Mental Health estimates 15% of all adults 18–74 years old suffer from depression in any given year.
      e. Etiology of depression
          1) Situational loss
          2) Genetic studies of manic-depressive illness
          3) Biochemical changes in depression, decreased catecholamines
      f. Types of depressive illness: diagnoses
          1) Manic-depressive disorder: a psychosis in which periods of elation alternate with periods of depression.

2) Involutional depression: a severe depression, psychosis, occurring in later decades of life. Two to three times as many women experience this illness as men. Loss often precedes the disorder. Symptoms include marked depression, weight loss, somatic complaints and/or delusions, extreme shame or guilt over supposed "bad" behavior. About 40% of patients recover without treatment. Many more are successfully treated with ECT or antidepressant drugs.

3) Reactive depression: generally a less severe form of depression secondary to unresolved loss, e.g., a death. May occur in any age group and both sexes. Symptoms include depressed feelings, withdrawal, poor sleep, and poor eating patterns, but do not include extreme guilt, delusions, etc. Treated with psychotherapy and drugs.

g. Nursing assessment and intervention
1) Assess priority problems and set goals
2) Provide physical care of patient: food, rest, bathing
3) Protect patient from suicide
4) Develop a supportive relationship, decreasing withdrawal
5) Provide for ways to increase self-esteem, and decrease feelings of helplessness and hopelessness
6) Allow for expression of feelings
7) Aid in resolution of grief, if needed

h. Medical treatment of depression
1) Medication: antidepressants
2) Somatic treatments: electroconvulsive therapy (ECT)

        a.   Nurses role: instruction and support of patient
        b) Method of treatment
        c) Contraindications for treatment
        d) Effects of treatment
   i. Prevention of depression: resolution of grief reactions

2. Mania
   a. Characteristic behaviors of hypomania include: marked activity, rapid speech, excitement, rapid but not thorough completion of tasks. Person is in touch with reality.
   b. Characteristic of mania include: hyperverbal, hyperactive, delusions, euphoria, aggressiveness, flight of ideas, psychotic thinking
   c. Psychodynamics of manic-depressive disorder: depression is the underlying problem and results from loss of dependent relationship.
   d. Incidence and prevalence: more common among northern Europeans and their descendants. Occurrence is 25 times more frequent among siblings or close relatives and occurs twice as frequently in women as in men.
   e. Types include: manic-type (long period of manic behavior and brief period of depression), depressed-type (long period of depression, brief mania) and cyclic-type (equal periods of depression and mania)
   f. Medical treatment: lithium
      1) Nursing responsibilities in lithium treatment
   g. Nursing assessment and intervention
      1) Assessment of priority problems and setting goals
      2) Assisting patient to set limits on his activity and verbalization
      3) Providing for adequate food, rest, and activity

           4) Aiding patient in maintaining good interpersonal relationships

D. *Schizophrenia*

1. Conceptions of schizophrenia
   a. E. Kraepelin: dementia praecox
   b. E. Bleuler: Schizophrenia (split mind) and the symptomatology of the four As-autism, ambivalence, affective impairment, associative looseness
   c. A. Meyer: deterioration of habits

2. Incidence and prevalence of disease
   a. Known in all cultures throughout history
   b. Schizophrenic patients in United States public mental hospitals equal to 150 per 100,000 population in 1955 or 1% of total United States population

3. Etiology of schizophrenia
   a. Biological theories
      1) Genetic factors: numerous studies of twins and families with schizophrenia indicate higher incidence when family history exists.
      2) Biochemical imbalance
         a) Transmethylation hypothesis (decreased MAO in platelets)
         b) Dopamine hypothesis (overactivity of dopamine synapses)
   b. Psychologic theories
      1) Early childhood deficits: Harry Stack Sullivan, Melanie Klien, Theodore Lidz
      2) Double-bind hypothesis: D. Bateson
      3) Learned behavior: Thomas Szasz

4. Symptomatology
   a. Affective impairment: inability to feel in a manner appropriate to situation (inappropriate or blunted)

b. Ambivalence: marked contradiction in feelings toward other persons or situation and unable to resolve conflict

c. Autistic ideas: unique to that person, e.g., neologism

d. Associative looseness: thoughts loosely connected, if at all, and not logical

e. Lack of attention

f. Other behaviors: ideas of reference, hallucinations, delusions, extreme negativism, withdrawal

5. Clinical subtypes

a. Catatonic: person manifests phases of stupor alternating with sudden periods of great excitement, shows "waxy flexibility," more frequent in young women; prognosis for recovery is good.

b. Paranoid: person manifests suspiciousness, delusions of persecution, hallucinations, ideas of reference, and often is hostile and negative; occurs later in life (30s or older) and in individuals who are rather intelligent and well-functioning persons before illness.

c. Hebephrenic (mind of youth): person manifests a rather insidious onset of schizophrenic symptoms of delusions, hallucinations, inappropriate affect—often silly. Occurrence is at adolescence, among young people who are rather withdrawn and shy; disorder progresses slowly and prognosis is poor.

d. Simple: person manifests marked disturbance of emotion, interest, and activity; hallucinations and delusions are rare; there is a slow impoverishment of personality; occurrence is at adolescence; some become vagrants, prostitutes, or delinquents. Prognosis: limited.

e. Chronic: a variety of schizophrenic symptoms occur but none predominate; hallucinations, delusions occur, affect is flat; diagnosed after repeated acute psychotic episodes.

6. Prognostic types: reactive (rapid onset, good prognosis) vs process (slow onset, poor prognosis)

7. Nursing assessment and intervention
   a. Social model of care: milieu therapy
      1) Providing structure for patient's day to decrease regression and to deal with reality
      2) Providing recreation, socialization to decrease withdrawal and increase pleasure
      3) Provide for decision-making, community activity, self-governance to increase self-esteem
      4) Provide for good nutrition, rest, hygiene
      5) Decrease suspiciousness, act openly and with consistency, keep promises
   b. Psychological model of care
      1) Establish a working relationship
      2) Deal with termination from the beginning
      3) Help decrease anxiety and deal with reality
      4) Help patient to give up psychotic defenses, substituting more appropriate coping mechanisms
      5) Provide for one-on-one therapy, and progress to group therapy
   c. Biologic model of care
      1) Phenothiozine drug treatment, e.g., with Thorazine
         a) Purpose of medication: antipsychotic, antianxiety
         b) Rapid tranquilization with oral or IM injections, e.g., Thorazine 50 mg q1hr until drowsy for extremely confused, excited, psychotic patients
         c) Usual tranquilizer administration is in oral dosages during the day, e.g., Thorazine 100 mg p.o. t.i.d. (dose and medication varies markedly with size and condition of the patient) and is, of course, ordered by a physician

        d) Nursing considerations: observe for side reactions, initially hypo- or hypertension, slowed pulse, lowered basal rate, sleepiness, dry mouth and nasal congestion, antiemetic. Larger doses produce motor retardation, muscular hypotonia, unsteady gait, other parkinsonian effects.

          (i) Warn patient regarding potentiating effects of alcohol, barbiturates, and other drugs.

          (ii) Protect skin of patients from sun, protect nurses skin from contact with medication solution.

        e) Treatment of parkinsonian side effects with anticholinergic medication, e.g., benztropine (Cogentin), trihexyphenidyl (Artane), etc.

      2) Somatic treatments: electroconvulsive therapy

    d. Community treatment and prevention

      1) Working with families

      2) Day programs

      3) Aftercare

E. Personality disorders

  1. Definition: character traits stable over time

  2. Prevalence: 7% of United States population

  3. Types of personality disorder

    a. Paranoid personality

      1) Characteristic behavior: suspiciousness, fearful of attack, shy, or aggressive

      2) Nursing responses/intervention

        a) Permit freedom of choice and movement

        b) Be a "safe" person, not taking sides

   b. Schizoid personality
       1) Characteristic behavior: withdrawn,
          lonely, empty
       2) Nursing response/intervention
          a) Provide careful limited contact
              as a bridge to other social rela-
              tionships
   c. Passive-aggressive personality
      1) Characteristic behavior: two types
         a) Passive-aggressive: late, avoidant, co-
             vertly hostile
         b) Passive-dependent: oral, demanding,
             insatiable
      2) Nursing response: supportive, but set
         limits
   d. Obsessive-compulsive personality
      1) Characteristic behavior: rigid, perfection-
         istic, indecisive, critical
      2) Nursing response: respect individual's
         autonomy, help regain control
   e. Hysterical personality
      1) Characteristic behavior: seduction, pro-
         vocative, egocentric
      2) Nursing responsive: supportive, "mater-
         nal" noncompetitive response
   f. Borderline personality
      1) Definition: person's behavior on a con-
         tinuum between neurosis and schizo-
         phrenia
      2) Characteristic behavior varies from
         a) Somewhat regressed, childlike (neu-
             rotic)
         b) Angry, depressed, weak self-identity
             (core)
         c) Withdrawn, intellectualizing, poor self-
             identity ("as if")
         d) Inappropriate behavior, poor self-
             identity, anger, depression (psychotic)

    3) Nursing intervention
      a) Prevent manipulation or "splitting" of staff
      b) Provide safe environment
      c) Set consistent limits
      d) Deal openly with termination and other situations resulting in patient anger

  g. Antisocial personality (sociopathic)
    1) Characteristic behaviors
      a) Unable to relate fully to others but appears pleasant and charming
      b) Impulsive, seeks immediate gratification, not anxious
      c) Commits antisocial acts but feels no guilt and does not learn by experience
    2) Theories of causation
      a) Inadequate learning and control during early childhood
      b) Evidence of brain damage
    3) Criminal activity: 40% of prison population but responsible for 80–90% of crimes
    4) Treatment: group therapy in prison or long-term inpatient facility may help. Otherwise, limited treatment

  h. Sexual deviations dangerous to self or others: rape, autoerotic death

F. *Organic mental disorder*

  1. Acute confusional states (delirium)
    a. Definition: temporary, usually reversible alteration of the brain chemistry/physiology. This is a global syndrome affecting many brain functions.
    b. Symptoms: confusion, hallucinations, progressive loss of consciousness; need to differentiate from schizophrenia

    c. Causes
      1) Drug overdosage or drug reaction, delerium tremens
      2) Salt and water imbalance secondary to surgery, dehydration, heat stroke
      3) Endocrine disorder: hypoglycemia or acidosis in diabetes, hepatic failure
      4) Infections: meningitis
      5) Head trauma, concussion, seizures
    d. Nursing intervention
      1) Assessment of cause is crucial; careful history
      2) Collaborate with medical treatment to correct cause
      3) Provide for safety of patient
      4) Prevention of recurrence: education of patient, family

2. Subactue amnestic syndrome

This syndrome progresses from an acute cause to a subacute state. The syndrome may clear and recovery occurs, or it may become chronic, or the patient may die. The syndrome is potentially reversible. No clouding of consciousness.

    a. Definition: a long-term, partially reversible disorder with known cause. This is a focal syndrome affecting primarily memory.
    b. Symptoms: progressive memory loss, some confusion, disorientation, confabulation
    c. Causes
      1) Korsakoff's syndrome: a dysmnesic (poor memory) syndrome, which sometimes follows acute delerium. It is characterized by marked memory loss, confusion, and confabulation—making up stories. The syndrome is associated with alcoholism and vitamin B_1 deficiency.

    2) Severe head trauma or brain tumor: with subsequent injury or loss of brain tissue, the brain injury or tumor may result in memory loss, confusion, disorientation. If injury is not too severe, individual will recover.

    3) Cerebrovascular disorders: transient ischemic attacks (TIAs), atherosclerosis, and hypertension all produce some altered cerebral function. With decreased cerebral blood flow there is progressive memory impairment, poor intellectual functioning, confusion, disorientation, and emotional lability. Early in the disease process these behaviors are reversible, later they become chronic.

    4) Other causes that are less frequently seen include metabolic disorder, e.g., Addison disease, thyroid disease; bacterial infections of the central nervous system; neurologic disorders, e.g., multiple sclerosis, etc.

  d. Nursing intervention
    1) Assessment of cause
    2) Collaborating in medical treatment of disease process
    3) Assisting patient with memory aids
    4) Maintaining safe environment

3. Chronic organic mental syndrome
  a. Definition: a gradual general deterioration of intellectual ability and of personality (dementia); nonspecific cause. This is a global syndrome affecting many aspects of function.
  b. Disorders
    1) Alzheimer's disease: a progressive mental deterioration of the brain with progressive memory loss, personality changes, increased agitation, and emotional distress. Cause unknown and may occur as

early as aged 40 or 50 (presenile dementia) or as late as aged 70. Course is 2-5
years, and there is no recovery.
2) Huntington's chorea: a genetically in-
herited disease that has a progressive
degenerative course, beginning in middle
life. Personality changes occur first and
then a gradually worsening dementia.
3) Pick's disease: more rare than Alzheimer's
disease. Initially attention span is decreased and then memory fails. Patient
becomes more talkative but is hard to
understand. Intellectual and physical de-
bilitation occur later resulting in paralysis
or seizures.
c. Symptoms
1) Progressive loss of memory (recall) and
inability to retain new information
2) Increasing disorientation in (1) time;
(2) later, place; (3) finally, person
3) Difficulty in abstract thinking
4) Gradual loss of socialization, regression,
increased emotional lability
d. Nursing intervention
1) Preventive aspects, education of family
and public
2) Provide memory aids, familiar environment to reduce confusion
3) Support patients ability to socialize and
relate, deal with feelings
4) Provide safe environment, maintain physical status of patient—food, rest, lighting,
other physical safety factors
5) Provide support, instruction, physical assistance to family

G. *Childhood psychiatric disorders*

1. Atypical child (infantile autism)

a. Definition: the child who lives in a totally subjective world
b. Occurrence: symptoms occur after birth or at about the age of 2 or 3 years
c. Cause: unknown, possible constitutional or functional deficit
d. Characteristic behavior
   1) Lack of affect, unresponsive to parents and others, very withdrawn
   2) Unaware of physical environment
   3) Hyperactive, bizarre behavior
   4) Ritual activity and play, infantile
   5) Impaired verbalization
   6) Average intelligence
e. Nursing intervention
   1) Client requires help in bathing, eating, physical care, moving toward self-help
   2) Increase client's socialization
   3) "Teach" through reinforcement of more appropriate behavior

2. Childhood schizophrenia
   a. Cause: Genetic factors interacting with environmental ones
   b. Characteristic behavior (see Table 8)
      1) Grossly impaired relations with others
      2) Impaired sense of identity
      3) Preoccupation with objects
      4) Abnormal perceptions, hallucinations
      5) High anxiety
      6) Limited verbalization
      7) The older the child the more behavior resembles adult schizophrenia
   c. Nursing intervention
      1) Provide a safe environment
      2) Decrease social withdrawal
      3) Help child deal with anxiety
      4) Help child gain sense of personal identity

TABLE 8 Diagnostic Criteria for Schizophrenic Children

LEVEL OF IMPAIRMENT	DEFINITION	RATING
Very severe	No differentiation of important persons e.g., mother from others; makes no contact with anybody; no speech or gestural communication; total or near total avoidance of looking and listening; indiscriminate mouthing and smelling; near-total absence of self-care; no educability	1
Severe	Human preferences observable but misidentifications of important persons occur often; limited contact; speech and gestural communication below level of 3-year-old (echoic, pronouns confused, comprehensibility below 90%); mouthing and smelling still prominent; self-care below that of 3-year-old; minimal educability (at preschool level)	2
Moderate	Recognition of responses to important persons; contacting behavior (approaching, talking to others); speech and gestural communication above that of 3-year-old; responds to school education above grade 1; yet gross distortions of reality (body image, capacities, etc.) and psychotic behavior	3
Mild	Mild eccentricity and no friends but functions acceptably in relation to school (including community school and with or without special adjustment such as ungraded class or special tutoring) and in relation to the external environment; or no longer manifestly outlandish or bizarre relationship to people, school and the external environment but neurotic defenses present (e.g., obsessional or phobic)	4

TABLE 8   (cont'd)

LEVEL OF IMPAIRMENT	DEFINITION	RATING
Normal	By ordinary observation	5

SOURCE: Reprinted, with permission, from Goldfarb, W. *Growth and Change of Schizophrenic Children: A Longitudinal Study.* New York: John Wiley & Sons, 1974.

3. Behavior disorder of childhood
   a. Types of problems: eneuresis, encopresis, phobias in early childhood; and depression, anxiety, and social withdrawal or hyperactivity and aggressive behavior in later childhood
   b. Nursing intervention
      1) Consistent emotional support using verbal response and touch
      2) Consistent limit setting to help child experience a sense of control
      3) Help child maintain boundaries through appropriate verbalization and touch
      4) Working closely with family to aid learning new ways of relating to child

4. Behavior disorders of adolescence
   a. Four types: behavior may be unsocialized or socialized and aggressive or nonaggressive
   b. Nursing intervention
      1) Increase appropriate socialization with adolescent peer group
      2) Careful consistent limit setting with adolescent participating in making rules
      3) Help client to verbalize and work through feelings verbally rather than acting out
      4) Stop client's antisocial behavior, preventing harm to self or others
      5) Assist person in building self-identity and self-esteem

6) Collaborate in family therapy to help families learn new ways of relating and problem solving

H. *Developmental disabilities*

1. Definition: developmental diability is a severe chronic disability due to physical or mental impairment, or both, and results in substantial limitations in three or more of the following: self-care, learning, mobility, self-direction, capacity of independent living and for economic self-sufficiency, and requires extended treatment

2. Etiology of mental retardation
   a) Genetic conditions: chromosomal, e.g., Down's syndrome; or errors in metabolism, e.g., phenylketonuria
   b. Acquired conditions: prenatal, e.g., rubella; perinatal, e.g., anoxia; postnatal, e.g., infection

3. Diagnosis is based on
   a. Measured intelligence (IQ)
   b. Social adaptive behavior (see Table 9)

4. Prevalence of mental retardation is 0.3% of United States population; most common developmental disability

5. Levels of retardation
   a. Mild: needs special education, but can learn, can work, and be self supporting (IQ 55–69)
   b. Moderate: can care for self, develops social skills, does routine tasks, can work in sheltered workshop (IQ 40–54)
   c. Severly retarded: requires services throughout life, vary in their ability to care for self (IQ 24–39)
   d. Profoundly retarded: requires ongoing nursing and medical services, may do limited self-care with help (IQ less than 25)

TABLE 9 Characteristic Behavior by Level of Mental Retardation and Developmental Stage

DEVELOPMENTAL STAGE	PROFOUNDLY RETARDED	SEVERELY RETARDED	MODERATELY RETARDED	MILDLY RETARDED
Stage 1: Maturation and development (birth to 5 years)	Sensorimotor capabilities virtually absent, needs total nursing care	Minimal speech, motor abilities poor, little communication, little self-help training possible	Can communicate, has little social awareness, trainability in self-help, needs supervision	May be normal in communication and social skills, minimal sensorimotor deficiency
Stage 2: Training and education (6–20 years)	Slight motor development reached, limited training in self-help possible	May communicate, can be trained in hygienic habits	Can learn social and occupational skills, academic level no higher than second grade, may move freely in limited areas	Academic skills to sixth-grade level possible, social awareness may be fostered

TABLE 9 (cont'd)

DEVELOPMENTAL STAGE	PROFOUNDLY RETARDED	SEVERELY RETARDED	MODERATELY RETARDED	MILDLY RETARDED
Stage 3: Social and vocational adequacy (21 years and over)	May develop rudimentary speech pattern, self-care capabilities do not preclude nursing care	Can aid in self-care but only under total supervision, can protect self in structured, monitored environment	Can do unskilled work in sheltered workshop, needs supervision for most stressful circumstances	Minimum self-support possible with social and vocation skills, stress requires support

SOURCE: Adapted from U.S. Department of Health, Education, and Welfare, *Mental Retardation Activities* Washington, D.C.: Government Printing Office, 1983, p. 2.

6. Nursing intervention
   a. Assessment of child and family
      1) Note appearance of any developmental lags in child
      2) Explore patterns of sleep, eating, elimination, play, temperature, social interaction in client
      3) Explore with family members regarding parental involvement with child, sibling interaction, family interaction
      4) Use observation, interviewing, and appropriate tools, e.g., Denver Developmental
      5) Explore family response to diagnosis of mental retardation (often one of shock, followed by grief reaction)
      6) Nurse must develop understanding of how crisis affects family.
   b. Intervention with child and parents
      1) Counsel parents regarding diagnosis
      2) Provide parents with ongoing teaching related to child growth and development
      3) Provide help in planning activities of daily care
      4) Provide protection from life-threatening problems and instruct family
      5) Support relief of stress on caretakers. Use opportunities for educating public regarding handicapped
      6) Identify program choices for child. Learn what services are available
      7) Evaluate care
   c. Primary prevention through health education and well-child care

APPENDIX

Glossary

Acrophobia: Fear of high places.

Acting out: Expressions of unconscious emotional conflicts or feelings of hostility or love in actions, rather than words. The individual is not consciously aware of the meaning of such acts.

Addiction: Dependence on a chemical substance to the extent that physiological dependence is established. The latter manifests itself as withdrawal symptoms (the abstinence syndrome), when the drug is withdrawn.

Adolescence: A chronological period beginning with the physical and emotional processes leading to sexual and psychosocial maturity, and ending at an ill-defined time when the individual achieves independence and social productivity.

Affect: A person's emotional feeling tone and its outward manifestations.

Affective disorder: Any mental disorder in which a disturbance of affect is predominant (including depressive neurosis, major affective disorders, and psychotic depressive reaction).

Aggression: A forceful physical, verbal, or symbolic action. May be appropriate and self-protective, including healthful self-assertiveness, or inappropriate to the situation.

Agitated depression: A psychotic depression accompanied by constant restlessness.

Agitation: Severe restlessness; a major psychomotor expression of emotional tension.

Agoraphobia: Literally, fear of open places; in practice, fear of physically leaving one's home.

Many of the definitions in this glossary are reprinted, with permission, from *Psychiatric Glossary*. Washington, D.C.: American Psychiatric Association, 1975.

Akathisia: Inability to sit down because the thought of doing so causes severe anxiety. Also may be a psychotropic drug side effect.

Al-Anon: Organization of relatives of alcoholics operated in many communities within the structure of Alcoholic Anonymous.

Alcoholics Anonymous (AA): Group of former alcoholics who collectively assist other alcoholics in learning to cope without using alcohol.

Alcoholism: Chronic disease manifested by repeated drinking that produces injury to the drinker's health or to his social or economic functioning.

Alienation: The state of estrangement the individual feels in cultural settings he views as foreign or unacceptable.

Ambivalence: Coexistence of two opposing drives, desires, feelings, or emotions toward the same person, object, or goal. These may be conscious or partly conscious.

Amnesia: Pathological loss of memory; forgetting. The phenomenon in which an area of experience is forgotten and becomes inaccessible to conscious recall.

Anal character: A personality type that manifests excessive orderliness, miserliness, and obstinacy.

Anger: A feeling of displeasure, dislike, or anxiety aroused by a perceived threat to oneself, one's possessions, or significant others.

Anhedonia: Lacking in interest or pleasure in acts which are normally pleasurable. May be an early sign of schizophrenia.

Anomie: Apathy, alienation, and personal distress resulting from the loss of goals previously valued.

Anorexia nervosa: A syndrome marked by severe and prolonged inability to eat, with marked weight loss, amenorrhea (or impotence), and other symptoms resulting from emotional conflict and biological changes.

Antabuse (disulfiram): Drug used in the treatment of alcoholism. It blocks the normal metabolism of alcohol and produces increased blood concentrations of acetaldehydes which cause very unpleasant reactions, including pounding of the heart, shortness of breath, nausea, and vomiting.

Anxiety: Apprehension, tension, or uneasiness that stems from the anticipation of danger, the source of which is largely unknown or unrecognized.

Apathy: Disinterest or lack of attention to self and environment.

Association: Relationship between ideas or emotions.

Aura: A premonitory, subjective sensation (e.g., a flash of light) that often warns the person of an impending headache or convulsion.

Autism: Form of thinking marked by extreme self-absorption and egocentricity, in which objective facts are obscured, distorted, or excluded in varying degrees.

Autistic thinking: Self-centered thinking from which reality tends to be excluded.

Autoeroticism: Sensual self-gratification. Characteristic of, but not limited to, an early stage of emotional development.

Behavior: The actions of a person or persons.

Behavior therapy: Any treatment approach designed to modify the patient's behavior directly rather than to correct the dynamic causation.

Benzodiazepines: A group of chemically related antianxiety drugs.

Biofeedback: A training program designed to develop an individual's ability to control the autonomic nervous system.

Bisexuality: Sexually oriented to both males and females.

Blocking: Sudden inability to recall that which is familiar.

Blunting: Dulling of emotional response.

Castration: Removal of the sex organs. In psychological terms, the fantasized loss of the penis.

Castration anxiety: Due to fantasized danger or injuries to the genitals and/or body.

Catatonic state: Characterized by immobility with muscular rigidity or inflexibility, and, at times, excitability.

Catchment area: Used in psychiatry to delineate a geographic area for which a mental health facility has responsibility.

Catharsis: The therapeutic release of ideas through a "talking out" of conscious material accompanied by the appropriate emotional reaction.

Cathexis: Attachment, conscious or unconscious, of emotional feeling and significance to an idea or object, most commonly a person.

Cerea flexibilitas: The "waxy flexibility" often present in catatonic schizophrenia, in which the patient's arm or leg remains passively in the position in which it is placed.

Cerebral arteriosclerosis: Hardening of the arteries of the brain, sometimes resulting in an organic brain syndrome that may be either primarily neurologic in nature or primarily mental, or a combination of both.

Character: The personality trait or behavioral style of a person.

Character defense: Any character or personality trait which serves an unconscious defensive purpose.

Character disorder: A personality disorder manifested by a chronic and habitual pattern of reaction that is maladaptive, in that it is relatively inflexible, limits the optimal use of potentialities, and often provokes the very counterreactions from the environment that the subject seeks to avoid.

Cholinergic: Activated or transmitted by acetylcholine.

Clang association: A type of thinking in which the sound of a word, rather than its meaning, gives the directions to subsequent associations.

Claustrophobia: Fear of closed places.

Cognitive: Referring to the mental process of comprehensive judgment, memory, and reasoning, as contrasted with emotional and volitional processes.

Commitment: A legal process for admitting a mentally ill person to a mental hospital. The legal definition and procedures vary from state to state.

Community health center: A health service delivery system first authorized by the Federal Mental Retardation Facilities and Community Mental Health Centers Construction Act of 1963, to provide a coordinated program of continuing mental health care to a specific population.

Compensation: A defense mechanism, operating unconsciously, by which the individual attempts to make up for real or fantasized deficiencies.

Complex: A group of associated ideas that have a common strong emotional tone.

Compulsion: An insistent, repetitive, intrusive, and unwanted urge to perform an act that is contrary to the person's ordinary wishes or standards.

Compulsive personality: A personality characterized by excessive adherence to rigid standards (inflexible, over-conscientious).

Confabulation: The filling in of memory gaps with made-up stories.

Confidentiality: Responsibility of an agency and its employees to keep all records, reports, correspondence, and interactions confidential and accessible to authorized individuals.

Conflict: A mental struggle that arises from the simultaneous operation of opposing impulses, drives, or external (environmental) or internal demands.

Confusion: Disturbed orientation in respect to time, place, or person.

Conscience: The morally self-critical part of the self, encompassing standards of behavior, performance, and value judgments.

Conscious: That part of the mind or mental functioning of which the content is subject to awareness or known to the person.

Conversion: A defense mechanism, operating unconsciously, by which intrapsychic conflicts that would otherwise give rise to anxiety are instead given symbolic external expression.

Convulsion disorder: Primarily the centrencephalic seizures, grand mal, and petit mal and the focal seizures of Jacksonian and psychomotor epilepsy.

Coping: Ability to problem-solve and deal with life stressors and crises.

Coping mechanisms: Ways of adjusting to environmental stress without altering one's goals or purposes; includes both conscious and unconscious mechanisms.

Countertransference: The therapist's partly unconscious or conscious emotional reaction to his patient.

Crisis intervention: Short-term treatment for assisting people to cope with a stressful situation.

Death instinct (Thanatos): In Freudian theory, the unconscious drive toward dissolution and death; coexists with and is in opposition to the life instinct (Eros).

Decompensation: Deterioration of existing defenses, leading to an exacerbation of pathological behavior.

Defense mechanism: Unconscious intrapsychic process serving to provide relief from emotional conflict and anxiety.

Deja vu: Sensation that what one is seeing one has seen before.

Delirium: Acute reversible mental state characterized by confusion and altered, possibly fluctuating, consciousness due to an alteration of cerebral metabolism with delusions, illusions, and/or hallucinations.

Delirium tremens: Acute and sometimes fatal brain disorder caused by withdrawal or relative withdrawal from alcohol, usually developing in 24–96 hours.

Delusion: A firm, fixed idea not amenable to rational explanation; maintained against logical argument, despite objective contradictory evidence.

Delusions of grandeur: Exaggerated ideas of one's importance or identity.

Delusions of persecution: Ideas that one has been singled out for persecution.

Delusions of reference: Incorrect assumptions that certain causal or unrelated events or the behavior of others apply to oneself.

Dementia: Irreversible mental state characterized by decreased intellectual function, personality change, impairment of judgment, and often changes in affect.

Dementia praecox: Obsolete descriptive term for schizophrenia.

Denial: Defense mechanism, operating unconsciously, used to resolve emotional conflict and allay anxiety by disavowing thoughts, feelings, wishes, needs, or external reality factors that are consciously intolerable.

Dependence: The mental and physical state of being dependent upon a drug in order to achieve a feeling of wellbeing.

Dependency needs: Vital needs for mothering, love, affection, security, and warmth; may be a manifestation of regression when they reappear openly in adults.

Depersonalization: Feelings of unreality or strangeness concerning either the environment or the self or both.

Depression: When used to describe mood, depression refers to feelings of sadness, despair, and unhappiness. As such, depression is universally experienced and is a normal feeling state.

Deprivation, emotional: A lack of adequate and appropriate interpersonal and/or environmental experience, usually in the early developmental years.

Deterioration: Worsening of a clinical condition, usually expressed as progressive impairment of function.

Detoxification: Treatment by use of medication, diet, rest, fluids, and nursing care to restore physiological functioning after it has been seriously disturbed by the overuse of alcohol, barbiturates, or other addictive drugs.

Disorientation: Loss of awareness of the position of the self in relation to space, time, or other persons.

Displacement: A defense mechanism, operating unconsciously, in which an emotion is transferred from its original object to a more acceptable substitute, used to allay anxiety.

Dissociation: A defense mechanism, operating unconsciously, through which emotional significance and affect are separated and detached from an idea, situation or object.

Double bind: A type of interaction in which one person demands a response to a message containing mutually contradictory signals, while the other is unable either to comment on the incongruity or to escape from the situation.

Drive: Basic urge, instinct, motivation.

Drug dependence: Habituation to, abuse of a chemical substance.

Drug interaction: The effects of two or more drugs being taken simultaneously, producing an alteration in the usual effects of either drug taken alone.

Dysarthria: Difficulty in speech production due to incoordination of speech apparatus.

Dysphoria: Disorder of mood.

Dystonia: Impaired or disordered muscle tone.

Echolalia: Pathological repetition of words.

Echopraxia: Pathological repetition, by imitation, of the movements of another.

Ecology: Study of relations between organisms and their environments, especially the study of relations among human beings, their environment, and human institutions.

ECT (electroconvulsive treatment): A form of psychiatric treatment in which electric current is administered to the patient and results in a loss of consciousness or a convulsive or comatose reaction to alter favorably the course of the illness.

Ego: In psychoanalytic theory, one of the three major divisions in the model of the psychic apparatus, the others being the id and superego. The ego represents the sum of certain mental mechanisms, such as perception and memory, and specific defense mechanisms.

Ego ideal: That part of the personality that comprises the aims and goals of the self; usually refers to the conscious or unconscious emulation of significant figures with whom the person has identified.

Electra complex: An infrequently used term describing the pathological relationship of a woman with men, based on unresolved developmental conflicts partially analogous to the Oedipus complex in the man.

Emotion: A feeling such as fear, anger, grief, joy, or love which may not always be conscious.

Empathy: An objective and insightful awareness of the feelings, emotions, and behavior of another person, their meaning, and significance.

Encopresis: Incontinence of feces.

Enuresis: Incontinence of urine.

Epilepsy: A disorder characterized by periodic motor or sensory seizures or their equivalents and sometimes accompanied by a loss of consciousness or by certain equivalent manifestations; may be idiopathic (no known organic cause) or symptomatic (due to organic lesions).

Euphoria: An exaggerated feeling of physical and emotional well-being not consonant with apparent stimuli or events.

Exhibitionism: A man exposing his genitals to women or girls in socially unacceptable situations.

Existential psychiatry: A school of psychiatry evolved from orthodox psychoanalytic thought; stresses the way in which man experiences the phenomenological world about him and takes responsibility for his existence.

Extrapsychic: That which takes place between the psyche (mind) and the environment.

Extrapyramidal system: The portion of the central nervous system responsible for coordinating and integrating various aspects of motor behavior or bodily movements.

Fabrication: Made up events to fill in gaps in memory.

Fainting: Temporary loss of consciousness.

Family therapy: Treatment of more than one member of the family simultaneously in the same session. The treatment may be supportive, directive, or interpretive.

Fantasy: An imagined sequence of events or mental images (for example, daydreams).

Fear: Emotional and physiological response to recognized sources of danger; to be distinguished from anxiety.

Fetishism: A sexual deviation characterized by attachment of special meaning to an inanimate object (or fetish) which serves, usually unconsciously, as a substitute for the original object or person.

Fixation: The arrest of psychosexual maturation. Depending on degree, it may be either normal or pathological.

Flat affect: Dull or nonexpressive emotional tone or response.

Flight of ideas: Verbal skipping from one idea to another. The ideas appear to be continuous but are fragmentary and determined by chance or temporal associations.

Folie à deux: A condition in which two closely related persons, usually in the same family, share the same delusion.

Forensic: Pertaining to legal considerations.

Free association: In psychoanalytic therapy, spontaneous, uncensored verbalization by the patient of whatever comes to mind.

Free-floating anxiety: Pervasive apprehension or tension which cannot be attributed to a specific cause.

Fugue: Personality dissociation characterized by amnesia and involving actual physical flight from the customary environment or field of conflict.

Functional disorder: A disorder in which the performance or operation of an organ or organ system is abnormal, but not as a result of known changes in structure.

General paresis: An organic brain syndrome resulting from a chronic syphilitic infection. Detectable with laboratory tests of the blood or spinal fluid.

General systems theory: A theoretical framework that views events from the standpoint of the "systems" involved in the event. Systems are groups of organized, interacting components.

Gestalt psychology: A school of psychology that emphasizes a total perceptual configuration and the interrelations of its component parts.

Globus hystericus: A hysterical symptom in which there is a disturbing sensation of a lump in the throat.

Grandiose: Referring to delusions or feelings of fame, power, or other extraordinary self-perception.

Grief: Normal, appropriate emotional response to an external and consciously recognized loss; usually self-limited and gradually subsides within a reasonable period of time.

Group dynamics: Process of interaction in a small group.

Gynecomastia: Abnormal development of the mammary glands in the male; may secrete milk.

Habeas corpus: Legal term most commonly used to describe a petition which asks a court to decide whether confinement of any sort has been accomplished with due process of law.

Hallucination: A false perception in the absence of an actual external stimulus; may be induced by emotional and other factors such as drugs, alcohol, and stress.

Homeostasis: Self-regulating biological processes which maintain the equilibrium of the organism.

Homosexual panic: An acute and severe attack of anxiety based upon unconscious conflicts involving homosexuality.

Homosexuality: Sexual orientation toward persons of the same sex; not a psychiatric disorder, as such.

Hyperactivity: Increased or excessive muscular activity seen in diverse neurological and psychiatric disorders.

Hyperkinesis: Increased muscular movement.

Hyperventilation: Overbreathing associated with anxiety and marked by reduction of blood carbon dioxide, subjective complaints of lightheadedness, faintness, tingling of the extremities, palpitation, and respiratory distress.

Hypnosis: Induced dissociative state.

Hypnotic: Any agent that induces sleep. While sedatives and narcotics, in sufficient dosage, may produce sleep as an incidental effect, the term *hypnotic* is appropriately reserved for drugs employed primarily to produce sleep.

Hypochondriasis: Preoccupation with one's state of health.

Hypomania: Psychopathological state and abnormality of mood falling somewhere between normal euphoria and mania; characterized by increased happiness, optimism, mild to moderate pressure of speech and activity, and a decrease in the need for sleep.

Hysteria: Illness resulting from emotional conflict and often characterized by the use of the defense mechanisms of dissociation and conversion.

Id: In Freudian theory, that part of the personality structure which harbors the unconscious instinctual desires and striving of the individual.

Ideas of reference: Incorrect interpretation of casual incidents and external events as having direct reference to one's self.

Identification: A defense mechanism, operating unconsciously, by which an individual patterns himself after another.

Identity crisis: A loss of the sense of the sameness and historical continuity of one's self and inability to accept or adopt the role the subject perceives as being expected of him by society; often expressed by isolation, withdrawal, extremism, rebelliousness, and negativity.

Idiopathic: Disease without recognizable cause; those of spontaneous origin.

Illusion: Misinterpretation of a real experience.

Impulse: Psychic striving; usually refers to an instinctual urge.

Inappropriate affect: Emotional response or feeling tone which seems unrelated or in opposition to the situation—for example, a person laughing at a funeral.

Incompetency: Determination that a person is not psychologically fit to stand trial. People are competent to stand trial when they (1) understand the nature of the charge they face and the consequences that might occur from conviction and (2) are able to assist the attorney in their own defense.

Incorporation: Primitive defense mechanism, operating unconsciously, in which the psychic representation of a person, or parts of him, are figuratively ingested.

Infantilism: Condition in which the mind and body make slow development; failure to attain adult characteristics.

Informed consent: A client's consent to treatment based on adequate knowledge and understanding of the treatment plan.

Inhibition: Unconscious defense against forbidden instinctual drives.

Insight: Self-understanding of one's attitudes and behavior.

Instinct: Inborn drive for either self-preservation or sexuality.

Intellectualization: The utilization of reasoning as a defense against confrontation with unconscious conflicts and their stressful emotions.

Intelligence: Capacity to learn and to utilize appropriately what one has learned.

Interpretation: The process by which the therapist communicates to the patient understanding of a particular aspect of his problems or behavior.

Interview: Systematic interpersonal method of gathering information.

Insomnia: Inability to fall asleep and difficulty staying asleep, including early morning awakening.

Intrapsychic: That which takes place within the psyche or mind.

Introjection: A defense mechanism, operating unconsciously, whereby loved or hated external objects are taken within oneself symbolically. The converse of projection. May serve as a defense against conscious recognition of intolerable hostile impulses.

Introversion: Preoccupation with one's self; a turning inward of one's thoughts.

Involutional psychosis: Psychiatric disorder occurring during the middle years (menopause).

Isolation: A defense mechanism, operating unconsciously, in which an unacceptable impulse, idea, or act is separated from its original memory source, thereby removing the emotional charge associated with the original memory.

Kleptomania: Compulsion to steal.

Korsakoff's psychosis: A disorder of central nervous system metabolism due to a lack of vitamin B_1 (thiamine) seen in chronic alcoholism. Characterized by confabulation and grossly impaired memory function with deficient new learning ability.

La Belle indifference: Literally, "beautiful indifference"; seen in certain patients with hysterical neurosis, conversion type, who show an inappropriate lack of concern about their disabilities.

Labile: Pertaining to rapidly shifting emotions.

Labile affect: Rapidly shifting changes in mood and emotion.

Latent content: The hidden (unconscious) meaning of thoughts or actions, especially in dreams or fantasies.

Latent homosexuality: A condition characterized by unconscious homosexual desires.

Latency period: Developmental phase between childhood and adolescence; usually between 7 and 10 years.

Left bundle branch block: Cardiac conduction defect in which the nervous connection in the left branch of the bundle of His is obstructed so that one ventricle contracts independently of the other.

Lesbian: A homosexual woman.

Libido: The psychic drive or energy usually associated with the sexual instinct.

Lithium carbonate: The particular lithium salt usually used in the treatment of acute manic states and in the prevention of future episodes in individuals with recurrent affective disorders, which are bipolar (both mania and depression occasionally occurring).

Loosening (of associations): A thinking disorder or disturbance in associations, in which thinking becomes overgeneralized, diffuse, and vague, progressing unevenly toward a goal and generally failing as an adequate vehicle of communication with others.

LSD (lysergic acid diethylamide): A potent drug that produces psychotic symptoms and behavior.

Magical thinking: A person's conviction that thinking equates with doing.

Major affective disorders: A group of psychoses characterized by severe disorders of mood—either extreme depression or elation or both—that do not seem to be attributable entirely to precipitating life experiences.

Malingering: Deliberate simulation or exaggeration of an illness or disability that in fact is nonexistent or minor in order to avoid an unpleasant situation or to obtain some type of personal gain.

Mania: Formerly used as a nonspecific term for any kind of "madness." Currently used as a suffix, with any number of Greek roots, to indicate a morbid preoccupation with some kind of idea or activity and/or a compulsive need to behave in some deviant way.

Manic-depressive psychosis: A major affective disorder characterized by severe mood swings and a tendency to remission and recurrence.

Manifest content: The overt or remembered content of a dream or fantasy, as contrasted with latent content, which it conceals and distorts.

Masochism: Pleasure derived from physical or psychological pain inflicted either by one's self or by others.

Masturbation: Genital manipulation for the purpose of sexual stimulation.

Melancholia: Severe depression.

Mental health: A state of being, relative rather than absolute, in which a person has effected a reasonably satisfactory integration of his instinctual drives.

Mental retardation: Significantly below average intellectual functioning, which may be present at birth or become evident later in the developmental period, and is always characterized by impaired adaptation in one or all of the areas of learning, social adjustment, and maturation.

Mental status: The level and style of functioning of the psyche, used in its broadest sense to include intellectual functioning, as well as the emotional, attitudinal, psychological, and personality aspects of the subject.

Metacommunication: Messages about a communication pertaining to both the relationship and informational aspects.

Methadone: A synthetic narcotic. It may be used as a substitute for heroin, producing a less socially disabling addiction, or it may be used to aid the withdrawal from heroin.

Migraine: A syndrome characterized by recurrent, severe, and usually one-sided headaches, often associated with nausea, vomiting, and visual disturbances.

Milieu: Environment.

Milieu therapy: Socioenvironmental therapy in which the attitudes and behavior of the staff of a treatment service and the activities prescribed for the patient are determined by what the patient's emotional and interpersonal needs are presumed to be.

Monoamine oxidase (MAO) inhibitors: A group of antidepressant drugs that inhibit certain brain enzymes and raise the level of serotonin.

Mutism: Refusal to speak for conscious or unconscious reasons.

Nanogram: Unit of mass (weight) of the metric system, being one one-billionth gram. Abbreviated ng. Called also millimicrogram.

Narcissism: Self-love as opposed to object love (love of another person or object).

Narcolepsy: Condition in which a person is overcome by an uncontrollable desire to sleep.

Narcotic: Any opiate derivative drug, natural or synthetic, that relieves pain or alters mood.

Neologism: A new word and condensed combination of several words coined by a person to express a highly complex idea often related to his conflicts.

Nervous breakdown: A nonmedical nonspecific euphemism for a mental disorder.

Neurasthenia: Neurosis characterized by complaints of chronic weakness, easy fatigability, and exhaustion.

Neurosis: An emotional maladaptation arising from an unresolved, unconscious conflict. The anxiety is either felt directly or modified by various psychological mechanisms to produce other, subjectively distressing symptoms.

Object: Psychoanalytic term meaning person.

Object relations: The emotional bonds that exist between an individual and another person, as contrasted with his interest in, and love for, himself.

Obsession: A persistent, unwanted idea or impulse that cannot be eliminated by logic or reasoning.

Occupational therapy: An adjunctive therapy that utilizes purposeful activities as a means of altering the course of illness.

Oculogyric crisis: Attack of involuntary deviation and fixation of the eyeballs, usually upward.

Oedipus complex: Attachment of the child to the parent of the opposite sex, accompanied by envious and aggressive feelings toward the parent of the same sex.

Opisthotonus: Arched position of the body with feet and head on the floor caused by a tetanic spasm.

Oral stage: Developmental stage during the first year of life.

Organic brain syndrome: Any mental disorder associated with or caused by disturbance in the physiological functioning of brain tissue at any level of consciousness—structural, hormonal, biochemical, electrical, etc.

Orientation: Awareness of one's self in relation to time, place, and person.

Orthostatic hypotension: Drop in blood pressure when a person arises from a sitting or standing position. Often occurs when phenothiazine drugs are taken.

Overcompensation: A conscious or unconscious process in which a real or imagined physical or psychological deficit inspires exaggerated correction.

Panic: Acute, overwhelming anxiety; can be life-threatening due to exhaustion.

Paranoid: An adjective applied to individuals who are overly suspicious.

Paranoid ideation: Type or form of thinking or thoughts not based on reality.

Parasympathetic nervous system: That part of the autonomic nervous system that controls the life-sustaining organs of the body under normal, danger-free conditions.

Paresis: Weakness of organic origin; incomplete paralysis.

Partial hospitalization: A psychiatric treatment for patients who require hospitalization but not on a full-time basis (day hospital, night hospital, weekend hospital).

Passive-aggressive: Aggressive behavior manifested in passive ways, such as pouting, procrastination, stubbornness.

Passive-dependent personality: A disorder manifested by marked indecisiveness, emotional dependency, and lack of self-confidence.

Pedophilia: A sexual deviation involving sexual activity with children as the objects.

Perception: Process of being aware of; receiving sensory messages.

Perioral tremor: Tremor around the mouth.

Perseveration: Tendency to emit the same verbal or motor response again and again to varied stimuli.

Personality: The characteristic way in which a person behaves; the ingrained pattern of behavior that each person evolves, both consciously and unconsciously, as his style of life or way of being, in adapting to his environment.

Personality disorders: A group of mental disorders characterized by deeply ingrained maladaptive patterns of behavior, generally lifelong in duration and consequently often recognizable by the time of adolescence or earlier.

Perversion: An imprecise term used loosely to designate sexual variance.

Phallic stage: Period from about 2½ to 6 years during which sexual interest, curiosity, and pleasurable experiences center around the penis in boys, and in girls, to a lesser extent, the clitoris.

Phenothiazines: Group of psychotropic drugs that chemically have in common the phenothiazine configuration but that differ from one another through variations in chemical radicals.

Phobia: An obsessive, persistent, unrealistic, intense fear of an object or situation.

Photosensitivity: Sensitive to light.

Physical dependence: Physiological need to take drugs or alcohol.

Pleasure principle: The psychoanalytic concept that man instinctually seeks to avoid pain and discomfort and strives for gratification and pleasure.

Porphyria: Porphyrin in the blood; a rare metabolic disorder characterized by acute abdominal pain and neurological disturbances. May be precipitated by excessive use of barbiturates and other drugs.

Posturing: Positioning of the body; often seen in psychotic individuals where they position themselves in atypical poses.

Prevention: In traditional medical usage, the prevention of a disorder. The modern trend is to broaden the meaning of prevention to encompass also the amelioration, control, and limitation of disease. (Often categorized as primary, secondary and tertiary.)

Prevention, primary: Measures taken to prevent the onset of a mental disorder.

Prevention, secondary: Measures taken to limit or treat early a disease process.

Prevention, tertiary: Measures taken to reduce impairment or disability following a disorder.

Priapism: Abnormal, painful, and continued erection of the penis, usually without sexual desire.

Primary gain: The relief from emotional conflict and the freedom from anxiety achieved by a defense mechanism.

Primary process: In psychoanalytic theory, the generally unorganized mental activity characteristic of unconscious mental life. Seen in less disguised form in infancy and in dreams.

Privileged communication: Certain kinds of communications, between persons who have a special confidential relationship, that according to the laws of evidence in some jurisdictions may not be divulged.

Problem-oriented record: A simple, conceptual framework to expedite and improve the medical record. The record is structured to contain four logically sequenced sections: (a) the data base, (b) the problem list, (c) the plans, and (d) the follow-up.

Projection: A defense mechanism, operating unconsciously, whereby that which is emotionally unacceptable in the self is unconsciously rejected and attributed (projected) to others.

Psychiatric nursing: Interpersonal process between nurse and client(s) designed to help clients maintain and promote their level of psychological functioning.

Psychoanalysis: Psychological theory of human development and behavior and a system of psychotherapy originally developed by Sigmund Freud.

Psychodrama: Technique of group psychotherapy in which individuals express their own or assigned emotional problems in dramatization.

Psychological dependence: Craving or emotionally perceived need for an abused substance.

Psychomotor excitement: Generalized physical and emotional overactivity in response to internal and/or external stimuli, as in hypomania.

Psychomotor retardation: A generalized slowing of physical and emotional reactions.

Psychophysiological disorders: A group of disorders characterized by physical symptoms that are caused by emotional factors and that involve a single organ system, usually under autonomic nervous system control.

Psychosexual development: Generally, a term encompassing all of the influences from prenatal life onward, including biological, cultural, and emotional, that affect the sexuality of the individual throughout the life cycle.

Psychosis: A major mental disorder of organic or emotional origin in which the individual's ability to think, respond emotionally, remember, communicate, interpret reality, and behave appropriately is sufficiently impaired so as to interfere grossly with his capacity to meet the ordinary demands of life.

Psychosurgery: Surgical intervention to sever fibers connecting one part of the brain with another or to remove or to destroy brain tissue with the intent of modifying or altering disturbances of behavior, thought content, or mood for which no organic pathological cause can be demonstrated by established tests and techniques.

Psychotherapy: A generic term for the treatment of mental and emotional disorders based primarily upon verbal or nonverbal communication with the patient.

Rationalization: A defense mechanism, operating unconsciously, in which the individual attempts to justify or make consciously tolerable, by plausible means, feelings, behavior, and motives that would otherwise be intolerable.

Reaction formation: A defense mechanism, operating unconsciously, wherein attitudes and behavior are adopted that are the opposites of impulses the individual harbors either consciously or unconsciously.

Reality principle: In psychoanalytic theory, the concept that the pleasure principle, which represents the claims of instinctual wishes, is normally modified by the inescapable demands and requirements of the external world.

Regression: The partial or symbolic return to more infantile patterns of reacting.

Remotivation: A group treatment technique administered by nursing service personnel in a mental hospital; of particular value to long-term withdrawn patients by way of stimulating their communication skills and interest in their environment.

Repression: A defense mechanism, operating unconsciously, that banishes unacceptable ideas, affects, or impulses from consciousness or that keeps out of consciousness what has never been conscious.

Retardation: Slowing down of mental and physical activity; most frequently seen in severe depression.

Ritual: Any psychomotor activity sustained by an individual to relieve anxiety.

Sadism: Pleasure derived from inflicting physical or psychological pain or abuse on others.

Schizophrenia: A group of disorders, usually of psychotic proportion, manifested by characteristic disturbances of thought, mood, and behavior.

School phobia: Term used when a child, usually in the elementary grades, unexpectedly and without apparent reason, strenuously refuses to attend school because of some irrational fear.

Secondary gain: The external gain that is derived from any illness, such as personal attention and service, monetary gains, disability benefits, and release from unpleasant responsibility.

Secondary process: In psychoanalytic theory, mental activity and thinking characteristic of the ego and influenced by the demands of the environment.

Sedative: A broad term applied to any agent that quiets or calms or allays excitement.

Self-concept: A person's notions and beliefs about personal worth and value.

Self-esteem: An individual's personal judgment of his own worth obtained by analyzing how well his behavior conforms to his self-ideal.

Senile dementia: A chronic organic brain syndrome associated with generalized atrophy of the brain due to aging.

Sensorium: Consciousness.

Separation anxiety: The fear and apprehension noted in infants when removed from their mother (or surrogates) or when approached by strangers.

Sexual deviation: The direction of sexual interest toward objects other than persons of the opposite sex and/or toward sexual acts not associated with coitus.

Sibling: Full brother or sister.

Sibling rivalry: The competition between siblings for the love of a parent or for other recognition or gain.

Situational: Unexpected and unplanned event affecting a person's or group's ability to maintain homeostasis.

Socialization: The process by which society integrates the individual and the way in which the individual learns to become a functioning member of that society.

Sociopath: An unofficial term of antisocial personality.

Status epilepticus: Rapid succession of epileptic attacks without regaining consciousness during the intervals.

Sublimation: A defense mechanism, operating unconsciously, by which instinctual drives, consciously unacceptable, are diverted into personally and socially acceptable channels.

Substitution: A defense mechanism, operating unconsciously, by which an unattainable or unacceptable goal, emotion, or object is replaced by one that is more attainable or acceptable.

Succinylcholine: A potent drug used intravenously in anesthesia as a skeletal muscle relaxant.

Suicide: Actions undertaken by a person which if effectively carried out will result in death.

Superego: In psychoanalytic theory, that part of the personality structure associated with ethics, standards, and self-criticism.

Suppression: Conscious effort to control and conceal unacceptable thoughts, impulses, feelings, and acts.

Tangentiality: Unrelated to or not addressing the present situation.

Tardive dyskinesia: Untoward effect, appearing after long-term use of antipsychotic drugs, with muscle involvement about the face, neck, and trunk, leading to spasms, ticks, eye signs, and speech disturbances.

Therapeutic community: A term of British origin, now widely used, for a specially structured mental hospital milieu that encourages patients to function within the range of social norms.

Therapeutic window: The narrow range of blood levels at which a medication is effective when blood levels both above and below the therapeutic range are ineffective.

Tolerance: Need to increase the dosage of a drug to achieve the desired state.

Torticollis: Stiff neck caused by spasmodic contraction of neck muscles drawing the head to one side with chin pointing to the other side.

Transference: The unconscious assignment to others of feelings and attitudes that were originally associated with important figures (parents, siblings) in one's early life.

Transsexual: A disturbance of gender identity in which the person feels a lifelong discomfort with his or her own sex and a compelling desire to be of the opposite sex.

Transvestitism (transvestism): Sexual pleasure derived from dressing or masquerading in the clothing of the opposite sex.

Trauma: An extremely upsetting emotional experience that may aggravate or contribute to a mental disorder.

Tricyclics: Group of chemically related antidepressant medications.

Unconscious: That part of the mind of mental functioning of which the content is only rarely subject to awareness.

Undoing: A defense mechanism, operating unconsciously, in which something unacceptable and already done is symbolically acted out in reverse, usually repetitiously, in the hope of relieving anxiety.

Voyeurism: Sexually motivated and often compulsive interest in looking at or watching others and, particularly, looking at genitals.

Withdrawal symptoms: Physical and mental effects of withdrawing drugs from patients who have become habituated or addicted to them.

Word salad: A mixture of words or phrases that lack comprehensive meaning or logical coherence, commonly seen in schizophrenic states.

2

Commonly Prescribed Drugs

This chapter lists, in table form, the most commonly prescribed drugs used in treating adult clients. Along with each drug's major action, therapeutic action and effects, and commonly prescribed dose and route, the text that follows each given drug further outlines the drug's nursing implications, untoward and allergic reactions, and precautions in administration.

Sources used in compiling the information for this chapter are: 1. Kastrup, E. K. (ed.): *Facts and Comparisons: Drug Information.* Philadelphia: J. B. Lippincott, updated monthly; 2. AMA Department of Drugs, in cooperation with the American Society for Clinical Pharmacology and Therapeutics: *AMA Drug Evaluations,* 4th Revised Ed. Chicago: American Medical Association, 1980; and 3. Drug manufacturer inserts (information supplied with each drug by the manufacturer).

DRUG CATEGORY	MAJOR ACTION	THERAPEUTIC ACTION AND EFFECT	COMMONLY PRESCRIBED DOSE AND ROUTE
ANTIBIOTICS			
1. Ampicillin	Broad spectrum bactericidal	Treatment of genitourinary, respiratory, and GI tract infection	Respiratory: 250 mg q.i.d.
			GU, GIT, and other: 500 mg q.i.d.
		Treatment of gonorrhea	Routes include IM, IV, and p.o. (capsule and suspension). Choice of route depends on severity
			Gonorrhea dosage: 3.5 g ampicillin and 1 g probenicid in a single oral dose

Culture and sensitivity reports should be initiated before drug therapy. Contraindicated in anyone with previous sensitivity to penicillin and some patients showing sensitivity toward cephalosporins, if allergic reaction was pronounced. Ampicillin is also contraindicated in infections caused by penicillinase-producing organisms, i.e., *Pseudomonas aeruginosa*, *Klebsiella pneumoniae*, and some strains of *Escherichia coli*. A minimum of 10 days of antibiotic therapy is suggested, especially when treating beta-hemolytic streptococci. Ampicillin, being a semisynthetic penicillin, is stable in the presence of gastric acid and is well absorbed from the GI tract. This is not the case with penicillin G. Darkfield examinations should be done to rule out syphilis before initiating therapy for gonorrhea. If syphilis is suspected, appropriate parenteral penicillin therapy also should be used. In the event that syphilis is not treated, patients treated for gonorrhea with ampicillin should have follow-up serologic tests for syphilis each month for 4 months to detect syphilis that may have been masked by the ampicillin treatment. Adverse reactions include overgrowth of nonsusceptible organisms, including the fungi responsible for sudden vaginal infections; nausea, vomiting, diarrhea, glossitis, and stomatitis. Some blood dyscrasias have been noted during penicillin therapy but appear to be reversible upon discontinuation of the drug and are believed to be a hypersensitivity phenomena. A classic skin rash has been reported fairly frequently in hypersensitivity reactions. It usually does *not* develop within the first week of therapy, and when it does appear, it may cover the entire body including the soles, palms, and oral mucosa. It is erythematous, mildly pruritic, and maculopapular.

| 2. **Keflex** (cephalexin) | Broad spectrum bactericidal | Treatment of respiratory tract infections, otitis media, skin and skin structure infections caused by staphylococci and/or streptococci, bone infections, and genitourinary tract infections | 250–500 mg orally q.i.d. Comparable cephalosporins are also available for IV and IM use |

Culture and sensitivity reports should be initiated before drug therapy. It is contraindicated in patients with known allergy to the cephalosporin group of antibiotics. There is approximately 5% crossover in allergic response in patients allergic to penicillin therefore the nature of allergy is important, i.e., difficulty in breathing with past penicillin treatment might also indicate a possible problem with Keflex. Antibiotics should be taken for 7–10 days to prevent relapse or a superinfection that may no longer be susceptible to this drug. Instruct the patient not to stop taking this drug until all gone. False-positive C&A test for glucose in the urine may occur. Testape or Ketodiastix should be used instead. Diarrhea is the most frequent side effect—rarely severe enough to warrant cessation of therapy.

DRUG CATEGORY	MAJOR ACTION	THERAPEUTIC ACTION AND EFFECT	COMMONLY PRESCRIBED DOSE AND ROUTE
CARDIOVASCULAR DRUGS			
1. Digoxin (Lanoxin)	Cardiotonic	Treatment of heart failure, atrial fibrillation, atrial flutter, PAT	Maintenance dose after digitalization is usually 0.125–0.25 mg q.d. to q.o.d.
		Increases cardiac output, strengthens cardiac muscle tone, reduces ventricular rate, slows heart rate, slows conduction through the AV node	Available as tablet, pediatric elixir, injectable Lanoxin (pediatric and adult)
			May be given p.o., IV or IM
			Dosing should be modified for individual sensitivity, renal function, and associated conditions

Digoxin is *one* of the cardiac glycosides derived from the digitalis leaf. The term digitalis is used to designate a whole group of drugs with similar cardiac effects varying mainly in onset and duration of actions. Contraindications: ventricular fibrillation, hypersensitivity to drugs in this family. Although allergy to digoxin may occur rarely, it may or may not limit the use of other digitalis derivatives. Each member must be tried with caution.

Incomplete heart block may progress to complete if digoxin is given. The drugs in this family are not interchangeable. If a patient is on digoxin therapy, he must remain taking that drug until his doctor makes changes. Serious arrhythmias and toxicities can result from inappropriate switching of digitalis glycosides. Serum electrolytes and BUN and/or serum creatinine should be assessed periodically. Hypercalcemia, hypomagnesemia, hypokalemia, and renal impairment may predispose a patient to digitalis toxicity. Likewise, digoxin may be ineffective in a patient with too low a calcium level because calcium affects contractility and excitability of the heart in a manner similar to digoxin. Quinidine causes a rise in serum digoxin concentration. In some patients with sick sinus syndrome, digoxin may worsen the bradycardia. It is common practice to prescribe oral potassium to patients on digoxin and diuretic regimens because of the potential for potassium depletion with resulting digoxin toxicity and/or arrhythmias. Periodic serum digoxin levels will expose toxicity. Although patients' tolerance for the drug varies greatly, blood concentrations of 2 ng/L or higher are associated with toxic levels.

Adverse reactions include: toxicity; PVCs—bigeminal or trigeminal, ventricular tachycardia, AV dissociation, accelerated junctional rhythm, and atrial tachycardia; excessive slowing of the pulse, anorexia, nausea, vomiting, weakness, headache, and blurred vision. A "halo effect" may be noted when looking at lights. The lamp or bulb will appear to have a halo of light surrounding it. In children, any arrhythmia or change in cardiac conduction should be assumed to be a consequence of the drug. The GI tract disturbances in children and infants are less reliable. Attention must be given to bioavailability of the drug when switching from the IV to p.o. route. Frequently digitalization (a loading dose used to bring the body stores of the drug to an effective level rapidly) is obtained through the IV route, while the oral route is used for maintenance therapy.

| 2. Hydrochloro-thiazide | Diuretic antihypertensive | Controls high blood pressure by decreasing fluid volume when used alone or in combination with other antihypertensives | 25–100 mg orally q.d. (for antihypertensive) |
| | | As adjunctive therapy in edema of CHF, hepatic | |

DRUG CATEGORY	MAJOR ACTION	THERAPEUTIC ACTION AND EFFECT	COMMONLY PRESCRIBED DOSE AND ROUTE
2. Hydrochloro-thiazide (cont'd)		cirrhosis, and corticos-teroid and estrogen therapy	
		Also useful in edema due to various forms of renal dysfunction	

Hydrochlorothiazide does not affect *normal* blood pressure; it works by causing a loss of Na^+ and Cl^-, which take water with them, resulting in a secondary loss of K^+ and $HCO3^-$. Therefore, patients must be instructed to take potassium supplements in the form of a drug or food (bananas or orange juice). It is contraindicated in patients allergic to sulfonamides; also in anuria or oliguria. It is not for standard use in edema of pregnancy. Insulin requirements of diabetics may change and latent diabetes mellitus may become manifest. Depleted K^+ levels make patients more sensitive to toxic effects of digitalis and can result in death producing arrhythmias.

DRUG CATEGORY	MAJOR ACTION	THERAPEUTIC ACTION AND EFFECT	COMMONLY PRESCRIBED DOSE AND ROUTE
3. Inderal (propranolol)	Beta-adrenergic receptor-blocking agent, antihyper-tensive, antianginal antiarrhythmic, migraine prophyl-axis; also hyper-	Decreases cardiac output, heart rate, and blood pressure Slows tachyarrhythmias: 1. PAT 2. Sinus tachycardia	*Oral*: Hypertensive: 40 mg q.i.d. Antianginal: 20–40 mg t.i.d. to q.i.d. Antiarrhythmic: 10–30 mg q.i.d. Migraine: 20–40 mg q.i.d.

trophic subaortic stenosis and phenochromocytoma

3. Thyrotoxicosis tachycardia
4. Atrial fibrillation
5. Atrial flutter
6. Persistant atrial extrasystoles (PACs)
7. Tachyarrhythmias associated with digitalis toxicity
8. Resistant tachyarrhythmias during anesthesia

May reduce O_2 requirements of heart

IV:
1–3 mg with careful monitoring

When administered IV, the dosage is markedly reduced because in oral administration a large portion of the drug is destroyed by the liver before reaching the bloodstream (first-pass effect). Contraindicated in: (1) bronchial asthma, (2) allergic rhinitis, (3) sinus bradycardia and greater than first-degree heart block, (4) CHF, unless this is secondary to tachycardia which can be treated with Inderal, (5) cardiogenic shock, (6) right ventricular failure secondary to pulmonary hypertension, (7) patients on certain psychotropic drugs and within 2 weeks of taking these drugs. Inderal therapy should not be halted abruptly as exacerbation of angina and, in some cases, myocardial infarction, may result; therefore, the drug should be tapered. In surgical patients, except for pheochromocytoma, Inderal should be held for 48 hours before surgery because beta-blockade impairs the ability of the heart to respond to reflex stimuli. Can be used in conjunction with digitalis; however, the effects are additive in depressing the AV conduction. Can only be used for *prophylaxis* of migraine; of no use once the headache has started.

DRUG CATEGORY	MAJOR ACTION	THERAPEUTIC ACTION AND EFFECT	COMMONLY PRESCRIBED DOSE AND ROUTE
4. Procardia (nifedipine)	Calcium ion antagonist or slow channel blocker	Selectively inhibits influx of Ca^{++} ions into cardiac muscle and smooth muscle without changing Ca^{++} levels. Results in relaxation and prevention of coronary artery spasm; reduction of oxygen utilization Uses: 1. Vasospastic angina 2. Chronic stable angina	10–20 mg t.i.d. oral capsule only A single dose should rarely exceed 30 mg Titration upward should proceed over 7–14 days so the physician can assess the response to each dosage level

No rebound effect has been noted upon discontinuation of the drug. However, it is probably better drug therapy to taper it off gradually. Nitroglycerin sublingual can be taken concurrently for acute episodes of angina. Careful monitoring of blood pressure during initiation of therapy is recommended because hypotension is a main side effect. Other side effects include: peripheral edema, dizziness, headache, nasal congestion, muscle cramps, tremor, palpitation, and joint stiffness. Occasional reports suggest concomitant administration of beta-blockers with Procardia may increase likelihood of CHF, severe hypotension, and exacerbation of angina. Procardia does not seem to affect the electrical conduction system of the heart, i.e., no slowing of AV conduction.

RESPIRATORY DRUGS

1. Aminophylline

Bronchodilator
Pulmonary
vasodilator
Smooth muscle
relaxant

Other actions
typical of xan-
thine derivatives:
coronary
vasodilator,
diuretic, cardiac
stimulant, cere-
bral stimulant,
skeletal muscle
stimulant

Indicated for the relief
and/or prevention of
symptoms of asthma and
reversible bronchospasm
associated with chronic
bronchitis and emphysema

100–315 mg t.i.d. to
q.i.d., orally

IV: Must be diluted
(25 mg/ml). If given
"push" this would be
500 mg/20 ml. May be
further diluted with IV
fluids, usually 500 mg/L.
Administration should
not exceed 25 mg/min.
Warm to room temper-
ature

IM: Adults, 500 mg as
required

Rectal: 250–500 mg
q.d. to b.i.d.

Should not be administered to patients with peptic ulcer disease since it may increase the volume and acidity of gastric secretions. Contraindicated in patients with history of hypersensitivity to aminophylline or theophylline. Should
not administer with other xanthine derivatives. Toxic synergism may occur with other bronchodilators of the sym-
pathomimetic family, i.e., epinephrine.

DRUG CATEGORY	MAJOR ACTION	THERAPEUTIC ACTION AND EFFECT	COMMONLY PRESCRIBED DOSE AND ROUTE
1. Aminophylline (cont'd)	Use with caution in patients with severe cardiac disease, hypertension, hyperthyroidism, or acute myocardial injury.		
	Adverse reactions include: nausea and vomiting, headache, tachycardia, flushing, gastrointestinal distress, dizziness, agitation, extrasystoles, increased respiratory rate, and urticaria.		
ENDOCRINE DRUGS			
1. Insulin 1. Regular 2. Semilente 3. NPH 4. Globin zinc 5. Lente 6. PZI 7. Ultralente	Pancreatic hormone	Treatment of diabetes mellitus—juvenile-onset	Dose is individualized for each patient based on blood and urine sugar concentrations, i.e., 30–60 mg NPH SQ q A.M. Insulin may be given SQ, IM, or IV (regular only) 1. Regular: fast-acting; duration 6 hr

2. Semilente: fast-acting; duration 12–16 hr (insulin zinc suspension, prompt)

3. NPH: intermediate-acting; duration 24 hr

4. Globin zinc: intermediate-acting; duration 18 hr

5. Lente: Insulin zinc suspension, intermediate-acting; duration 24 hr

6. PZI: long-acting; duration 36 hr

7. Ultralente: long-acting; duration 36 hr

Changing brands of insulin arbitrarily is unwise, unless the physician is monitoring the change with the patient. All U-100 insulin (100 U/ml) should be given with an insulin syringe bearing markings based on this concentration. Regular insulin should be clear and colorless and not used if it appears cloudy. It is the only insulin that can be injected intravenously, as the others are made up of suspended particles. Two types of insulin can be mixed in the same syringe for subcutaneous use. However, the same brand of syringe and the same order of mixing should always be consistent to eliminate the possibility of dosage error. The most common reaction to insulin is local swelling or redness and hardness. Scarring is not uncommon with long-term use. True hypersensitivity reactions, although rare, can occur, manifest by generalized rash, shortness of breath, rapid pulse, and drop in blood pressure. Insulin requirements change based on diet, exercise, stress, illness and other medications. The easiest way to test for insulin needs is urine sugar (C&A Keto-

DRUG CATEGORY	MAJOR ACTION	THERAPEUTIC ACTION AND EFFECT	COMMONLY PRESCRIBED DOSE AND ROUTE
1. Insulin (cont'd)		diastix, or Testape). Diabetic acidosis (hyperglycemia) usually comes on gradually with a drowsy feeling, flushed face, thirst, loss of appetite, heavy breathing, and rapid pulse (in more severe cases). Remedy is more insulin after blood sugar analysis confirms suspension. Diabetic acidosis can lead to coma. Insulin shock (hypoglycemia) comes on suddenly with a feeling of nervousness, fatigue, nausea, increased pulse rate, cold sweat, personality change, or confusion. Remedy is orange juice or sugar in some form. Beef insulin is obtained strictly from the beef pancreas. Pork insulin is obtained strictly from pork pancreas. Some products contain a mixture of these. Patients allergies to beef or pork products need to be considered. Pork insulin more closely resembles human insulin and seems to produce fewer reactions of the allergic nature. Storage of insulin is best done in a refrigerator (do not freeze); however, it will remain useful at room temperature for approximately 1 month. Mixing insulin suspensions is best done by rotating or rolling the vial between palms or fingers; shaking vigorously gets air bubbles in the product making exact measurement more difficult. Some patients become resistant to insulin over a period, requiring alarmingly large doses. This is due to antigens produced in the response to the beef or pork properties. The solution is to use 500 U/ml of pork insulin. The new human insulin, recently marketed may alleviate this problem.	
2. Diabinese (chlorpropamide)	Oral hypoglycemic agent	Treatment of diabetes mellitus—adult-onset; mild or moderately severe nonketotic which cannot be controlled by diet alone	Only available as oral tablets Moderately severe: 250 mg q.d. Mild: 100 mg q.d.

Severe: 500 mg q.d.

Occasionally b.i.d. usage is seen to alleviate symptoms of GI intolerance

The mode of action of Diabinese seems to be stimulation of synthesis and release of endogenous insulin. The potency is approximately six times that of tolbutamide (Orinase). There is now evidence that improvement in pancreatic cell function may occur with prolonged use. A past history of diabetic coma does not necessarily rule out successful control with Diabinese. Some patients, uncontrolled on other oral hypoglycemics, respond appropriately when switched to Diabinese. It is contraindicated in juvenile diabetes, brittle diabetes, diabetes complicated by ketosis, acidosis, diabetic coma, major surgery, severe infection, or severe trauma; also in pregnancy* and patients with serious impairment of hepatic, renal, and thyroid function. The action of barbiturates may be prolonged by concurrent use of Diabinese. Use cautiously in Addison disease—may see exaggerated hypoglycemic effect. In some patients, an Antabuse-like reaction may occur with alcohol ingestion. Since Diabinese is a sulfonamide derivative, caution must be used if patients demonstrate allergies to other sulfa drugs. Also concurrent use of antibacterial sulfonamide, phenylbutazone, salicylates, probenecid, warfarin or MAO inhibitors may result in potentiation of the hypoglycemic effect or on accumulation of sulfonylureas. During stress or hospitalization, the patient may need to be placed on insulin therapy temporarily. Hypersensitivity symptoms include pruritus, rash, jaundice, dark urine, light-colored stools, low-grade fever, sore throat, or diarrhea. If a progressive rise in alkaline phosphatase levels is noted, the drug should be discontinued. Diabinese has a somewhat higher incidence of adverse reactions than does Orinase. However, most are dose-related or transient and have responded to reduction or withdrawal of the medication.

Examples of these dose-related side effects are GI intolerance, weakness, and parethesias. Blood dyscrasias have been documented with Diabinese use but are generally benign and revert to normal following cessation of the drug.

---

*In pregnancy, higher levels of female hormones may cause greater glucose intolerance, and women previously taking oral hypoglycemics usually use insulin during this time. Also, there is potential danger to the fetus from the Diabinese.

DRUG CATEGORY	MAJOR ACTION	THERAPEUTIC ACTION AND EFFECT	COMMONLY PRESCRIBED DOSE AND ROUTE
3. Thyroid, USP	Replacement hormone therapy for: hypothyroidism, cretinism, myxedema, nontoxic goiter	Increases: 1. Metabolic rate of body tissues, i.e., O_2 consumption 2. Respiratory rate 3. Body temperature 4. Cardiac output 5. Heart rate 6. Blood volume 7. Rate of fat, protein, and carbohydrate metabolism 8. Enzyme system activity 9. Growth and maturation	Starting with very small doses, because hypothyroid patients are very sensitive to the hormone, very gradual increases should take place to reach the maintenance dose of 65 mg p.o. q.d. (capsules and tablets only) Dosage varies with the commercial product used, but all are based on 65 mg (1 gr) of thyroid, USP In the synthetic hormones, dosage in μg is equal to dosage in mg of the natural thyroid Some T^4 products are available in IM/IV forms;

used very rarely in myxedema coma or stupor

There are natural and synthetic thyroid hormones. The natural ones are derived from beef or swine, and standardized by iodine content. Synthetic ones are sometimes preferred because there is more uniform standardization of potency with these. Lack of thyroid in young children causes growth retardation (cretinism). Endogeneous thyroid secretion is suppressed if a normal individual (euthyroid) is given exogenous hormone in excess of the gland's secretion.

The anterior pituitary controls the secretion of thyroid from the thyroid gland by secreting TSH (thyroid-stimulating hormone), as a result of feedback from the amounts of circulating thyroid hormones. There are two thyroid hormones: T^4 and T^3. A commercial product is available that contains both of these in a 4:1 ratio. Each hormone is also available separately. T^4 is usually the treatment of choice for hypothyroidism because of its purity and prolonged duration of action. However, it has a slow onset, so if there is a need for rapidly correcting the hypothyroid state, T^3 may be preferred. Patients should know that replacement therapy is usually for life, except in transient hypothyroidism. They should not discontinue their medication except on the advice of their physician.

Partial loss of hair may occur in children initially started on therapy with a thyroid hormone, but this is temporary, and reverts to normal later on in therapy. This drug should never be used to treat obesity or infertility unless they are associated with hypothyroidism. Congenital hypothyroidism must be corrected after birth, as only small amounts of the hormone cross the placental barrier, making it possible for pregnant women to continue their thyroid therapy. In changing from one thyroid product to another, equivalent dosages must be given attention. Laboratory tests, T^3, and T^4 levels should be done at regular intervals for patients on long-term thyroid therapy to maintain effectiveness without toxicity. Other laboratory tests also utilized are: T^3 uptake resin, free thyroxine index, and serum TSH.

Many drugs affect these laboratory values; a few being: Dilantin, Inderal, barbiturates, steroids, Valium, estrogens, IV heparin, and insulin. Also, if thyroid therapy is started for patients on oral anticoagulants, a one-third reduction in anticoagulant dosage may be necessary because thyroid potentiates anticoagulant effects of the oral agents; however the opposite is not true. No adjustment need be made for patients already on maintenance thyroid dosages when oral anticoagulant therapy is started. Careful observation is required when catecholamines (e.g., epinephrine) are administered in patients with coronary artery disease, on thyroid therapy, because coronary insufficiency may develop. Thyroid increases a diabetic's need for insulin or oral hypoglycemic agents. Cholestyramine binds both T^3 and T^4

DRUG CATEGORY	MAJOR ACTION	THERAPEUTIC ACTION AND EFFECT	COMMONLY PRESCRIBED DOSE AND ROUTE
3. Thyroid, USP (cont'd)		in the intestine, thus impairing absorption. Thyroid may make patients more sensitive to digoxin and other cardiotonic glycosides, resulting in possible toxicity.	

Some commercial products contain tartrazine which may cause allergic reactions, including bronchial asthma. Although the incidence is low, it is frequently seen in individuals allergic to aspirin.

Persistence of hypothyroidism, in spite of adequate replacement therapy indicates either poor patient compliance, poor absorption, excessive fecal loss, or inactivity of the preparation. Intracellular resistance to thyroid hormone is rare. Adverse reactions, other than hyperthyroidism due to therapeutic overdosage, include: palpitation, tachycardia, angina pectoris, cardiac arrhythmias, cardiac arrest, tremors, headache, nausea, insomnia, nervousness, abdominal cramps, diarrhea, changes in appetite, menstrual irregularities, allergic skin reactions, weight loss, sweating, and intolerance to heat.

DRUG CATEGORY	MAJOR ACTION	THERAPEUTIC ACTION AND EFFECT	COMMONLY PRESCRIBED DOSE AND ROUTE
4. Prednisone	Replacement therapy for adrenocortical insufficiency	Treatment of:	Initial dosage may vary from 5–60 mg q.d. or q.o.d. depending on the disease state
	Anti-inflammatory	1. Endocrine disorders 2. Rheumatic disorders 3. Collagen diseases 4. Dermatologic diseases 5. Allergic states 6. Ophthalmic diseases 7. Respiratory diseases 8. Hematologic disorders 9. Neoplastic diseases	Prednisone is only available orally (tablets), but IV and IM dosage forms of *other* glucocorticoids are available

10. Edematous states
11. Gastrointestinal diseases
12. Nervous system disorders
    (multiple sclerosis)
13. Tuberculosis meningitis
14. Trichinosis with neurologic
    or myocardial involvement

Contraindications to prednisone use are systemic fungal infections, primarily. It must be used with caution in patients with ocular herpes. Immunizations, especially for smallpox, should be postponed if prednisone is being taken, because of possible neurologic complications and lack of antibody response. The use of prednisone in active tuberculosis should be restricted to cases of the fulminating or disseminated disease. If steroids are indicated in patients with latent tuberculosis, close observation is necessary as reactivation may occur. Patients on steroid therapy may require higher dosages during stressful circumstances. Steroids may mask some signs of infection, and new infection may appear.

There may be decreased ability to localize infection, while taking steroids. Prolonged use may produce posterior subcapsular cataracts, glaucoma with possible optic nerve damage, and enhancement of ocular infections due to fungi or viruses. All steroids increase calcium excretion. Large dosages may cause elevations of blood pressure, salt and water retention, and increased excretion of potassium. After long-term therapy, it is recommended that the drug be withdrawn gradually rather than abruptly, giving the adrenal gland a chance to take over secretion of endogenous glucocorticoids and preventing possible psychic derangements. Some psychic changes that may take place while on steroid therapy are: euphoria, insomnia, mood swings, personality changes, severe depression, and frank psychotic manifestations. Existing emotional instability or psychotic tendencies may be aggravated. Aspirin should be used cautiously in conjunction with steroids because peptic ulcer may result.

Alternate day therapy (ADT) is a dosage regimen that may provide the patient requiring long-term therapy with the beneficial effects of steroids while minimizing certain undesirable effects, including pituitary adrenal suppression, the cushingoid state, corticoid withdrawal symptoms, and growth suppression in children.

DRUG CATEGORY	MAJOR ACTION	THERAPEUTIC ACTION AND EFFECT	COMMONLY PRESCRIBED DOSE AND ROUTE
4. Prednisone (cont'd)			

Some common side effects of steroid therapy include: sodium and water retention, potassium loss, hypertension, muscle weakness, loss of muscle mass, osteoporosis, peptic ulcer, impaired wound healing, increased sweating, suppression of reactions to skin tests, protein catabolism, convulsions, headache, increased intracranial pressure, menstrual irregularities, cushingoid state, secondary adrenocortical and pituitary unresponsiveness, suppression of growth in children, increased requirements for insulin or oral hypoglycemics, glaucoma, cataracts, and exophthalmos.

NERVOUS SYSTEM DRUGS

DRUG CATEGORY	MAJOR ACTION	THERAPEUTIC ACTION AND EFFECT	COMMONLY PRESCRIBED DOSE AND ROUTE
1. Morphine	Analgesic	Uses: 1. Analgesic 2. Preoperatively to sedate and allay apprehension, facilitate induction of anesthesia, and reduce anesthetic dosage 3. Cancer pain control Effects: 1. Relief of pain 2. Respiratory depression	SQ ⎱ 10–15 mg q4 hr IM ⎰ IV: 2–10 mg IV q2–4 hr May also be administered as a continuous/infusion in 1 L of IV fluid for cancer patients, i.e., 30 mg/L titrated rate for pain usually approximately 2 mg/hr

p.o.: 10–15 mg q4 hr

3. Depression of cough center
4. Release of antidiuretic hormone
5. Activation of vomiting center
6. Pupillary constriction
7. Decrease in gastric, pancreatic, and biliary secretion
8. Reduction of intestinal motility
9. Increase in biliary tract pressure
10. Increased amplitude of ureteral contractions

Onset of action: 10–30 min
Duration: 4–5 hr

Morphine is contraindicated in persons exhibiting hypersensitivity to it and in convulsive states such as status epilepticus, tetanus, and strychnine poisoning because of its stimulating effect on the spinal cord. Use cautiously in patients with head injuries and increased intracranial pressure. Symptoms may be obscured, and the respiratory depressant effect may be markedly exaggerated. Morphine may mask the diagnosis of acute abdominal conditions. It should be given cautiously to elderly and debilitated patients and those with severe impairment of hepatic or renal function, hypothyroidism, Addison disease, prostatic hypertrophy, or urethral stricture. Hypoxic patients may pro-

DRUG CATEGORY	MAJOR ACTION	THERAPEUTIC ACTION AND EFFECT	COMMONLY PRESCRIBED DOSE AND ROUTE
1. Morphine (cont'd)		gress to apnea if morphine is used. There is an additive hypotensive effect when given with phenothiazines, i.e., promethazine (Phenergan) and chlorpromazine (Thorazine). Severe hypotension may result in postoperative patients because of inability to maintain blood pressure postanesthesia. Hypotension may also be exaggerated if morphine is given to patients having suffered severe blood losses. Morphine should be used with caution with atrial flutter and supraventricular tachycardia as they may worsen due to pulse rebound from hypotension. Additive effects occur when given with other CNS depressants. The use of morphine in obstetrics may prolong labor. It also passes the placental barrier and may depress respirations in the newborn. Morphine is highly addictive. Patients receiving 10 mg q4hr for 1–2 weeks exhibit mild withdrawal symptoms when the drug is removed. Overdose results in severe respiratory depression which may lead to apnea, hypotension, circulatory collapse, cardiac arrest, and death. Narcotic antagonists are the specific antidote. Adverse reactions include: nausea, vomiting, dizziness, lightheadedness, sedation, euphoria, dysphoria, constipation, and pruritus. Some of these side effects may be alleviated if the patient lies down. Effects are more prominent in ambulatory patients.	
2. Demerol (meperidine)	Analgesic Sedation	Uses: 1. Pain relief 2. Preoperative, support of anesthesia 3. Obstetric analgesic The latter two use parenteral form only	50 mg q3–4 hr IM, p.o., SQ, IV Available in 25 mg, 50 mg, 75 mg, 100 mg Dosages from 25–150 mg may be seen depending

on patient size
and circumstances

Demerol, 60–80 mg parenterally, is approximately equal in analgesic effect to 10 mg morphine. Onset of Demerol is slightly more rapid than morphine, but duration of action is slightly shorter. Demerol is significantly less effective orally than parenterally. It is contraindicated in hypersensitivity cases, patients receiving or having received (within 14 days) monamine oxidase inhibitors. Unpredictable, severe, and occasional fatal reactions occur in these patients. Drug dependence of the morphine type can occur with Demerol, as well as psychic dependence. Caution must be used when administering other CNS depressants, general anesthetics, phenothiazines, and tricyclic antidepressants. Demerol must be used with caution in patients with head injury, increased intracranial pressure, convulsions, and acute abdominal conditions, for the same reasons as morphine. Special risk patients also include those with impaired renal or hepatic function, hypothyroidism, Addison disease, prostatic hypertrophy, urethral stricture, atrial flutter, other supraventricular tachycardias, immediate postoperative patients, or those exhibiting large blood losses.

Demerol should be used with extreme caution in patients having an acute asthma attack, patients with chronic obstructive pulmonary disease or cor pulmonale, and in hypoxic or hypercapnia patients. Even usual therapeutic dosages may decrease respiratory drive while simultaneously increasing airway resistance.

Adverse reactions are many: respiratory depression, circulatory depression, dizziness, nausea, vomiting, sweating, sedation, euphoria, dysphoria, weakness, headache, agitation, tremor, uncoordinated muscle movements, transient hallucinations, disorientation, visual disturbances, dry mouth, constipation, flushed face, tachycardia, bradycardia, syncope, urinary retention, pruritus, skin rashes, wheal or flare over the vein at IV injection site, pain at injection site, biliary tract spasm, antidiuretic effect, and local tissue irritation. Signs and symptoms of overdosage are the same as for morphine. In the event of overdosage, narcotic antagonists, again, are the specific antidote but will precipitate acute withdrawal in patients physically dependent. In these patients, one-tenth to one-fifth the usual dosage of antagonist should initially be used. This is also true for morphine.

When used in obstetrics, Demerol crosses the placental barrier and can produce respiratory depression, but its shorter duration of action makes it more practical than morphine.

DRUG CATEGORY	MAJOR ACTION	THERAPEUTIC ACTION AND EFFECT	COMMONLY PRESCRIBED DOSE AND ROUTE
3. Valium (diazepam)	Tranquilizer	Uses: 1. Anxiety 2. Alcohol withdrawal 3. Skeletal muscle spasm 4. Convulsive disorders 5. Adjunct to anesthesia	2–10 mg b.i.d. to q.i.d. orally IM and IV dosage and frequency depends upon the condition treated

Valium passes the placental barrier and increases the risk of congenital malformation, especially during the first trimester of pregnancy. It is contraindicated in patients with known hypersensitivity to the drug or other members of its family, e.g., chlordiazepoxide. Librium, lorazepam (Ativan), oxazepam (Serax). It is also contraindicated in children under 6 months of age and in acute narrow-angle glaucoma (although it may be used in open-angle glaucoma if patients are receiving appropriate therapy). Valium is not of value in treating psychotic patients. Abrupt withdrawal of Valium in seizure patients may result in temporary increase in the frequency and/or severity of seizures. Use cautiously with CNS depressant drugs, especially alcohol. Withdrawal symptoms (similar to those noted with barbiturates and alcohol) have occurred following abrupt discontinuation of Valium. These are usually limited to patients who have received excessive dosage over a prolonged period; therefore, a gradual tapering off of the drug is recommended. Overdosage manifestations include: somnolence, confusion, coma, and diminished reflexes. Respiration, pulse, and blood pressure should be monitored, although in general these are not affected. Management of intentional overdosage should be based on the possibility of multiple agents having been ingested.

Precautions should be taken where renal or hepatic function is impaired. The smallest effective amounts should be used in elderly and debilitated patients.

The clearance of Valium can be delayed in association with cimetidine (Tagamet) administration. Most common side effects include: drowsiness, fatigue, and ataxia. Infrequently seen are: confusion, constipation, depression, dyplopia, headache, hypotension, incontinence, jaundice, nausea, change in libido, skin rash, slurred speech, urinary

retention, vertigo, blurred vision, and changes in salivation.
Paradoxic reactions include: acute hyperexcited states, anxiety, hallucinations, insomnia, rage, sleep disturbances, and muscle spasticity.

| 4. **Thorazine** (chlorpromazine) | Tranquilizer Antiemetic Antipsychotic | Uses: 1. Management of manifestations of psychotic disorders 2. Control nausea and vomiting 3. Relief of restlessness and apprehension before surgery 4. Relief of intractable hiccoughs 5. Treatment of severe behavioral problems in children | SQ: not recommended IV: only for severe hiccoughs, surgery and extreme psychosis (avoid injecting undiluted Thorazine into a vein) IM: slowly and deeply into upper, outer quadrant of buttock Oral: tablets spansule; liquid concentrate syrup Rectal: suppositories Usual dose: 25–100 mg b.i.d. to q.i.d. Dosage is based on patient and circumstances. Psychiatric patients may need up to 500–1000 mg/day in |

DRUG CATEGORY	MAJOR ACTION	THERAPEUTIC ACTION AND EFFECT	COMMONLY PRESCRIBED DOSE AND ROUTE
4. Thorazine (cont'd)			divided doses; there is little therapeutic gain to be achieved by exceeding 1000 mg for extended periods

Thorazine is contraindicated in comatose states, bone marrow depression, presence of large amounts of CNS depressants, and in patients demonstrating previous hypersensitivity reactions to this drug (and possibly other phenothiazine derivatives). Thorazine use should be avoided in children and adolescents whose signs and symptoms suggest Reye syndrome or other encephalopathy, including brain tumors. The extrapyramidal symptoms that can occur secondary to Thorazine may be confused with the CNS signs of these disease states. Thorazine may impair mental and /or physical abilities, especially during the first few days of therapy. Use with caution in patients with cardiovascular or liver disease and chronic respiratory disorders (i.e., asthma, emphysema) due to increased sensitivity to CNS effects. Elevated prolactin levels occur with Thorazine therapy; therefore use in breast cancer patients must be carefully evaluated, because one third of human breast cancers are prolactin-dependent in vitro. Thorazine does not intensify the anticonvulsant action of barbiturates as it does the CNS depressant actions. Therefore, dosage of anticonvulsant should not be lowered; instead, lower Thorazine dosages should be used. Thorazine tablets contain tartrazine, which may cause allergic reactions, including bronchial asthma in susceptible individuals. This is frequently seen in patients also allergic to aspirin. Use Thorazine with caution in patients who will be exposed to extreme heat, organophosphorous-insecticides, and persons receiving atropine or related drugs. Patients on long-term therapy should be evaluated periodically to see if their maintenance dosage can be lowered. No known psychic dependence or physical addiction occurs with Thorazine. There are, however, some symptoms upon abrupt withdrawal from high dosages that resemble those of physical dependence. Adverse reactions include: drowsiness, nausea, vomiting, tremors, and dizziness. These can be avoided by gradual reduction. Adverse reactions include: drowsiness, nausea, vomiting, jaundice, agranulocytosis, other hematologic disorders, hypotension, (mainly from the injectable route), nonspecific ECG changes, extrapyramidal symptoms resembling parkinsonism, persistent tardive dyskinesia (to which there is no known cure), mild urticaria, photosensitivity, cerebral edema, lactation, moderate breast engorgement, mild fever after large IM doses, dry mouth, nasal congestion, urinary retention, and catatoniclike states.

Rarely, on long-term therapy, skin pigmentations and oculocorneal and lens changes are seen.

| 5. **Ritalin** (methylphenidate) | Nervous system stimulant | Uses:
 1. Attention deficit disorders (previously known as minimal brain dysfunction— MBD)

 2. Narcolepsy
 3. "Possibly effective" for mild depression, apathetic or withdrawn senile behavior | Oral only (tablets)

 Adults: 20–30 mg daily in divided doses, b.i.d. to t.i.d. 30–45 min before meals

 Children: Start with 5 mg before breakfast and lunch. Make gradual increases weekly of 5–10 mg to obtain best results

 Daily dosages of above 60 mg are not recommended |

DRUG CATEGORY	MAJOR ACTION	THERAPEUTIC ACTION AND EFFECT	COMMONLY PRESCRIBED DOSE AND ROUTE

5. Ritalin (cont'd)

Ritalin may increase the hypotensive effect of guanethedine and must be used cautiously with pressor agents and MAO inhibitors. Periodic CBC, differential, and platelet counts are advised during prolonged use. Adverse reactions include: nervousness and insomnia (usually controlled by reducing the dosage and omitting the drug in the afternoon or evening); other reactions are: skin rash, fever, arthralgia, exfoliative dermatitis, anorexia, nausea, dizziness, palpitations, headache, drowsiness, blood pressure and pulse changes (both up and down), cardiac arrhythmias, abdominal pain, weight loss with prolonged therapy, leukopenia, anemia, and thrombocytopenic purpura. Rare instances of blurred vision have also been reported. Ritalin should be given cautiously to emotionally unstable patients, especially those with a history of drug dependence or alcoholism. Such patients may increase dosages on their own or parenterally abuse the drug leading to psychic dependence, marked tolerance, varying degrees of abnormal behavior, including frank psychosis. In these cases, careful supervision is required during withdrawal as severe depression and chronic overactivity can be unmasked.

Ritalin should not be used in children under 6 years of age. Where possible, drug administration should be interrupted occasionally to evaluate the patient for continued therapy. Drug treatment need not be indefinite and usually may be discontinued after puberty. There have been reports of suppression of growth in children on long-term therapy. Ritalin should not be used to treat severe depression, and in psychotic children, administration of Ritalin may exacerbate the symptoms. There is some clinical evidence that Ritalin lowers the seizure threshold. Safe concomitant use of anticonvulsants have not been established; therefore, in the presence of seizures, the drug should be discontinued. Ritalin may inhibit the metabolism of warfarin (Coumarin) anticoagulants, phenobarbital, phenytoin (Dilantin), primidone, phenylbutazone, and tricyclic antidepressants, creating a need for downward adjustments of these drugs, lest toxic levels build up.

Drug treatment is not indicated in all cases of attention deficit disorders; many factors must be considered. When the child's symptoms are associated with acute stress reactions, treatment with Ritalin is usually not indicated.

Contraindications include: marked anxiety, tension and agitation, glaucoma, and known hypersensitivity. Use cautiously in patients with high blood pressure.

URINARY TRACT DRUGS

1. Pyridium (phenazopyridine) | Topical analgesic for urinary tract | Relief of pain, burning, frequency, and other discomforts arising from irritation of the lower urinary tract mucosa from infection, trauma, surgery, endoscopic procedures, or passage of catheters | Oral (tablets only): 200 mg t.i.d. p.c.

Also available in 100 mg tablets

The contraindication is renal insufficiency. A yellow tinge of the skin or sclera may indicate accumulation of the drug due to impaired renal excretion. Patients should be told to expect a reddish-orange discoloration in the urine. Use of Pyridium in urinary tract infection is only for symptoms of discomfort. Proper antibacterial therapy should be included in the treatment.

Adverse reactions include: occasional gastrointestinal disturbance, methemoglobinemia, hemolytic anemia and renal and hepatic toxicity. All, with the exception of the GI disturbances, usually occur at overdosage levels. Treatment of methemoglobinemia includes methylene blue IV or ascorbic acid orally for prompt disappearance of the cyanosis, which is the diagnostic indicator.

2. Septra (trimethoprim-sulfamethoxazole) | Antibacterial | Uses: 1. Urinary tract infections 2. Acute otitis media | UTI (adults and children 88 lb or more): one Septra D.S. or two Septra tabs

DRUG CATEGORY	MAJOR ACTION	THERAPEUTIC ACTION AND EFFECT	COMMONLY PRESCRIBED DOSE AND ROUTE
2. Septra (cont'd)		3. Acute exacerbations of chronic bronchitis in adults 4. Shigellosis 5. *Pneumocystis carinii* 6. pneumonitis	q12 hr for 10–14 days UTI and acute otitis media (children): 8 mg/kg of trimethoprim; 40 mg/kg of sulfamethoxazole per 24 hr in two divided doses q12 hr for 10 days Shigellosis (adult): identical dosing as for UTI except for 5 days Shigellosis (children): identical dosing as for otitis media and UTIs except for 5 days Acute exacerbations of chronic bronchitis (adults): one Septra D.S. or two Septra tabs q12 hr for

14 days

Pneumonitis: 20 mg/kg
trimethoprim; 100 mg/kg sulfame-
thoxazole in divided doses
q6 hr for 14 days

Pneumonitis (over 70 lb):
one Septra d.s. tab or two
Septra tabs q6 hr for 14
days

Septra should not be used in infants under 2 months old, nor should it be used for treatment of streptococcal pharyngitis. Other contraindications include: hypersensitivity to sulfonamides or trimethoprim; patients with documented megaloblastic anemia due to folate deficiency; pregnancy at term and during nursing period, because sulfonamides pass the placental barrier and are excreted in milk of nursing mothers and may cause kernicterus in infants. Give Septra with caution to patients with impaired hepatic or renal function, folate deficiency, severe allergy or bronchial asthma, and in glucose-6-phosphate dehydrogenase deficient individuals. Adequate fluid intake must be maintained to prevent crystalluria and stone formation in the kidneys. It has been reported that septra may prolong the prothrombin time of patients receiving warfarin (Coumadin).

Because Septra may interfere with folic acid metabolism, use in pregnancy should be limited to cases where the overall benefit outweighs the risks.

Adverse reactions: multiple blood dyscrasias, various allergic reactions, gastrointestinal reactions, and CNS reactions, some of which are: agranulocytosis, aplastic anemia, hemolytic anemia, Stevens-Johnson syndrome, epidermal necrolysis, urticaria, serum sickness, photosensitivity, stomatitis, nausea, vomiting, hepatitis, diarrhea, headache, mental depression, hallucinations, muscle weakness, chills, and toxic nephrosis.

DRUG CATEGORY	MAJOR ACTION	THERAPEUTIC ACTION AND EFFECT	COMMONLY PRESCRIBED DOSE AND ROUTE
REPRODUCTIVE DRUGS			
1. Premarin (conjugated estrogens)	Replacement hormone	Uses: 1. Vasomotor symptoms of menopause 2. Atrophic vaginitis 3. Kraurosis vulvae 4. Female hypogonadism 5. Female castration 6. Primary ovarian failure 7. Breast cancer (palliative treatment) 8. Prostatic cancer (palliative treatment) 9. Postpartum breast engorgement 10. Probably effective for estrogen deficiency-induced osteoporosis	Available as tablets, vaginal cream, and Premarin IV (may also be given IM) Other estrogens (not Premarin) are available as pellets for SQ implant Dosage varies with condition being treated: 1. Vasomotor (menopause): 1.25 mg q.d. cyclic (3 weeks on, 1 week off) 2. Atrophic vaginitis and kraurosis vulvae: 0.3–1.25 mg or more q.d.; dose depends on tissue response; administer

cyclically

3. Female hypogonadism: 2.5–7.5 mg q.d. in divided doses for 20 days, rest 10 days

4. Female castration and primary ovarian failure: 1.25 mg q.d. cyclic

5. Breast cancer: 10 mg t.i.d. for 3 months

6. Prostatic cancer: 1.25–2.5 mg t.i.d.

7. Postpartum breast engorgement: 3.75 mg q4 hr x 5 doses or 1.25 mg q4 hr x 5 days

8. Osteoporosis (estrogen deficient): 1.25 mg q.d. cyclically

Premarin contains a mixture of estrogens, obtained exclusively from natural sources. Estrogens have been reported to increase the risk of endometrial cancer; and due to possible serious damage to offspring, estrogens should not be used during pregnancy. There is no evidence that estrogens are effective in treating threatened or habitual abortion. Acute overdosage of estrogens by young children have indicated that serious ill effects do not occur. Nausea is the most common symptom, with a possibility of withdrawal bleeding in females, as the drug levels drop off. Adverse

DRUG CATEGORY	MAJOR ACTION	THERAPEUTIC ACTION AND EFFECT	COMMONLY PRESCRIBED DOSE AND ROUTE

1. Premarin (cont'd)

reactions to estrogens are many, a few of which are: breakthrough bleeding, dysmenorrhea, amenorrhea during or after treatment, vaginal candidiasis, change of cervical erosion and in degree of cervical secretion, cystitislike syndrome; breast tenderness, enlargement, and secretion; nausea and vomiting, bloating, cholestatic jaundice, chloasma of skin which may persist even after the drug is discontinued, loss of scalp hair, hirsuitism, intolerance to contact lenses, headache, dizziness, migraine, mental depression, increase or decrease in weight, changes in libido, and finally, carbohydrate intolerance. Contraindications include: known or suspected breast cancer except in selected patients being treated for metastatic disease, known or suspected estrogen-dependent neoplasia, known or suspected pregnancy, undiagnosed abnormal genital bleeding, acute thrombophlebitis or thrombo-embolic disorders or past history of these with previous estrogen use.

Other warnings: a recent study reports a two- to threefold increase in the risk of gallbladder disease. Benign hepatic adenomas appear to be associated with the use of oral contraceptives (estrogen-containing). Although they are benign, they may cause death by rupturing with resulting abdominal hemorrhage. Some women taking Premarin experience increased blood pressure which in most cases, returns to normal when the drug is discontinued. Glucose tolerance may be lower, so diabetic patients should be monitored more closely, and estrogens may be poorly metabolized in patients with impaired liver function.

2. Depo-testosterone (testosterone cypionate)

Replacement hormone

Uses:
1. Eunichism; deficiency after castration
2. Male climacteric symptoms secondary to androgen deficiency;

Dosage varies with product being used:
1. Depo-testosterone is in oil and intended only for IM use
2. Other testosterone

forms available are: tablets for oral and buccal use; pellets for SQ implant; suspensions and solutions for IM use only

impotence due to testicular deficiency
3. Oligospermia

Dosage varies with condition being treated:
1. Eunichism: 200–400 mg q3–4 wk
2. Male climacteric symptoms: 200–400 mg q3–4 wk
3. Oligospermia: 100–200 mg q3–6 wk or 200 mg once a week for 6–10 weeks for suppression of spermatogenesis, which may be followed by increased production of sperm when the drug is withdrawn

DRUG CATEGORY	MAJOR ACTION	THERAPEUTIC ACTION AND EFFECT	COMMONLY PRESCRIBED DOSE AND ROUTE
2. Depo-testosterone (cont'd)		Testosterone is contraindicated in known or suspected carcinoma of the male breast, or prostatic, cardiac, hepatic, or renal decompensation; hypercalcemia; liver function impairment; prepubertal males; and elderly patients in whom overstimulation is to be avoided. Warnings: testosterone products should not be used interchangeably due to differences in duration of action. Because the prolonged action of Depo-testosterone, it should be used cautiously with organic heart disease or debilitation. Hypercalcemia may occur in immobilized patients. In this event, the drug should be discontinued. Adverse reactions include: priapism, acne, gynecomastia, excessive sexual stimulation, edema, hypersensitivity (including skin manifestations and anaphylactoid reactions), local irritation, and decreased ejaculatory volume. Depo-testosterone may increase sensitivity to oral anticoagulants.	
3. Oral contraceptives, e.g., Ortho-Novum	Contraception	Prevention of pregnancy	Cyclic administration of one pill a day for 21 days; none for 7 days then restart cycle

Start taking the first pill on day 5 of the menstrual cycle (day 1 is the first day of menstrual bleeding) |

Some packs contain 21 birth control pills and 7 sugar or iron pills, allowing the patient to take one pill every day, eliminating the possibility of forgetting to restart the cycle

Oral contraceptives (OCs) include both estrogen-progestin combinations and progestin only products. Ortho-Novum is an example of a combination product. It is thought that these products work by inhibiting ovulation through suppression of follicle-stimulating hormone and luteinizing hormone, as well as altering the cervical mucus and the endometrium in such a way that sperm penetration of the cervix and implantation of the fertilized ovum are hindered. The combination products seem to be slightly more effective than the progestin-only products. How to handle missed doses: if one tablet is missed, take it as soon as it is remembered or take two tablets the next day. If two consecutive tablets are missed, take two tablets daily for the next 2 days, then resume the regular schedule. Use additional forms of contraception for 7 days. If three consecutive tablets are missed, begin a new compact of pills starting 7 days after the last tablet was taken. Use additional forms of birth control for 14 days. While there is little likelihood of ovulation occurring after one missed dose, the possibility of spotting or bleeding is increased. Also, as more doses are missed, chances for ovulation rise. After several months on birth control pills, menstrual flow may be reduced to a point of virtual absence. This reduced flow is not indicative of pregnancy. However, if the menstrual period is missed altogether, the possibility of pregnancy should be ruled out, because birth control pills should not be taken if pregnancy is suspected. Postpartum contraception using OCs may be initiated immediately after birth in nonnursing mothers but are routinely started at the 6-week checkup. Nursing mothers should wait until the infant is weaned. Several products may be tried before effective results are obtained with minimal side effects. After the second month of therapy, breakthrough bleeding may indicate a need for a higher dosage. Other causes must also be considered. In progestin-only oral contraceptive failures, the ratio of ectopic to intrauterine pregnancy is higher than in women not taking OCs. This is probably because the drug is more effective in preventing intrauterine pregnancies. There is evi-

DRUG CATEGORY	MAJOR ACTION	THERAPEUTIC ACTION AND EFFECT	COMMONLY PRESCRIBED DOSE AND ROUTE

3. Oral contraceptives, etc. (cont'd)

dence of fertility impairment in women discontinuing OCs in comparison with women using other methods. The impairment does not seem to be related to duration of use and diminishes with time (30–42 months).

Drug interactions include: reduced efficacy and increased incidence of breakthrough bleeding have been reported with concurrent use of rifampin, barbiturates, phenylbutazone, phenytoin, primidone, carbamazepine, chloramphenicol, sulfonamides, nitrofurantoin, analgesics, tranquilizers, and antimigraine preparations. Oral contraceptives may decrease the effects of oral anticoagulants, anticonvulsants, tricyclic antidepressants, antihypertensives, vitamins, and hypoglycemic agents. Impairment of elimination of other drugs may occur including, Valium, caffeine, corticosteroids, Librium, phenytoin, phenylbutazone, imipramine, as well as others. This results in higher blood levels of these drugs.

Contraindications include: thrombophlebitis, thromboembolic disorders, history of deep vein thrombophlebitis, cerebral vascular disease, myocardial infarction, coronary artery disease, known or suspected breast cancer or estrogen-dependent neoplasia, undiagnosed abnormal genital bleeding, known or suspected pregnancy, past or present benign or malignant liver tumor.

There are numerous side effects and adverse reactions to OCs, the most common of which are: nausea, vomiting, elevated blood pressure, fluid retention, headache, bleeding irregularities, increase in existing fibroid size, depression, pyridoxine deficiency, folic acid deficiency, photosensitivity, tartrazine sensitivity, pulmonary embolism, stroke, thrombophlebitis, myocardial infarction, mesenteric thrombosis, breast enlargement, tenderness and secretion, skin rash, migraine, intolerance to contact lenses, weight change, changes in appetite, anemia, vaginitis, cystitis-like syndrome, backache, rhinitis, lupus erythematosus, rheumatoid arthritis, endometrial, cervical, and breast cancer, and increased risk of gallbladder disease. Benign and malignant hepatic adenomas have been associated with usage of OCs. Sudden abdominal pain may be indicative of rupture and hemorrhage of liver tumors.

Oral contraceptive users who also smoke, have a fivefold increased risk of fatal myocardial infarction than non-smoking users; and 10 to 12-fold increased risk compared with nonsmokers not using OCs.

The risk of thromboembolic disorders increases after the approximate age of 30. The use of OCs in women 40 and over is not recommended.

It is recommended that an alternate form of contraception be used for several months after discontinuing OCs, before intentionally becoming pregnant. There is some evidence of chromosomal abnormalities in aborted embryos conceived during this period.

Serious ill effects have not been reported with overdosage. As, with Premarin, nausea is the main symptom, and possibly withdrawal bleeding in females as blood levels drop with metabolism of the drug.

TOPICAL DRUGS

1. Mycolog ointment

(ingredients: nystatin, neomycin, gramicidin, triamcinolone)

Anti-inflammatory and antibiotic

Uses:
1. Cutaneous candidiasis
2. Superficial bacterial infections
3. Infantile eczema
4. Lichen simplex chronicus
5. Pruritus ani and pruritus vulvae
6. When complicated by candidial and/or bacterial infection:
   a) Eczematoid, stasis, nummular, contact or

Available as cream or ointment

Cream: rub into affected areas b.i.d. or t.i.d.

Ointment: apply a thin film to affected area b.i.d. or t.i.d.

May be used with an occlusive dressing

DRUG CATEGORY	MAJOR ACTION	THERAPEUTIC ACTION AND EFFECT	COMMONLY PRESCRIBED DOSE AND ROUTE
1. Mycolog ointment (cont'd)		seborrheic dermatitis b) Neurodermatitis c) Dermatitis venenata	
		Triamcinolone: provides anti-inflammatory, anti-pruritic, and vasocon-strictive actions	
		Neomycin and gramicidin: provide antibacterial activity	
		Nystatin: provides specific anticandidal activity	

Topical steroids should not be used in viral or fungal conditions of the skin, except for candidiasis. This preparation should not be applied in the external auditory canal of patients with perforated eardrums, nor should it be used ophthalmically. Topical steroids should not be used when circulation is markedly impaired. Mycolog is contraindicated in patients with hypersensitivity to any of the ingredients. Other precautions include the potential hazard of nephrotoxicity and ototoxicity from systemic absorption of neomycin when Mycolog is used in large amounts for prolonged periods in treating skin infections following extensive burns or trophic ulceration. Systemic absorption of the corticosteroid may occur under these same or similar conditions with resulting adverse reactions. As with any antibiotic preparation, prolonged use may result in overgrowth of nonsusceptible organisms, including fungi other than candida. Should this occur, suitable concomitant antimicrobial therapy must be initiated. If a favorable response is not obtained with this method, the Mycolog should be discontinued.

Adverse reactions include: hypersensitivity to neomycin (reactions to nystatin and topical gramicidin are rare). Ototoxicity and nephrotoxicity have been reported. Corticosteroids topically have produced burning sensations, itching, irritation, dryness, folliculitis, skin atrophy, secondary infection, striae, miliaria, hypertrichosis, acnelike eruption, maceration of the skin, and hypopigmentation.

GASTROINTESTINAL DRUGS

1. Mylanta — Antacid

Ingredients:
aluminum hydroxide
magnesium hydroxide
simethicone

Uses:
1. Symptomatic relief of GI discomforts associated with heartburn, acid indigestion, and sour stomach
2. Also indicated in hyperacidity associated with the diagnosis of peptic ulcer, gastritis, peptic esophagitis, gastric hyperacidity, and hiatal hernia

Mylanta neutralizes the

5–15 ml between meals and at bedtime

The amount and frequency of dosing depends on the needs of each patient

Except under the advice and supervision of a physician, do not administer more than 24 teaspoonfuls in a 24-hour period or use the maximum dose for more than 2 weeks

DRUG CATEGORY	MAJOR ACTION	THERAPEUTIC ACTION AND EFFECT	COMMONLY PRESCRIBED DOSE AND ROUTE
1. Mylanta (cont'd)		acidity (or; reduces the acidity) of the gastric contents and inhibits the activity of pepsin, a proteolytic enzyme	Frequent administration is necessary due to the rapid emptying of the gastric content

Liquid forms have more rapid onset and greater activity

Mylanta tablets are also available |

Mylanta is one of the lowest in sodium content of all the antacids, making it more useful for patients on sodium-restricted diets. Magnesium-containing products should be used with caution in patients with kidney disease. Aluminum ions inhibit spontaneous smooth muscle contraction, thus slowing gastric emptying; therefore should be used with caution in patients with gastric outlet obstruction. Simethicone, although controversial, has been reported to decrease gas build up. Magnesium usually has an irritability effect on the intestines, tending to cause diarrhea; however, aluminum tends to constipate, so Mylanta is designed to be balanced in this regard. There are some very important drug interactions: reduced absorption of tetracycline, digoxin, quinidine, phenytoin, Coumadin, oral iron products, and isoniazide. In general, it is best not to administer other oral drugs within 1–2 hours of antacid administration, because the gastric pH is altered such that drugs designed to be best absorbed in an acidic environment may not be as effective.

2. Pro-Banthine (propantheline)	Gastrointestinal anticholinergic	Use: Adjunctive therapy in treatment of peptic ulcer 1. Inhibits GI motility 2. Diminishes gastric acid secretion 3. Inhibits the action of acetylcholine	15 mg taken 30 min before meals and 30 mg at bedtime Smaller doses may be used for geriatric patients and for those of small stature

In the presence of high environmental temperatures, heat prostration can occur because of decreased sweating. Pro-Banthine may produce drowsiness or blurred vision. Diarrhea may be an early symptom of incomplete intestinal obstruction, especially in patients with ileostomy or colostomy; therefore, a complete understanding of all underlying GI conditions precludes usage of this drug. It is not advisable in obstructive diseases. Varying degrees of urinary hesitancy may be observed in patients with prostatic hypertrophy. In these patients, retention may be avoided by having the patient urinate at the time of taking the medication. Pro-Banthine should be used with caution in the elderly and all patients with autonomic neuropathy, hepatic or renal disease, hyperthyroidism, coronary heart disease, congestive heart failure, cardiac tachyarrhythmias, or hypertension. In patients with ulcerative colitis, large doses of Pro-Banthine may suppress intestinal motility to the point of paralytic ileus, which may precipitate or aggravate toxic megacolon, a serious complication of ulcerative colitis.

Adverse reactions include: drying of salivary secretions, decreased sweating, blurred vision, mydriasis, cycloplegia, increased ocular tension, urinary hesitancy, retention, tachycardia, loss of sense of taste, headache, drowsiness, weakness, dizziness, insomnia, nausea, vomiting, constipation, bloating, impotence, suppression of lactation, urticaria, anaphylaxis, and other skin manifestations of allergy.

Overdosage may produce a curarelike effect leading to muscle weakness and possible paralysis, as well as restlessness, excitement, psychotic behavior, flushing, fall in blood pressure, fever, respiratory failure, coma. The specific treatments include physostigmine IV up to a total of 5 mg (0.5–2 mg given at intervals, checking for reversal of symptoms) and chloral hydrate solution rectally or sodium thiopental (Pentothal) slow IV for control of the CNS excitement. Maintenance of respiration by artificial means may be necessary.

DRUG CATEGORY	MAJOR ACTION	THERAPEUTIC ACTION AND EFFECT	COMMONLY PRESCRIBED DOSE AND ROUTE
2. Pro-Banthine (cont'd)			

Pro-Banthine is contraindicated in: obstructive diseases of the GI tract, glaucoma, obstructive uropathy (prostatism), intestinal atony of elderly or debilitated, severe ulcerative colitis or toxic megacolon, hiatal hernia associated with reflux, unstable cardiovascular adjustment in acute hemorrhage, and myasthenia gravis.

Drug interactions are mainly of the excessive anti-cholinergic type when the following drugs are given concomitantly: belladonna alkaloids, synthetic and semisynthetic anticholinergic agents (i.e., antispasmodics, antiparkinsonian drugs), phenothiazine, tricyclic antidepressants, quinidine antihistamines, or procainamide.

Increased digoxin levels have been noted when Pro-Banthine is given concurrently with slow-dissolving digoxin tablets. This can be avoided by administering only the rapidly dissolving digoxin tablets by USP standards, while using Pro-Banthine.

DRUG CATEGORY	MAJOR ACTION	THERAPEUTIC ACTION AND EFFECT	COMMONLY PRESCRIBED DOSE AND ROUTE
3. Tagamet (cimetidine)	H_2-receptor antagonist	Effects: 1. Inhibits both daytime and nighttime basal gastric acid secretion 2. Inhibits gastric acid secretion stimulated by food, histamine, pentagastrin, caffeine, and insulin	Available as tablets, liquid, and injection Highest dose should not exceed 2400 mg/day Dosing: 1. Active duodenal ulcer: 300 mg orally q.i.d. with meals and at

3. Reduces total pepsin output as a result of the decrease in gastric juice
4. Inhibits the rise in the intrinsic factor although some is excreted at all times

Uses:
1. Short-term treatment of active duodenal ulcer
2. Prophylactic use in duodenal ulcer patients to prevent recurrence, and therefore prevent possible surgery
3. Short-term treatment of active benign gastric ulcer
4. Treatment of pathologic hypersecretory conditions
5. Intractable ulcers

bedtime
2. Prophylaxis of recurrent duodenal ulcer: 400 mg at bedtime (prophylactic treatment with higher or more frequent doses not improve effectiveness)
3. Active benign gastric ulcer: 300 mg orally q.i.d. with meals and at bedtime
4. Pathologic hypersecretory conditions: 300 mg orally q.i.d. with meals and at bedtime

In hospitalized patients that require injectable Tagamet, it may be given IM, IV push, or intermittent IV infusion; dosing is 300 mg q6 hr

DRUG CATEGORY	MAJOR ACTION	THERAPEUTIC ACTION AND EFFECT	COMMONLY PRESCRIBED DOSE AND ROUTE
3. Tagamet (cont'd)			IM Tagamet does not require diluting. Tagamet for IV push should be diluted in at least 20 ml and injected over a period of no less than 2 min. Intermittent IV administration is accomplished by diluting Tagamet 300 mg in 100 ml solution and infusing over 15–20 min

There are no known contraindications to the use of Tagamet, unless a patient has experienced a previous hypersensitivity reaction. Tagamet is not an anticholinergic drug.

Adverse reactions include: mild and transient diarrhea, dizziness, somnolence, and rash may occur in 1 in 100 patients; a few cases of headache, ranging from mild to severe, have been reported but cleared with withdrawal of the drug; rare reports of reversible arthralgia, myalgia, and exacerbation of joint symptoms in patients with preexisting arthritis; reversible states of confusion (agitation, disorientation, psychosis, anxiety, depression, and hallucinations) have been reported, generally in severely ill patients; mild gynecomastia has been reported in patients treated for 1 month or longer; an antiandrogenic effect has been documented with Tagamet, resulting in slightly lower sperm levels in some cases; reversible impotence has been reported in patients with pathologic hypersecretory disorders; decreased white blood cell counts have been documented, including agranulocytosis. However most of these patients were serously ill and received drugs and/or treatments, other than Tagamet, known to produce neutropenia; reversible alopecia has been reported; and rare cases of fever, interstitial nephritis, hepatitis, and pancreatitis which cleared on withdrawal of the drug.

Rare instances of cardiac arrhythmias and hypotension have been reported following the rapid administration of Tagamet by IV bolus.

Drug interactions include: Tagamet has been noted to reduce metabolism of the following drugs, resulting in higher blood levels: Coumadin, phenytoin, propranolol, Librium, Valium, lidocaine, and theophylline.

Symptomatic response to Tagamet therapy in active benign gastric ulcers does not preclude the presence of gastric malignancy.

Tagamet therapy cannot be recommended for children under 16 years of age, due to limited studies in this area.

The physician must weigh the possible benefits against the risks.

Human experience with gross overdosage is also limited. However, in a few cases, doses up to 10 g have not been associated with any untoward effects.

CHEMOTHERAPY DRUGS

| 1. Adriamycin (doxorubicin) | Cytotoxic anthracycline antibiotic | Uses: Produces regression in disseminated neoplastic conditions such as: 1. Acute lymphoblastic leukemia 2. Acute myeloblastic leukemia 3. Wilms tumor 4. Neuroblastoma | IV only: 60–75 mg/m² q21 days (m² refers to body surface area) or 30 mg/m² daily for 3 days, then repeat in 4 weeks

Lower doses need to be given in cases of elevated bilirubin, inadequate marrow reserves, or |

Commonly Prescribed Drugs 159

DRUG CATEGORY	MAJOR ACTION	THERAPEUTIC ACTION AND EFFECT	COMMONLY PRESCRIBED DOSE AND ROUTE
1. Adriamycin (cont'd)			impaired hepatic function
		5. Soft-tissue and bone sarcomas	It is recommended that Adriamycin be administered through a freely running IV
		6. Breast carcinoma	
		7. Ovarian carcinoma	
		8. Transitional cell bladder carcinoma	
		9. Thyroid carcinoma	
		10. Lymphomas of both Hodgkin and non-Hodgkin types	
		11. Bronchogenic carcinoma (small-cell histologic type)	

The mechanism of action appears to be related to its ability to bind to DNA and inhibit nucleic acid synthesis. Severe local cellulitis, vesication, and tissue necrosis will occur if Adriamycin is extravasated or infiltrates during administration. Redness and streaking along the vein proximal to the site of injection has been reported without extravasation. Infiltration and extravasation may occur with or without the accompanying stinging and burning and even if blood returns well on aspiration. Adriamycin must never be given IM or SQ. Serious irreversible myocardial toxicity with delayed congestive heart failure, unresponsive to treatment, may occur as the total dosage approaches 550 mg/m².

This cardiac toxicity may occur at lower cumulative doses in patients with prior mediastinal irradiation or with concurrent Cytoxan therapy. Acute life-threatening arrhythmias have been reported during or within a few hours of administration of Adriamycin. However at the present time, transient ECG changes consisting of T wave flattening, ST depression, and arrhythmias lasting up to 2 weeks after a dose are not considered indications for suspension of therapy. There is a high incidence of bone marrow suppression, primarily of leukocytes. Red blood cells and platelets should also be monitored, as they also may be depressed. Persistent and severe myelosuppression can result in superinfection and hemorrhage. Adriamycin may potentiate the toxicity of other anticancer therapies.

Like other cytotoxic drugs, Adriamycin may induce hyperuricemia due to rapid lysis of the neoplastic cells. Other adverse reactions include: nausea and vomiting (frequently), which may be alleviated by prior antiemetic therapy; reversible complete alopecia occurs in most cases; hyperpigmentation of nailbeds and dermal creases, primarily in children; stomatitis and esophagitis may occur 5–10 days after therapy; fever, chills, and urticaria have been reported occasionally; and anaphylaxis may occur. Patients should be warned that their urine will be red in color for 1–2 days after therapy.

Contraindications include patients who have marked myelosuppression as a result of previous chemotherapy or radiation, patients with preexisting heart disease, and those who have reached their maximum cumulative dose of Adriamycin.

Because Adriamycin is so caustic, precautions should be taken in handling to prevent contact with the skin.

2. **Cytoxan (cyclophosphamide)**

Alkylating agent

Uses:
1. Malignant lymphomas (stages III and IV)
   a) Hodgkin disease
   b) Follicular lymphoma
   c) Lymphocytic lymphosarcoma
   d) Reticulum cell sarcoma

Induction:
1. IV: 40–50 mg/kg given in divided doses over a period of 2–5 days; patients with compromised bone marrow function may require a reduction of the dose by one-third to one-

DRUG CATEGORY	MAJOR ACTION	THERAPEUTIC ACTION AND EFFECT	COMMONLY PRESCRIBED DOSE AND ROUTE

2. Cytoxan (cont'd)		e) Lymphoblastic lymphosarcoma
		f) Burkitt lymphoma
		2. Multiple myeloma
		3. Leukemias
		  a) Chronic lymphocytic leukemia
		  b) Chronic granulocytic leukemia (it is ineffective in acute blastic crises)
		  c) Acute myelogenous and monocytic leukemia
		  d) Acute lymphoblastic (stem cell) leukemia in children
		4. Mycosis fungoides (advanced)
		5. Neuroblastoma
			half
			2. Oral: 1–5 mg/kg/day
			Maintenance (several schedules have been used):
			1. 1–5 mg/kg p.o. daily
			2. 10–15 mg/kg IV every 7–10 days
			3. 3–5 mg/kg IV twice weekly
			Infrequently responsive malignancies:
			1. Carcinoma of the breast
			2. Malignant neoplasms of the lung
			Cytoxan may be given IM, IV, intraperitone-

(disseminated)
6. Adenocarcinoma of
the ovary
7. Retinoblastoma

ally, intrapleurally, as
an IV push, or as an IV
infusion using com-
patible diluents

Although it is classified as an alkylating agent, Cytoxan itself is not an alkylating agent or irritant. It interferes with the growth of susceptible neoplasms and, to some extent, normal tissues, but its mechanism of action is unknown. Cytoxan may interfere with normal wound healing. Modification of dosage should be considered for patients who develop bacterial, fungal, or viral infections. Varicella zoster infections appear to particularly dangerous when Cytoxan is given concurrently with steroid therapy or in patients with a recent history of steroid therapy. Under these same circumstances, other infections have been fatal. Adjustment of the dosage of both Cytoxan and steroids may be necessary for the adrenalectomized patient. Chronic administration of high doses of phenobarbital increases the rate of metabolism and the leukopenic activity of Cytoxan. If given during remission of acute lymphoblastic (stem cell) leukemia in children, Cytoxan is effective in prolonging its duration.

Cytoxan tablets contain tartrazine which may cause allergic reactions (including bronchial asthma) in susceptible individuals. Precautions should be taken in administering Cytoxan to the following patients: those with leukopenia, thrombocytopenia, tumor cell infiltration of bone marrow, previous x-ray therapy, previous therapy with other cytotoxic drugs, impaired renal function, and impaired hepatic function.

Other adverse reactions include: anorexia, nausea, vomiting (all common) which are related to dosage as well as individual susceptibility; sterile hemorrhagic cystitis, which can be severe and even fatal, and is probably due to metabolites in the urine; nonhemorrhagic cystitis and fibrosis of the bladder have also been reported (ample fluid intake and frequent voiding help prevent the development of cystitis); gonadal suppression resulting in amenorrhea or azoospermia has been reported in a number of patients; this side effect is quite possibly irreversible. It is not known to what extent Cytoxan affects prepubertal gonads. Alopecia is a frequent side effect. Regrowth of hair can be expected, although it may be a different color and/or texture. The skin and fingernails may become darker during therapy. Interstitial pulmonary fibrosis has been reported in patients receiving high doses over prolonged periods. Nephrotoxicity, including hemorrhage and clot formation in the renal pelvis have also been reported. A marked leukopenia is usually associated with induction dosages, but recovery begins after 7-10 days. Leukopenia is an expected side effect

DRUG CATEGORY	MAJOR ACTION	THERAPEUTIC ACTION AND EFFECT	COMMONLY PRESCRIBED DOSE AND ROUTE
2. Cytoxan (cont'd)	and ordinarily is used as a guide to therapy. Reversible thrombocytopenia and anemia may occur in a few patients. Unless the disease is unusually sensitive to Cytoxan, the largest maintenance dosage that can be reasonably tolerated is advised. The total leukocyte count is a good objective guide for regulating the maintenance dosage. Ordinarily, a leukopenia of 3000–4000 cells/cu mm can be maintained without undue risk of serious infection or other complications.		
	Secondary malignancies have developed in some patients treated with Cytoxan alone or in association with other antineoplastic drugs. In some cases, the secondary malignancy is detected several years after Cytoxan therapy was discontinued.		
3. Fluorouracil (5-fluouracil; 5-FU)	Antimetabolite	Palliative management of carcinoma of colon, rectum, breast, stomach, and pancreas in patients considered incurable by surgery or other means	IV only 12 mg/kg IV daily for 4 successive days. The daily dosage should not exceed 800 mg. Then, if no toxicity is observed, 6 mg/kg on the 6th, 8th, 10th, and 12th days, unless toxicity occurs. Therapy is discontinued at the end of the 12th day, even if

no toxicity has become apparent. No drug is given on days 5, 7, 9, or 11.

Poor risk patients or those in an inadequate nutritional state: 6 mg/kg daily for 3 successive days. Then, if no toxicity, 3 mg/kg on the 5th, 7th, and 9th day. No drug is given on days 4, 6, or 8. Dose should not exceed 400 mg.

Maintenance therapy: Where no toxicity has been observed after initial course of therapy, the following maintenance schedules may be used:
1. Repeat dosage of first course q30 days after the last day of the previous course of

DRUG CATEGORY	MAJOR ACTION	THERAPEUTIC ACTION AND EFFECT	COMMONLY PRESCRIBED DOSE AND ROUTE
2. Cytoxan (cont'd)			treatment 2. When toxic signs resulting from the initial course of therapy have subsided, administer a maintenance dosage of 10–15 mg/kg/wk as a single dose. Do not exceed 1 g/wk The amount of drug to be used should take into account the patient's reaction to the previous course and should be adjusted accordingly. All dosages are based on patients' actual weight. However, the estimated lean body mass (dry weight) is used if the pa-

tient is obese or if there has been sudden weight gain due to edema.

No dilution required for administration

5-FU interferes with the synthesis of DNA and to a lesser extent, inhibits the formation of RNA; since both of these are essential for cell growth, 5-FU provokes unbalanced growth and therefore, death of the cell. The DNA and RNA deprivation are most marked on those cells that grow rapidly and take up the drug at a more rapid pace (i.e., cancer cells). 5-FU is contraindicated in patients in poor nutritional state, those with depressed bone marrow function, and those with serious infections. The daily dose of 5-FU should not exceed 800 mg, and it is recommended that the patient be hospitalized during the first course of treatment. The drug should be given with caution to patients with impaired renal and hepatic function, as well as patients having received high doses of pelvic radiation, those having previously used alkylating agents and those with metastatic involvement of the bone marrow. The drug is not intended as an adjuvant to surgery, and fatalities may be encountered in patients in relatively good condition. The toxicity of 5-FU will be increased by any therapy that adds to the stress of the patient, interferes with nutrition, or depresses bone marrow function. Therapy is to be discontinued promptly when any one of the following signs of toxicity appears: the first visible sign of stomatitis or esophagopharyngitis; WBC under 3500, or a rapidly falling WBC; intractable vomiting, diarrhea, gastrointestinal ulceration, and bleeding; platelets under 100,000; hemorrhage from any site. Other adverse reactions include: anorexia, nausea and vomiting (common); leukopenia usually follows every adequate course of therapy but usually returns to normal by the 30th day; alopecia and dermatitis are seen in a substantial number of cases, both are generally reversible; dry skin and fissuring have also been noted; photosensitivity, photophobia, lacrimation, epistaxis, euphoria, acute cerebellar syndrome (which may persist), nail changes, loss of nails, and myocardial ischemia have all been documented.

Intravenous administration should be done carefully in an effort to avoid extravasation. Although fluorouracil solution may discolor somewhat in the ampule during storage, the potency and safety are not adversely affected.

DRUG CATEGORY	MAJOR ACTION	THERAPEUTIC ACTION AND EFFECT	COMMONLY PRESCRIBED DOSE AND ROUTE
4. Oncovin (vincristine)	Antineoplastic	Uses: 1. Acute leukemia 2. Also useful in combination with other oncolytic agents in: Hodgkin disease, lymphosarcoma, reticulum cell sarcoma, rhabdomyosarcoma, neuroblastoma, Wilms tumor	IV only Adults: 1.4 mg/m^2 weekly (m^3 refers to body surface area) Children: 2 mg/m^2 weekly May be injected either directly into the vein or into the tubing of a running IV Various dosage schedules have been used

There are no actual contraindications to the use of Oncovin, but precautions must be used in administering to patients with preexisting neuromuscular disease when other neurotoxic drugs are being used, in the presence of leukopenia, or complicating infection. The most common adverse reaction is hair loss; the most troublesome reactions are neuromuscular in origin.

Leukopenia, neuritic pain, constipation, and difficulty in walking may occur after therapy. They are of shorter duration after a single weekly dose is given than if the drug is given in divided doses. Other side effects include: sensory loss, parethesia, slapping gait, loss of deep tendon reflexes, and muscle wasting. In addition, constipation and paralytic ileus may occur, particularly in young children. The ileus will reverse itself upon discontinuation of the drug and with symptomatic care. Constipation may take the form of upper-colon impaction. On physical examination, the rectum is empty, but the patient may be experiencing colicky pain. A flat film of the abdomen reveals this condition, which usually responds to high enemas and laxatives. A routine prophylactic regimen against constipation is recommended for all patients on this drug. Other adverse reactions include: fever, weight loss, footdrop, ataxia, cranial nerve manifestations, paresthesia and numbness of the digits, polyuria, dysuria, oral ulceration, headache, vomiting and diarrhea; there does not appear to be any significant effect on the platelets or red blood cells; convulsions, frequently with hypertension have been reported in a few patients.

Frequently there is a sequence in the development of the neuromuscular side effects. Initially only sensory impairment and paresthesia appear, then with continued treatment neuritic pain develops, and later motor difficulties.

If central nervous system leukemias are diagnosed while on Oncovin, other oncolytic agents must be used, because Oncovin does not appear to pass the blood-brain barrier.

Acute uric acid nephropathy has also been reported with Oncovin, as with other chemotherapeutic agents.

All side effects seem to be reversible and are related to dosage. The mechanism of action of Oncovin is unknown; however, it is thought to cause an arrest in the mitotic division at the stage of metaphase in cell reproduction.

PART II

Nursing Self-Assessment and Review

3

Review Questions

A. BASIC CONCEPTS OF NURSING PRACTICE IN MENTAL HEALTH

1. Theories of Personality and Psychosocial Development and Their Application

1. In Sullivan's theory of interpersonal growth and development, which of the following is true?
   A. Socialization is less important than biologic changes
   B. Personality development proceeds through the prototoxic, parataxic, and syntaxic modes of perception
   C. Sexuality is a major emphasis
   D. Anxiety is mastered in childhood

2. During a routine visit to the clinic, a mother requests your help in understanding her infant's psychosocial development. The baby has been seen by a doctor and no physical problems are apparent. Upon questioning, you find that when the baby was 3 months old his father became critically ill. The mother began working and felt inadequate in this role. The baby seemed to change gradually from a happy, attentive child to an irritable, cranky baby. In explaining H. S. Sullivan's ideas about normal development, you both agree that
   A. the baby's formula is inappropriate and should be changed
   B. the manifested behavior is common in small babies and will soon disappear
   C. the baby is "testing" his mother and should be allowed to "cry it out" so he will not be spoiled
   D. anxiety in the mother is perceived by the infant, influencing his self-image and behavior

3. Sally, aged 19, and Bill, aged 20, have been married 1 year. About 6 months ago they came to you for marital therapy because of Bill's apparently insatiable need for sex, regardless of Sally's feelings. Recently, Bill recognizes Sally's sexual desires as being as important as his own. According to Sullivan's theory, Bill is at what stage of interpersonal development at this time in his life?
   A. Maturity, concerned about life's meaning
   B. Late adolescence, developing an enduring intimate relationship
   C. Self-actualization, achieving self-fulfillment
   D. Civilized identity, achieving involvement and cooperation

4. Joan Anderson is admitted into the psychiatric unit of the local hospital in a state of hysteria. According to Sullivan, Joan probably has
   A. an unconscious conflict between her id and superego
   B. an inability to deal with her excess amounts of unchanneled energy
   C. been in a "double-bind" situation for most of her life
   D. an unresolved conflict with a significant person

5. According to Freudian theory, psychosexual stages of growth and development occur in which order?
   A. Oral, anal, phallic, latency, and genital
   B. Sensory, muscular, locomotor, latency, and adulthood
   C. Exploration, experimentation, manipulation, and collaboration
   D. Conscious, unconscious, and preconscious

6. According to Freudian theory, defense mechanisms are
   A. unconscious, intrapsychic processes that protect the ego from anxiety
   B. conscious intrapsychic processes that protect the ego from anxiety
   C. preconscious processes that distort reality
   D. conscious processes that distort reality

7. The id, according to Freud, is characterized by
   A. conscious thoughts and feelings
   B. perceptual reality
   C. delayed gratification
   D. unconscious, instinctual forces

8. According to Freud, the ego is characterized by
   A. substituting pleasure for reality
   B. directing the motor activity of the body
   C. a sense of conscience
   D. analyzing unconscious feelings

9. According to Freud, the superego is characterized by
   A. working cooperatively with the id
   B. primarily conscious thoughts and feelings
   C. rules that direct thoughts, feelings, and actions
   D. primarily unconscious thoughts and feelings

10. Marie Smyth is a tall, skinny 12-year-old who comes to the attention of the school nurse because of disruptive behavior. Her parents were divorced when Marie was an infant and since then, according to her mother, Marie has been unmanageable, overly protective of everything that she claims as her own, and insulting to her peers and everyone at home. Using Erickson's theory of personality development, it may be that Marie
    A. is in the industry-vs-inferiority stage and does not like to work
    B. has not successfully resolved the crisis of trust-vs-mistrust stage and manifests her unresolved conflict
    C. is in the initiative-vs-guilt stage and wants to experiment with what she can do by herself
    D. has not successfully resolved the crisis of the intimacy-vs-role diffusion stage and manifests her unresolved conflict

11. Mrs. Jones, a 65-year-old woman, is seen at a geriatric community clinic. She says that life has no meaning, yet she fears death; she manifests despair. As a psychiatric nurse, operating from Erikson's framework, you would say that Mrs. Jones' despair
    A. results from a disturbance in her relations to self and others
    B. is a conditioned response which is reinforced by her environment
    C. is stimulated by irrational thinking and an erroneous belief system
    D. is motivated by failure to achieve ego integrity

12. You agree to work with Jordan Wood, a psychiatric patient who has been hospitalized for several months. In reviewing his treatment, you become aware that Jordan readily remembers his dreams and seems fascinated by their content. Using Jung's theory, assessing Jordan's dreams
    A. reveals past sources of psychic problems
    B. challenges erroneous belief systems
    C. helps to identify the environmental factors that reinforce neurotic or psychotic behavior
    D. reveals current difficulties and future strivings

13. During an initial interview, nurse therapists may encourage clients to discuss the past because knowledge of previous experience is necessary to understand the present. This approach reflects which model of care?
    A. Social
    B. Psychologic
    C. Behavioral
    D. Biologic

14. A patient is admitted to the emergency room for chest pain. Tests show no organic basis for the pain. During an interview the consultation-liaison nurse discovers that the patient's wife of 30 years died 2 weeks ago of a myocardial infarction. The nurse explains his physical symptoms are related to grieving for his wife and they agree to meet to further discuss his situation. Which model of care does this nursing approach represent?
    A. Social
    B. Psychoanalytic
    C. Behavioral
    D. Interpersonal

15. Mr. Billings is referred for group therapy in the outpatient unit of a general hospital. The group therapy is based on client-centered theory in which the main emphasis is on
    A. social interaction which encourages control
    B. the identification and support of effective coping mechanisms
    C. individual responsibility for the course and direction of therapy
    D. etiology, diagnosis, and prognosis

16. In a psychodynamic framework of therapy, which of the following factors is NOT used in assessing your client?
    A. Dreams
    B. Past experiences
    C. Reinforcement schedules
    D. Free association

17. Parents bring their 10-year-old son to a mental health clinic and report that his behavior has become very erratic and, at times, destructive. A physical examination reveals no organic problems. The nurse therapist initiates a program of operant conditioning. Which of the following therapeutic principles is implicit in this form of therapy?
    A. Self-understanding is the critical element in effective therapy
    B. Adaptive behaviors have never been learned
    C. An extensive review of the client's past life is necessary for therapy to begin
    D. Internal stimulation is the controlling factor in behavior

18. Sylvia Wright, a 27-year-old patient on the psychiatric unit, occasionally talks as if she is a computer being controlled by outside forces. Together, she and her nurse agree that every time she talks "crazy," the nurse will not respond and will even ignore her. On the other hand, when she speaks "normally" the nurse will respond, sharing Sylvia's interest. Basically, this planned response pattern is based on the principle that
   A. inappropriate modes of behavior can be modified by systematically altering their consequences
   B. verbalization is a critical aspect of therapy
   C. the support the nurse provides for a client makes her feel that something is being done for her
   D. the intellectual understanding of symptoms can help clients to terminate undesirable behavior

19. Mrs. Miller experiences overwhelming fears whenever she must ride in a bus or an automobile. Because she needs transportation to and from work each day, her anxiety level remains very high. She comes to the mental health center for help. Together you plan a program to desensitize the stimuli that are arousing her anxiety. The major features of this desensitization program are
   A. hierarchy construction and relaxation training
   B. sharing of perceptions, feelings, meanings, and values
   C. self-exploration and assessment of self-esteem
   D. developmental history and its relationship to the symptoms

20. Mr. Green was buried for 2 days in sand and mud when a tunnel in which he was working collapsed. He was not seriously injured, but was hospitalized for treatment of minor abrasions and dehydration. He is disturbed by fantasies and behaves in an indifferent manner. In planning daily visits with Mr. Green using Rogers' approach, the focus of communication should be on
   A. the causes of his present behavior
   B. any topic that the patient wishes to talk about
   C. topics that are distracting
   D. the prognosis for his improvement

21. As a reality therapist you have been working with Jean Hunt for several weeks. Jean has a history of consistently becoming friendly with attractive young men and, as soon as the relationship becomes serious, she terminates the friendship without understanding why she behaves in this fashion. Once this topic emerges, you ask her to evaluate her behavior in terms of
    A. her problems and her feelings about them
    B. her feelings about the men with whom she has been involved
    C. the social acceptability and personal benefit of this behavior
    D. the people, things, and events which motivate this behavior

22. Since Mrs. Brown had a hysterectomy her husband sleeps in a separate room and makes no attempt at intercourse. She and her husband begin rational-emotive therapy. After several weeks in therapy, Mr. Brown still does not view his wife as a woman because she has lost her uterus. In evaluating the progress made to date, it appears that Mr. Brown
    A. has not reached the stage of sexual maturity required for a harmonious marital relationship
    B. is manifesting repressed feelings and wishes
    C. prefers to retain his illogical thinking rather than accepting the work and discipline required for change
    D. is overly dependent upon his wife for gratification and self-esteem

23. Mr. Arnold has a stroke which leaves him with right-sided weakness. His daughter, Mary, visits him daily, feeds him, and does all she can for him. You and the other nurses on the unit have been helping him to become more independent, with considerable success, until Mary arrives each day. In a conversation with her, she says she feels guilty because she was on vacation when her father became ill, that he did not want her to take an out-of-state vacation, and that she thinks he blames her for his condition because he had lain on the kitchen floor for several hours before help arrived. Using Ellis's theory of rational-emotive therapy you conclude that
   A. Mary needs to tell herself that she is not to blame for her father's condition
   B. Mary should have planned for someone to stay with her father while she was on vacation
   C. Mary will not be able to be an active participant in her father's convalescence
   D. Mr. Arnold wants Mary to care for him and will not allow himself to be self-sufficient while she is present

24. Mary Jo, 21, had been sleeping with her boyfriend for 1 year, aware of her mother's strong disapproval. Three weeks ago her mother had a heart attack and died suddenly. Mary Jo became depressed and functionally incapacitated. She was admitted to the hospital for an electrolyte imbalance and psychosomatic problems. The psychiatric nurse assigned to her care was Adlerian in her theoretical approach. The nurse's intervention in a one-to-one therapeutic relationship involves regular conferences working with Mary Jo to
   A. differentiate between feelings and behaviors
   B. prescribe behavioral changes
   C. reeducate her to healthier goals
   D. develop desensitization exercises

25. Ellie, aged 16, was playing table tennis in the psychiatric unit when she noticed her nurse therapist talking and laughing with another patient. She went into a tantrum, shouting and crying. The nurse understood that Ellie had never felt affection and approval from her parents. Following Horney's directive approach the nurse
    A. enters into a discussion with Ellie about her behavior
    B. challenges her to a game of table tennis, allowing her to cope with the situation
    C. sets limits on Ellie's table tennis privileges
    D. tells Ellie to be quiet or leave the room

26. Anticipatory guidance is a useful nursing measure for preparing individuals to deal more effectively with developmental crises. An example of anticipatory guidance is
    A. providing emergency assistance to a family whose child was killed in a home fire
    B. referring an abused woman to a spouse abuse program
    C. counseling a young mother about the meaning of negativistic behavior in 2-year-olds
    D. establishing a trusting relationship with the person who is in crisis

27. One characteristic of neurotic feelings and behavior is
    A. vivid recall of past life events
    B. the occurrence of a loss within the past 2 years
    C. an overemphasis on safety
    D. a disrespect for the law

28. The general goals of care for a psychotic client differ from goals for a neurotic client. Which one of these goals would be appropriate for a psychotic client?
    A. Help the client to recognize rigid and/or repetitious behavior
    B. Discuss with the client his frustration and feelings of guilt over his fantasies
    C. Control distorted thought perceptions with proper medication
    D. Help the person to learn from past mistakes

2. Coping/Defense Mechanisms

29. Defense mechanisms function primarily to
    A. increase the person's conscious awareness
    B. prevent development of psychosis
    C. protect the ego
    D. consistently free the person from anxiety

30. The defense mechanism in which feelings connected to a thought, memory, or experience are excluded from awareness is
    A. regression
    B. isolation
    C. repression
    D. rationalization

31. Nancy, aged 15, is having a temper tantrum because she was not invited to the school dance. Which defense mechanism is Nancy using?
    A. Regression
    B. Repression
    C. Denial
    D. Isolation

32. Ms. L., a new graduate, is consistently late for work. She says that she just overslept. In talking with Ms. L. which approach is most appropriate?
    A. "Ms. L, your excuses are no longer acceptable. Why are you so irresponsible?"
    B. "Come on, Ms. L., you can come up with something more convincing, can't you?"
    C. "Ms. L., your behavior is causing a problem on the unit. Can we talk about some possible reasons for it?"
    D. "Ms. L., you're fired."

33. Dr. S., a short, unattractive man, is causing a problem on the nursing unit with his aggressive demands that the nurses obey his orders. Aware that Dr. S. is using the defense mechanism of compensation, the head nurse's most appropriate reply is which of the following?
    A. "Act your age and be polite."
    B. "You are not the only physician we have to listen to."
    C. "I realize that your orders are important; otherwise you would not be so insistent."
    D. "Your patients aren't the only ones who are sick."

34. Mrs. A., 35, has been married for 12 years. Because she and her husband have been unable to have children, she has been an active volunteer in the newborn nursery. Which defense mechanism is Mrs. A. using?
    A. Sublimation
    B. Compensation
    C. Regression
    D. Repression

35. At the end of her orientation, Ms. Q. tells the head nurse she cannot be expected to assume evening charge. The head nurse realizes Ms. Q. is using projection when Ms. Q says which of the following?
    A. "I'm capable of being in charge, but I'm too new."
    B. "You've expected too much of me and it isn't fair."
    C. "I'm afraid of the responsibility. Perhaps 1 more week will help me feel more secure."
    D. "I know I've learned everything; I don't have to prove it."

36. Don K., aged 15, has a diagnosis of adolescent adjust-
    ment reaction. He is admitted to the unit because of
    family abuse, especially by his mother. Upon seeing her
    walk down the corridor Don yells out, "Here comes
    the old bat now." Don is using the defense mechanism of
    A. condensation
    B. identification
    C. projection
    D. displacement

37. Mr. D., aged 20, is seen in the outpatient clinic for a
    paralysis of his right arm. He tells you, "I had a fight
    with my father and would have hit him but I couldn't
    move my arm." In caring for him you understand that
    Mr. D.'s symptom represents which coping mechanism?
    A. Suppression
    B. Displacement
    C. Conversion reaction
    D. Undoing

38. Mr. P. has just been informed that he has cancer of the
    prostate. When his wife comes in he tells her that he will
    be going home in a few days. Which defense mechanism
    is Mr. P. using?
    A. Denial
    B. Repression
    C. Suppression
    D. Compensation

39. Mrs. A., an attractive 40-year-old woman, admitted for
    treatment of cervical cancer, is causing concern among
    the staff because of her angry behavior toward the male
    staff. The head nurse observes that when the female
    staff takes care of Mrs. A., she demands to know where
    the males are. Which defense mechanism is Mrs. A. using?
    A. Reaction formation
    B. Repression
    C. Introjection
    D. Regression

40. Mrs. L. has a bag of unwashed coffee cups under her bed and refuses to give them up, stating she must keep them so no one else will use them. The nurse understands that Mrs. L.'s behavior represents the defense mechanism of
    A. Displacement
    B. Suppression
    C. Regression
    D. Denial

41. As the nurse enters Mrs. B.'s room, she hears Mrs. B. slam the phone down screaming, "I hate you!" Upon seeing the nurse, Mrs. B. yells, "You're so rude, you're always interrupting me when I'm talking to my husband." Which defense mechanism is Mrs. B. using?
    A. Displacement
    B. Denial
    C. Projection
    D. Rationalization

42. The nurse observes Mrs. W. compulsively washing her hands at frequent intervals. Which statement demonstrates the nurse's understanding of the defense mechanism used?
    A. "Mrs. W., stop that handwashing at once."
    B. "Mrs. W., everyone will see there is something wrong with you."
    C. "Mrs. W., here is some lotion to lessen the effect of the handwashing on your hands."
    D. "Mrs. W., do you think your hands are dirty?"

43. Mr. X., newly diagnosed with diabetes, screams insulting remarks to the nurse who refuses to let him eat the candy bar brought in by his mother. The next morning Mr. X. apologizes profusely, telling the nurse how much he appreciated her actions. Mr. X. is utilizing the defense mechanism of
    A. rationalization
    B. undoing
    C. repression
    D. projection

44. The nurse observes that Mr. S., recovering from an appendectomy, has no visitors. He says that no one appreciates his special sense of humor and interests. What coping mechanism is Mr. S. using?
   A. Fantasy
   B. Rationalization
   C. Sublimation
   D. Compensation

45. Mrs. K. insists that she cover her bed with her dead daughter's sheets. She tells the nurse, "Jane's room at home is exactly the way it was when she died; these are her sheets and I must use them so I can feel close to her." Which defense mechanism is Mrs. K. using?
   A. Introjection
   B. Projection
   C. Displacement
   D. Undoing

46. The nurse observes that Mrs. S., a hysteric, uses regression as a way of dealing with her anxiety, as is evident when Mrs. S. says which of the following?
   A. "Don't bother me. I can take care of myself."
   B. "You're to blame for my ill health; do something."
   C. "I can't feed myself. You must help me."
   D. "If I felt better, I could take care of myself."

47. The primary coping mechanism used by the client with a phobia is
   A. displacement
   B. projection
   C. suppression
   D. repression

48. In planning nursing intervention with the patient with a conversion reaction the nurse should
    A. focus on the impairment and the limitation it sets on the patient
    B. insist that the patient attend physical therapy each day
    C. encourage the patient to participate in unit activities
    D. tell the patient to grow up, there is nothing wrong with him

3. Communication Skills

49. During an interview the patient wrings her hands, speaks in an unsteady voice and her eyes are brimming with tears. When the nurse asks what she is feeling, the patient replies, "Oh nothing." In validating her impressions with the patient, the nurse would recall the principle that the
    A. patient's words must be taken seriously
    B. body never lies—the patient is lying
    C. patient's nonverbal communication contradicts her verbal message
    D. patient's nonverbal communication is unconscious

50. During an interview the patient fidgets with her rings, avoids eye contact with the nurse, and gives vague answers to the nurse's questions. To assess what seems like resistance to the nurse, an appropriate nursing action is to
    A. ignore these nonverbal cues and keep the patient engaged in conversation
    B. explore the meaning of her verbal and nonverbal behavior with the patient
    C. tell the patient you find her fidgeting and vague answers annoying
    D. end the interview and reschedule it only if the patient promises to cooperate better

51. A nurse who experiences anger when interviewing a depressed patient who complains that people always mistreat him is
    A. experiencing a countertransference response
    B. feeling the anger a depressed patient will not allow himself to feel
    C. angry at the patient
    D. is depressed herself and overidentifying with the patient

52. During the course of an interview, a patient tells a nurse he has just lost his leg due to an automobile accident, his father died last year, and he fears he will lose his girl friend due to the amputation. The nurse would describe the theme of the interview process as
    A. dependence
    B. grief
    C. loss
    D. guilt

53. Nurse: "How are you today, Mrs. Q.?"
    Patient: "Who would feel anything but rotten in my position?"
    In assessing this interaction the nurse would recognize that
    A. her opening comment stalled the communication process
    B. the patient has a right to be depressed
    C. she should not ask the patient a direct question
    D. the patient is afraid of probing by the nurse

54. Nurse: "What do you think about the situation with your husband, Mrs. K.?"
    Mrs. K.: "I'm so sad. I cannot believe he would leave me for another woman."
    Nurse: "Sad? I'd be furious if I were you."
    Mrs. K.: "I really do not feel angry, just very sad."
    In analyzing this interaction, the nurse recognizes she is using which barrier to communication when she questions the patient's sadness?
    A. Giving reassurance
    B. Changing the subject
    C. Being judgmental
    D. Challenging

55. Ms. X. realizes that during an initial interview she was judging a patient's sincerity in seeking treatment when he admitted substance abuse for the past 10 years. This patient reminded her of an alcoholic uncle to whom her family always referred as "weak." In planning an on-going treatment plan with the patient, the nurse must
    A. base her feelings on objective patient data
    B. acknowledge how her feelings influence client behavior and care
    C. remember that no drug addict can be trusted
    D. ask another nurse to assume responsibility for this client's care

56. In evaluating the benefit of an initial therapeutic interview, it is most important to determine
    A. the level at which both nurse and patient understood what was said
    B. how much the nurse and patient were able to develop the patient's future plans
    C. the quality of the nursing diagnosis developed
    D. the amount of historical data obtained from the client

57. A patient to whom the nurse has been assigned for the past month is leaving the hospital today. They have been discussing termination for the past few days. During their final interview the patient asks the nurse to visit him after discharge. The most appropriate nursing action is to
   A. talk about how the patient has dealt with other terminations
   B. gratefully accept his invitation
   C. explain gently that hospital policy prohibits her from fraternizing with patients
   D. joke her way out of answering directly

4. Group and Family Therapy

58. Mr. Jones comes to the mental health clinic requesting group therapy. On the initial interview the nurse finds that Mr. Jones has abruptly terminated his individual treatment and is convinced that his wife is a member of the Central Intelligence Agency. Which nursing action assumes priority at this time?
   A. Immediate referral to an interactional outpatient group
   B. Contact the former therapist without the patient's knowledge
   C. Suggest that the former therapist be involved in the decision about group therapy
   D. Contact the patient's wife

59. Ms. Swift contacts the clinic asking that she be allowed to join a therapy group. She says she is having difficulty communicating her ideas to colleagues and supervisors at work. She drops out of the group after two sessions stating that it is making her worse. Your evaluation of the situation is that
   A. the group leader probably ignored her
   B. Ms. Swift was inadequately oriented to the group
   C. the focus on communicating inner thoughts and feelings frightened Ms. Swift
   D. Ms. Swift did not like the other patients

60. A patient is considering group therapy in addition to individual treatment but is unsure of the reasons for which such a move might be indicated. It is important for the nurse group leader to discuss with this patient his
    A. feelings of being blocked with his individual therapist
    B. willingness for self-disclosure
    C. need to meet an eligible mate
    D. fear of consensual validation

61. In screening clients for selection as group members, the most important factor for the nurse to assess is the individual's
    A. ability to give time to the group
    B. willingness to attend the group regularly
    C. ability to verbalize feelings
    D. meeting the established selection criterion

62. Which criterion is most important in assessing a client's appropriateness for a therapy group experience?
    A. Similarity in age, adaptation style, and education level related to other potential group members
    B. Conflicted feelings about intimacy
    C. Degree of satisfaction with himself and the opinions others hold of him
    D. Ability to describe symptoms, seek and give advice with definite opinions

63. Sally Smith enters an ongoing therapy group. After the first four sessions, she telephones the nurse therapist and indicates she does not want to continue. The most appropriate nursing action is to
    A. tell the client on the phone that the initial attendance at group therapy is stressful for most patients
    B. arrange for an interview to discuss the reasons for the patient's wishing to terminate
    C. tell the patient that she must attend one more session to terminate from the group
    D. refer her to another group

64. During a group therapy session members remain silent or speak only to the nurse. To establish more member interaction, the nurse should
    A. reflect her observation about group communication patterns
    B. share her personal feelings about their silence
    C. confront members about their silence
    D. choose a topic and ask each person's opinion regarding the topic

65. Ms. A., nurse group leader, is criticized by the group for not being more directive. One member asks angrily if they are in a group to listen to each other or to get advice from an expert. She does not get defensive. After several meetings, group members begin to share more fully and actually seek each other's opinions and advice. Ms. A. would base her process comments on the knowledge that the group has moved from the
    A. initial phase to the termination phase
    B. working phase to the termination phase
    C. orientation stage to the conflict stage
    D. cohesive phase to the working phase

66. Ms. R. is aware that Mr. Q. is a powerful group member in a relatively passive group. He monopolizes group time and asks for special treatment such as trying to engage her in conversation outside the group and asking permission to come 10 minutes late to each session. The best strategy for dealing with such a group member where there has been no group confrontation is to
    A. make sure she treats every group member equally
    B. wait until the group raises Mr. Q.'s behavior as an issue
    C. ask other group members how they experience Mr. Q.'s monopolizing group time when it occurs
    D. take Mr. Q. aside and tell him how she perceives his behavior

67. The nurse is aware that a patient in her activity group is very self-conscious about his drawing. During the next group she plans to have the members sketch a self-portrait. It would be most appropriate for her to
   A. excuse the patient from the group
   B. ask him to attend but observe only
   C. ask the group how they feel about drawing as part of a warm-up exercise
   D. include a statement about not expecting artistic excellence as part of her general instructions about the group task

68. Mr. R., nurse group leader, realizes that Ms. T. has not spoken in the group for 3 weeks when she expressed anger at Mr. R. for being late and other group members jumped to his defense. To analyze this situation most effectively the leader would
   A. ask Ms. T. to speak since she has not said a word in 3 weeks
   B. ignore Ms. T. until she feels ready to speak
   C. observe Ms. T. for nonverbal cues before intervening
   D. review the sequence of events leading to Ms. T.'s silence with the group and ask the group to deal with her behavior

69. Ms. S.'s therapy group is very angry today, talking about how selfish people are and saying there is no one you can really trust. As group leader, it would be most appropriate for Ms. S. to suggest that
   A. there is little feeling of trust in the group
   B. what group members feel is realistic
   C. people cannot be as difficult as the group makes them out to be
   D. she is trustworthy as a group leader

70. A patient is being scapegoated in Mr. K.'s activity group. He is afraid that the patient or others will leave the group and there will be physical violence within the group. For the next session the most effective plan would be to
   A. state there will be no physical acting-out in the group
   B. exclude the scapegoated patient from the group to give everyone a chance to cool down
   C. speak with the patient individually and ask that he discontinue the behavior which is promoting his being scapegoated
   D. stop all group activity and express concern about scapegoating

71. Ms. T., who has attended a therapy group for 2 years, announces it is time for her to terminate with the group. Readiness to terminate would be most evident by the patient's
   A. ability to arrive at that decision
   B. progress over time in the group
   C. expressed reasons for leaving
   D. ability to relate to others in a nondefensive way

72. During the final session of a group that Ms. X. has led for 2 months, members are all discussing future plans. One group member expresses feelings of sadness that the group is ending and anger that no one acts as if they care it is ending. The nurse group leader supports this group member's comments because the group must recognize that
   A. denial and repression are common defenses against feelings of sadness and loss when a group terminates
   B. this member has never been able to express her feelings so clearly
   C. reaction formation and repression are common defenses against sadness and loss when a group terminates
   D. the patient has expressed an insight that she as the leader wishes she had said

73. Mrs. Gilbert calls the clinic asking for counseling for her son who has been arrested for drunken driving. She says there has been much conflict at home among the parents and two children. The nurse suggests family therapy. During the first interview it is most important to
    A. assess each person's view of the problem
    B. specifically address the son in trouble
    C. document the need for individual members to begin supplemental therapy
    D. assess the son's appropriateness for an adolescent therapy group

74. In interviewing the Sanford family, the nurse notes that individual members appear oblivious to how other members respond to them and are unresponsive to each other. Additional assessment data that would be important to document include
    A. the existence of a family secret that is being protected and hidden
    B. extent of maternal control
    C. roles assumed by each family member
    D. provision for teaching self-care to members

75. Mr. Wood is an abstinent alcoholic. He and his wife have been in couples therapy for several weeks and the nurse notices certain behavioral patterns. Mrs. Wood consistently steps in to manage most situations for the couple while Mr. Wood does not get involved in defining any of these areas. This interactional pattern probably results from
    A. Mrs. Wood's accommodation to her husband's alcohol problem
    B. a balance in the marriage established through an overadequate–inadequate reciprocity
    C. Mr. Wood's passive nature
    D. Mrs. Wood's need to protect her husband

76. The Rand family is terminating from a family treatment contract. Disagreements over what to do about the pregnancy of their unmarried adolescent daughter precipitated the therapy. The initial crisis was resolved and family functioning is stabilized. Which concept do the Rands need to understand in future interactions with their daughter?
    A. Emotional cutoff
    B. Double-bind communication
    C. Withdrawal
    D. Triangulation

77. The family therapy technique in which the therapist instructs family members to do consciously what they are doing unconsciously is called
    A. Freezing
    B. Paradoxical injunction
    C. Role playing
    D. Sculpting

5. Psychosocial and Mental Status Assessment

78. Biologic theories and research in psychoses indicate that psychoses are primarily related to
    A. brain lesions
    B. genetic disorders
    C. biochemical factors
    D. physiologic malfunctions

79. In interviewing a family for an initial assessment the 16-year-old daughter says, "My parents just don't know what life is about. They live in the Dark Ages." The father says, "She is just like her mother, takes drugs to escape the first sign of stress," and the mother says, "My daughter is a good girl who has just gotten mixed up with the wrong kind of kids. That's the only reason she has been using drugs." In hearing these statements you would conclude that
    A. family conflict seems to be the underlying problem
    B. differing perceptions account for these differences in opinion
    C. this family is essentially normal
    D. the mother and daughter need referral to a drug treatment center

80. Information regarding a client's thought processes could best be assessed by observing his
    A. general appearance
    B. communication patterns
    C. family support systems
    D. attitudes

81. During an interview a young man says, "My mother is one of the kindest, most helpful women alive; she has always helped our friends, neighbors, and the people with whom she works." Upon hearing this you would listen for cues that indicate
    A. the son felt neglected by his mother
    B. what his father thought about the mother's actions
    C. the mother's educational preparation and career choice
    D. whether or not the mother does for others to avoid her family

82. In completing a mental status evaluation it is essential to ask questions about the client's social background. Questions about the level of education completed and past employment are asked to
    A. determine if the person's vocabulary is consistent with educational level and career choice
    B. establish rapport in a nonthreatening manner
    C. determine where the person's interests and abilities lie
    D. determine if the person will need vocational rehabilitation services

83. In completing a mental status evaluation it is helpful to ask questions to evaluate memory. Asking a client to repeat ten digits both forward and backward is a means of evaluating
    A. recent memory
    B. remote memory
    C. immediate recall
    D. immediate recall and recent memory

84. During a mental status examination a client begins a meaningless repetition of your words, which is known as
    A. word salad
    B. flight-of-ideas
    C. echolalia
    D. neologism

85. The first step in planning psychiatric nursing intervention is to
    A. make a thorough assessment of the client
    B. complete a family history
    C. develop goals and objectives for nursing action
    D. establish rapport with the client

6. Social, Legal, and Ethical Aspects of Mental Health Nursing

86. Mrs. Johnson describes feelings of loneliness and isolation yet is functioning effectively in her job as a legal secretary. A primary prevention approach would be to
    A. encourage her to see a physician to receive antidepressant treatment
    B. recommend that she begin group therapy to discuss her feelings with people having similar needs
    C. ask her to identify potential areas of involvement in her church or neighborhood
    D. suggest that she take a relaxing vacation to get away from job pressures

87. Mrs. Beck seems depressed and stays in bed for long periods each day. In explaining to Mr. Beck the role of secondary prevention in her treatment you tell him to
    A. bring his wife to see a counselor
    B. immediately take his wife to a mental health facility
    C. have her committed
    D. take her to a physician for antidepressant medication

88. Mrs. Soo is returned to a group home following a 6-month stay in the state hospital. She attends a weekly group session, takes her medication regularly, and is working part time in a sheltered workshop. To what extent has she met the goals of tertiary prevention?
    A. She has most likely met the goals since she is functioning at a reasonable level of adaptation
    B. She has not met the goals since she is being housed in a very supportive setting
    C. Too little information is provided to make this determination
    D. We do not know exactly what Mrs. Soo's goals are

89. Mr. Smith is a 42-year-old man who becomes tearful at work. The nurse at his plant thinks he needs mental health counseling and refers him to a community mental health center. In deciding where to refer him, the nurse must be knowledgeable about the concept of catchment which involves
   A. how old he is
   B. where he lives
   C. how long he has had the symptoms
   D. what his family support system is like

90. You recommend to your staff that a community assessment be completed to determine the range and scope of resources in your area. To begin a community assessment you need to
   A. collect all pertinent information yourself and share this with the staff
   B. focus on client needs rather than provider preferences
   C. determine what data to gather, then decide what is missing
   D. first determine who the recipients of the services are

91. Mrs. Jones, a community leader, comes to the community mental health center complaining about the paucity of services for discharged psychiatric patients. She says patients are discharged into her neighborhood and seem to have no support. An appropriate strategy is to
   A. talk to her about leading a group to lobby for basic changes in public policy for mental health
   B. explain that with limited appropriations there will be little or no aftercare for this population
   C. share with her the many positive things which are being done
   D. ask for her suggestions about programs in her neighborhood

92. Since Mr. Stevens has been hospitalized for depression and a suicide attempt you have received numerous calls from his employer asking specific questions about his progress. The most appropriate nursing action is to
    A. provide the employer with limited information, assuring him that Mr. Stevens will soon be back to work
    B. explain that you cannot discuss Mr. Stevens' condition with him because this information is confidential
    C. refer the employer to Mr. Stevens' physician for answers
    D. answer the employer's questions with factual information

93. Mrs. Sands is referred to the mental health center in a state of acute agitation which she attributes to the fact that her 15-year-old daughter has run away from home and has been gone for 6 weeks. After seeing Mrs. Sands once you recommend that her family come to the next session because in crisis intervention
    A. a crisis state is self-limiting and the family needs to understand what to expect from Mrs. Sands
    B. you want to explain to the family that they should ignore the daughter's behavior
    C. massive amounts of anxiety are present and Mrs. Sands may not be hearing correctly
    D. a crisis state rarely affects only one member of the family system

94. Mrs. Jackson is brought to the psychiatric hospital in a state of acute agitation. She has been unable to do anything for the past several days except cry, pace, and wring her hands. She refuses admission to the hospital yet her family is unable to deal effectively with her. Which kind of admission would be tried first?
    A. Voluntary
    B. Formal commitment
    C. Emergency involuntary admission
    D. Foster home placement

95. Mrs. Jones calls the mental health center and hysterically tells the intake worker that her husband is manic-depressive and during his present manic episode he has been spending excessive amounts of money. She asks the nurse what she can do. The most appropriate nursing action is to
    A. recommend that she bring her husband to the center immediately for voluntary admission
    B. explain how she can begin the emergency commitment procedure if Mr. Jones refuses to accept voluntary admission
    C. refer her to a state hospital to immediately hospitalize her husband
    D. recommend that she hide all of her husband's money and credit cards

96. Mr. Simon is hospitalized for a manic episode. He becomes irate because he could not make business calls from the hospital. To decrease his anger with this limitation and protect him from business consequences, an appropriate nursing action is to
    A. deny him telephone privileges until his mania subsides
    B. ask Mrs. Simon to make the calls
    C. allow him to call in your presence after rehearsing what he will say
    D. make the calls for him and keep a log for his later review

97. You have been working with Mrs. Adams for several weeks. She is getting ready for discharge and you find that the goals you would recommend for her are not consistent with those she has chosen for herself. What action would be most appropriate?
    A. Allow Mrs. Adams to pursue her own goals, since she knows herself better than you do
    B. Establish the goals which seem most fitting and convey these to Mrs. Adams in an emphatic fashion
    C. Discuss your concern about her goals and attempt setting mutually satisfactory goals
    D. Talk with her physician about her apparent lack of readiness for discharge

B. PSYCHOPHYSIOLOGIC DISORDERS

98. The nurse recognizes that hostility is typically present in clients with psychophysiologic disorders, and that reaction formation is a characteristic manner of dealing with the hostility. She knows that in her interaction with the patient he will appear to be
    A. angry and resentful
    B. cool and aloof
    C. depressed and sad
    D. friendly and helpful

99. The plan of nursing care and nursing interventions are determined to a large extent by the theoretical model adopted by the nurse. Thus a nurse using the social model of care would assist the patient to develop goals in harmony with the premise that
    A. mental illness results from faulty social and interpersonal relationships
    B. when the person loses touch with himself and his values he becomes ill
    C. culture determines the definition, origin, and treatment of disease
    D. distorted verbal and/or nonverbal communications produce illness

100. A nurse who is helping a patient to understand the role of stress in causation of disease using Selye's model would NOT include the premise that
    A. stressors can be physical, emotional, social, and developmental
    B. living causes stress, and we can learn to minimize its adverse effects
    C. the entire body responds to stress, including individual organs and tissues
    D. only serious disease or injury causes stress

101. A nurse is preparing to teach a client about his psychophysiologic illness. She is basing the instruction on the premise that all illness results from a combination of psychologic, physiologic, and sociologic stressors. This model is known as the
    A. multicausal model
    B. specificity model
    C. nonspecific stress model
    D. individual response specificity model

102. According to the behavioral model certain maladaptive behaviors are learned and contribute toward the client's illness. Using this model, a nurse helps the client plan for discharge by
    A. assisting him to gain insight into traumatic early-life experiences
    B. designing a program for learning social skills
    C. emphasizing the importance of following the physician's orders
    D. identifying habits that need to be changed

103. Which of the following patient behaviors indicates that the nurse is effectively helping him resolve dependency needs?
    A. Attempting to get the nurse to assume a parental role
    B. Beginning to make decisions for himself
    C. Presenting many requests and questions to the nurse
    D. Exhibiting attention-seeking behavior

104. A nurse returns from a follow-up home visit to a client and charts her observations. Which of the following statements best illustrates client evaluation based on a nursing model?
   A. "There has been a significant improvement in communication between family members."
   B. "The patient has replaced several poor health habits that were contributing to her illness."
   C. "The client is carefully following the prescribed activity and medication regimen."
   D. "There has been a marked improvement in the use of adaptive behaviors to deal with stressors."

Situation (Questions 105–109): Anna Martinez, 16 years old, is admitted to the unit for the third time during a severe asthmatic attack.

105. During the initial assessment the nurse notes all of the following EXCEPT
   A. bronchial spasm
   B. difficult inspiration
   C. hyperventilation
   D. production of mucus

106. After initially assessing Anna, which intervention would the nurse institute first?
   A. Reduce the anxiety and stress
   B. Reduce the pain or discomfort
   C. Identify the type of asthma
   D. Provide for oxygen needs

107. Anna tells the nurse that she has been under the care of two different physicians before this admission. She tells the nurse that she is taking all of the medications listed below. Which medication is contraindicated for Anna at this time?
   A. Phenobarbital
   B. Epinephrine
   C. Beclomethasone
   D. Aminophylline

108. In developing a discharge plan for Anna, interventions are planned for the factors that are involved in Anna's disease. Which of the following is NOT implicated in asthma?
   A. Allergic sensitivity
   B. Genetic predisposition
   C. Dependency needs
   D. Decreased stimulation of the autonomic nervous system

109. Anna is ready for discharge. Anna knows that her prognosis depends upon her
   A. adherence to the desensitivity program
   B. response to group psychotherapy
   C. resolution of underlying emotional conflict
   D. acceptance and understanding of the disease process

Situation (Questions 110–117):   Bob Taylor is a 35-year-old insurance executive admitted with a provisional diagnosis of peptic ulcer.

110. The nurse knows that patients suffering from psycho-physiologic conditions typically
   A. are highly motivated to modify their behavior
   B. have insight into the psychologic aspect of their illness
   C. have difficulty establishing warm personal relationships
   D. respond well to long-term psychotherapy

111. Mr. Taylor wants to know why he became ill. The nurse should include information about all of the following EXCEPT
   A. genetic predisposition to gastric hypersecretion
   B. high levels of stress in life experiences
   C. strong oral-dependent needs
   D. unsatisfied independence needs

112. Mr. Taylor's physician tells him that he is a type A personality. Which of the following statements by Mr. Taylor best represents this personality type?
   A. "What I really need is a vacation."
   B. "There is never enough time to do everything."
   C. "My wife and I enjoy quiet evenings at home."
   D. "I'm not the kind of guy to take my work home."

113. In developing a nursing care plan with Mr. Taylor, the most important goal is that the patient
   A. recognizes he is under stress and needs help
   B. receive detailed instruction regarding proper dietary habits
   C. adhere strictly to the prescribed medication regimen
   D. develop a hobby that will facilitate displacement of his aggression

114. In helping Mr. Taylor set goals, which would be INAPPROPRIATE?
   A. Identifying and sharing feelings
   B. Limiting social engagements
   C. Identifying support persons
   D. Accepting that adults need friends

115. Mr. Taylor tells the nurse that he often feels frustrated. An important nursing goal is to help him recognize his basic need for
   A. independence and freedom
   B. power and authority
   C. love and attention
   D. rest and recreation

116. The best indication that Mr. Taylor's care plan is working would be his
   A. decreased feelings of restlessness
   B. idealized work ethic
   C. increased need to achieve
   D. tendency toward aggression

117. Four categories of medication are used in the treatment of peptic ulcer. Mr. Taylor is started on cimetidine (Tagamet). This medication is classified in which of the following groups?
    A. Anticholinergic
    B. Histamine antagonist
    C. Hyposecretory
    D. Mucosal barrier fortifier

Situation (Questions 118–127):   Sharon, 16, is admitted to a psychiatric unit in the hospital with a diagnosis of anorexia nervosa.

118. The history of a patient with anorexia nervosa is characterized by
    A. preoccupation with food
    B. excessive exercise routines
    C. "tomboyish" behavior
    D. ambivalence toward parents

119. Based on principles of operant conditioning, Sharon is placed on a strict regimen of supervised eating activities. Repeatedly she is found attempting to vomit after meals. Which of the following measures would be appropriate?
    A. Bed rest for 1 hour after meals
    B. Close staff supervision for a minimum of 30 minutes after meals
    C. No bathroom privileges immediately after meals
    D. Requiring that she eat again if she vomits

120. When interviewing Sharon, the nurse would most likely find that before any significant weight loss Sharon experienced
    A. listlessness
    B. diarrhea
    C. amenorrhea
    D. increased oral intake

121. On the second day of hospitalization, Sharon refuses to eat lunch stating, "How do you expect me to eat when I don't like the food?" Which is an appropriate reply by the nurse?
    A. "You haven't been eating properly lately; I'm sure your food preferences will change if you make an effort to eat all that is served to you."
    B. "Your past eating behaviors have shown that you do not use good judgment in food selection; therefore, we need to make decisions for you at this time."
    C. "I'm not sure if you really do not like the food or if this is an attempt to avoid eating."
    D. "You may have some input in selecting foods that you like and we will help you plan your meals so that you do not get fat."

122. During the third day of hospitalization, the nurse observes Sharon's parents bringing in a small bag of apples for her. In keeping with the regimen of eating activities which states no extra food other than that provided by the hospital, which action by the nurse is most appropriate?
    A. Place the apples in the refrigerator and give them to Sharon only at mealtimes
    B. Send the apples home with the parents and reinforce the instruction that no food is to be brought in by others
    C. Remove the apples and notify Sharon's physician
    D. Allow the apples to remain on this occasion, but remind her parents that they are not to bring in any other foods in the future

123. On the fourth day of hospitalization, the nurse finds Sharon arguing with other patients during breakfast and lunch. As a result, she does not finish her meals in the allotted 30 minutes. Which of the following interventions would exemplify the nurse's understanding of Sharon's behavior?
    A. Staff member will sit alone with Sharon at a separate table and encourage her to eat
    B. Sharon will eat meals alone at a time when other patients are not eating
    C. Staff member will sit alone with Sharon at a separate table and only respond to nonargumentative statements
    D. Staff member will sit with Sharon at a table and monitor her conversation with other patients

124. Sharon is on a regimen whereby she earns certain privileges by performing activities identified as conducive to her recovery. At the end of the second week, she has gained more than the required weight and is requesting that the nurse give her extra time out of her room. Which of the following actions is appropriate?
    A. Rigidly adhere to the regimen and deny the request
    B. Check to see if in some way Sharon has managed to falsely register a weight gain
    C. Discuss the request with the team as to its reasonableness and proceed accordingly
    D. Inform Sharon that she will have to wait for the doctor to make the decision

125. Which one of the following statements by Sharon would be considered as a positive move toward health?
    A. "Since I have been gaining weight while in the hospital, that must mean nothing was really wrong with me in the first place."
    B. "I forgot today was the one for me to be weighed; I guess I was just caught up in ceramics class."
    C. "Look how fat that other patient is; too bad she doesn't have control over her weight as I do."
    D. "I have decided to go to evening classes and study gourmet cooking after I am discharged."

126. The nurse has begun discussing discharge plans with Sharon. Which of the following plans suggested by Sharon indicates the greatest progress as to the understanding of her anorexic behavior?
    A. Quitting school and getting a job in a local fast-food chain to prove she can handle food
    B. Returning to school and strengthening the involvement with peers which she had developed before becoming anorexic
    C. Quitting school, moving back with her family, and getting a private tutor
    D. Returning home, attending school, and beginning a comprehensive fitness program to distract her preoccupation with food

127. During Sharon's hospitalization, she and her family have been in family therapy. The ability to successfully deal with conflict is an obvious issue with them. In one session, her parents begin to argue on a point about child-rearing practices and her father tries to draw Sharon into the conversation. Which statement by Sharon would evidence personal growth and understanding of the argumentative process between her parents?
   A. "I feel that is something you and Mom have to work out first."
   B. "I ought to have something to say since I'm the victim of your childrearing."
   C. Sharon asks the therapist, "What do you think I should do?"
   D. "I don't know why you are arguing about this anyway—you've done OK with me."

C. ANXIETY REACTIONS

128. Mr. Smith comes into the emergency room in a high level of anxiety. Which one of the following would the nurse expect to find on physical examination of Mr. Smith?
   A. Constricted pupils
   B. Hypotension
   C. Peripheral vasodilitation
   D. Dyspnea

129. David Johnson comes into the emergency room complaining of overwhelming fears that something is grossly wrong with him. He is tense and has palpitations, hypertension, and dizziness. A diagnosis of acute anxiety reaction is made and the medical doctor writes a referral for a psychiatric consult. How will the nurse best plan to assist David in this crisis state?

A. Monitor vital signs every 15 minutes to follow his physiologic response to the anxiety

B. Assist in the collection of data and specimens to invalidate a diagnosis of a physical disorder

C. Request that he focus on filling out the emergency room questionnaires to help him organize his thoughts

D. Request that he remain in an isolated cubicle until the psychiatric liaison nurse arrives

130. Mr. Jones comes into the psychiatric emergency room in a state of amnesia. No physical cause can be found. According to Freudian theory, amnesia is the result of

A. a basic conflict between the desire to express and the desire to prevent the expression of unconscious fantasies

B. culture placing too much emphasis on shame and guilt as a way of teaching individuals how to function in the society

C. an inability of an individual to change behavior at will and in accordance with societal pressures

D. the inability of the individual to meet such needs as affection, attention, approval, and recognition from others

131. Henry Johnson has a high-stress job at a stock-marketing firm. He recently has been experiencing heart palpitations and angina attacks. Which of the following behaviors would indicate that he understands the relationship of his symptoms and his life-style?
    A. Setting priority goals for his work each day and staying at work until he accomplishes them
    B. Allowing those who work for him to make more independent decisions
    C. Requesting diet counseling to reduce his intake of sugar, salt, and fats
    D. Writing a list of life-style changes that will promote healthful living

132. Mrs. James is admitted into a psychiatric unit with a chief complaint of "feeling anxious, nervous, and on edge." The nurse observes that she continually washes her hands in what appears to be a prescribed pattern. Which one of the following actions would help the nurse achieve the goal of decreasing her anxiety and helping her to adjust to the unit?
    A. Keeping her environment calm and approaching her in a quiet manner
    B. Interrupting her each time she starts the handwashing
    C. Directing her attention to more pleasurable and less purposeful activities
    D. Discussing with her the absurdity of the repetitious actions

133. Mrs. Jones, while waiting for her family to visit, begins pacing the hall, repeatedly asking the nurse what time it is, prodding her to quickly complete her assignment. The nurse begins to feel irritable and jumpy. The nurse can intervene effectively if she recognizes
    A. the patient's need for seclusion
    B. her own developing anxiety
    C. her need to leave the patient alone
    D. the patient's medication needs to be increased

134. Mrs. Rose is admitted to the hospital complaining of paralysis in both legs. No medical reason can be found for this disorder and the psychiatric liaison nurse believes that Mrs. Rose is suffering from a conversion reaction. Which one of the following would be important to consider when writing the initial plan of care for Mrs. Rose?

A. Continually repeating to Mrs. Rose that the paralysis is psychologic, not physical

B. Excluding her family because there is little connection between the paralysis and family dynamics

C. Continuously being aware that the paralysis has symbolic and unconscious meaning to Mrs. Rose

D. Remembering that Mrs. Rose is probably experiencing a lot of shame and guilt because of the paralysis

135. Mrs. Smith, a patient with a conversion reaction, has improved. Which nursing actions would be most effective in helping Mrs. Smith continue to increase her self-esteem?

A. Provide opportunities for Mrs. Smith to become a more effective parent

B. Assign Mrs. Smith as a group leader

C. Provide opportunities for Mrs. Smith to experience success in accomplishments

D. Help Mrs. Smith understand that her problems are not socially acceptable

136. Mrs. Evans was driving the car involved in an accident in which her 6-year-old daughter was killed. She cannot recall any events pertaining to the accident. Which defense mechanism is Mrs. Evans using?

A. Suppression

B. Repression

C. Reaction formation

D. Undoing

137. Mrs. Anderson has many physical complaints. Complete physical examination and laboratory studies have ruled out any organic basis for Mrs. Anderson's complaints. However, Mrs. Anderson continues to present new physical complaints to the nurse. In addition to listening matter-of-factly, which of the following nursing actions offers Mrs. Anderson the best alternative for reducing her anxiety?
    A. Showing Mrs. Anderson the laboratory reports
    B. Identifying that emotion which one senses as being expressed by Mrs. Anderson's behavior
    C. Asking her to describe her symptoms in detail
    D. Encouraging her to focus on topics outside herself

138. Mrs. Jones, a 20-year-old housewife with a fear of spiders, is to begin a program of desensitization and relaxation techniques. Which documentation by the nurse indicates that the program was successful in changing Mrs. Jones's phobic response?
    A. "Mrs. Jones attained muscle relaxation."
    B. "Mrs. Jones was exposed to situations she feared."
    C. "Mrs. Jones identified levels of anxiety she experienced."
    D. "Mrs. Jones relaxed and did not become anxious in the presence of spiders."

139. Mrs. Jacks, a 30-year-old accountant, complains of paralysis of the upper right extremity to which she appears indifferent. Neurologic examinations are negative. As she begins to improve she asks the nurse, "What if I should develop paralysis again?" At this time it is most important for Mrs. Jacks to
    A. explore what she usually does when she is anxious
    B. identify what meaning the paralysis has for her
    C. describe situations that upset her
    D. recognize when she is feeling anxious

140. A client arranges and rearranges objects on a nearby table as she describes her family to the nurse. The client states, "I know this appears foolish, but I can't seem to stop what I am doing." Which type of reaction does the client's behavior represent?
   A. Conversion reaction
   B. Hysteric reaction
   C. Obsessive-compulsive reaction
   D. Phobic reaction

141. In obsessive-compulsive behavior psychologic discomfort is reduced
   A. through repetitive stereotyped actions
   B. through contemplation
   C. by redirecting energy to the environment
   D. through physical activity

142. Which nursing action is most effective in helping a client reduce dependence on rituals for relief of anxiety?
   A. Requesting that the client change his ritualistic routine
   B. Planning activities for the client that will prevent self-preoccupation
   C. Seeking out and spending time with the patient
   D. Setting limits on the client's ritualistic behavior

143. Mrs. Jordan, a compulsive overeater, asks the nurse which therapeutic approach would help her achieve a relatively successful alteration in her eating patterns. Which approach would be recommended?
   A. Desensitization
   B. Behavior modification
   C. Psychoanalysis
   D. Gestalt therapy

144. Miss Peterson, an attractive 18-year-old college freshman, has an intense fear of becoming obese that is undiminished with a 20-lb weight loss. Her present weight is 99 lb. She tells the nurse that whenever she eats she feels guilty. She continues to lose weight on a high-caloric diet. In developing a nursing care plan for Miss Peterson, which goal is most appropriate?
   A. Establishing a therapeutic nurse-client relationship
   B. Exploring family dynamics
   C. Weighing the patient weekly
   D. Maintaining a strict behavior modification program

145. Mrs. White, a widowed mother of three children, is having difficulty falling asleep because she is anxious about her oldest son leaving to join the Air Force. Chlordiazepoxide (Librium) 50 mg, when needed, has been prescribed. In teaching Mrs. White about her condition and treatment, what is most important for her to know?
   A. The medicine takes effect immediately after ingestion
   B. The medication will not help her sleeping problem but will make her more comfortable
   C. Sedation is an expected side effect
   D. Psychotherapy is unnecessary as her symptoms will abate after her son leaves

146. The nurse will know that the client understands the use of chlordiazepoxide to handle his overwhelming anxiety when the client can
   A. repeat back the dosage and route of the medication
   B. state that alcohol potentiates the action of the drug
   C. recall the action of the medication
   D. state the reasons for which the medication should be taken

147. Mrs. Little was hospitalized for removal of a breast cyst and placed on diazepam (Valium) 5 mg three times a day. At her 8-week follow-up visit, she indicates she could never have managed without medication and wants the prescription refilled. What action would assume priority at this time?
    A. Assessing the client's means of coping when she feels uneasy
    B. Assessing the client for drug dependence
    C. Exploring the client's feelings about the operation
    D. Suggesting to the physician that the medication be reordered

D. AFFECTIVE DISORDERS/DEPRESSION

148. Mr. Smith comes to the local health clinic complaining of headaches and insomnia. His wife of 31 years died 4 months ago. Which of the following combination of symptoms would alert the nurse to the need for psychiatric evaluation and treatment of a severe depression?
    A. History of recent loss, lack of pleasure in activities
    B. Sadness, crying spells
    C. Early morning awakening, recent 20-lb weight loss
    D. Lack of concentration, pervasive feelings of fagitue

149. Mike is a 17-year-old, depressed patient admitted to the hospital after breaking up with his girl friend. Which aspects of his mental status would be most important to document?
    A. Mood and affect
    B. Psychomotor behavior
    C. Suicidal ideation
    D. Judgment and insight

150. In differentiating between anxiety and depression in a client, which observation is accurate?
    A. Discussing problems leads to improvement for the depressed but not for the anxious patient
    B. The anxious patient feels better in the evening, the depressed patient does not
    C. In contrast to the depressed patient, the anxious patient has difficulty enjoying activity
    D. The depressed patient desires sleep, but it is not satisfying, while the anxious patient generally feels better after sleep

151. Which therapeutic approach focuses upon resolving the depressed patient's painful feelings?
    A. Psychologic
    B. Biologic
    C. Behavioral
    D. Social

152. Mr. Owens, a 76-year-old retired engineer, is admitted with the diagnosis of bipolar disorder, depressed. Which of the following aspects of his nursing history would be most important to document?
    A. Previous suicide attempts
    B. Sleep pattern
    C. Weight loss or gain
    D. Level of functioning

153. A common delusion in a person with a major depressive episode is a belief that
    A. one is Jesus Christ
    B. the radio is broadcasting one's thoughts
    C. one is being persecuted because of his worthlessness
    D. voices are controlling one's thoughts and actions

154. Mrs. Allen is hospitalized for psychotic depression following her son's death from leukemia 2 months ago, after which she was forced to sell her house. She cries frequently and tends to arouse sympathy in others. To meet your nursing goal of providing empathy, you would first
   A. recognize your own need and wish to nurture Mrs. Allen
   B. frequently reassure her that she will survive this crisis period
   C. communicate your acceptance of her need to cry
   D. establish a regular daily meeting time to help Mrs. Allen ventilate her hurt feelings

Situation (Questions 155–158): Helen is a 15-year-old high-school student with numerous somatic complaints including migraine headaches, dysmenorrhea, and undiagnosed intermittent abdominal pain. A diagnosis of psychopathologic depression is made.

155. Biochemical changes are thought to be the basis for Helen's depression. Research indicates a probable biochemical cause of depression is
   A. increased catecholamines
   B. decreased calcium
   C. decreased testosterone
   D. reduced norepinephrine

156. In obtaining Helen's health history, which response would be most indicative of depression?
   A. "I don't know why I feel so bad all the time."
   B. "I make A's and B's in all my classes."
   C. "I am active in two clubs and have several girl friends and a 'steady.'"
   D. "God is punishing me for not making all A's."

157. Since Helen's stay in the hospital will be limited, the plan for care should include all of the following EXCEPT
    A. teaching the client practices that will increase her independence and self-care
    B. planning a 10-session nurse-patient therapy program
    C. encouraging increased socialization with an expanded social group
    D. helping set realistic goals, focused on positive activities

158. Chlordiazepoxide (Librium) 10 mg three times a day is prescribed for Helen. Which response indicates she is experiencing the desired effect in the early stage of treatment?
    A. Relaxation and drowsiness
    B. Urticaria and rash
    C. Vertigo and syncope
    D. Menstrual irregularities

159. Mrs. Merry, aged 57, is placed on chlorpromazine (Thorazine) 400 mg/day to control her agitation resulting from an involutional psychotic depression. Her plan of care should include
    A. placing the patient in seclusion until her agitation subsides
    B. monitoring blood pressure
    C. observing for physiologic dependence
    D. forcing fluids with each dose

160. Mr. Jones is admitted to the hospital with a diagnosis of psychotic depression. Because of his concurrent hypertension, the medication recommended to treat his depression is
    A. chlordiazepoxide hydrochloride
    B. imipramine hydrochloride
    C. phenelzine sulfate
    D. chlorpromazine

161. Mr. Adams is a 53-year-old business executive recently admitted to the hospital with a diagnosis of depression. You have identified the goal of raising Mr. Adams' self-esteem as assuming priority. Which plan of care would be most appropriate in meeting this goal?
   A. Teach Mr. Adams and his family what is known regarding depressive illness
   B. Contract with Mr. Adams to participate in milieu activities
   C. Help Mr. Adams accept his illness and need for hospitalization
   D. Set simple, realistic goals with Mr. Adams to help him experience success

Situation (Questions 162–167): Joan, a 45-year-old female, is admitted to the unit for depression. She states her depression began 2 years ago, when she stood on the shore and watched while her husband and two sons overturned their fishing boat and drowned. Since that time, she has been unable to "keep her house, take care of her affairs, or mix with people."

162. What information determines that Joan is experiencing depression rather than grief?
   A. Her feeling of true loss
   B. Her feeling of helplessness
   C. Her inability to function
   D. The duration of time

163. As Joan relates her nursing history, which of the following was most therapeutic in helping her with the work of grieving following the drowning?
   A. She was told she must be strong now, since she had many things to do
   B. "My husband and sons begged me to go fishing with them but I didn't want to."
   C. "I didn't do anything but stand on the shore, pointing and weeping."
   D. She can barely remember the funeral, although the doctor refused to medicate her

164. Joan is crying as she emerges from her room. Which response is most therapeutic?
   A. "What are you crying about now?"
   B. "Cheer up, Joan, you have a lot to live for."
   C. "Let's go over there and I'll stay with you."
   D. "Let's play Ping-Pong with the others and you'll feel better."

165. Joan is receiving electroconvulsive therapy (ECT) twice weekly. Following ECT, the nurse would NOT expect Joan to exhibit
   A. hypotension
   B. amnesia
   C. agitation
   D. immediate recall

166. Tranylcypromine (Parnate) 10 mg b.i.d. is prescribed for Joan. The patient should be taught
   A. that if she does not have problems with food in 2 weeks, she can eat anything
   B. to arise from the supine position gradually
   C. that taking hot showers and baths helps people relax
   D. to begin a vigorous activity program

167. Foods that may cause a serious adverse reaction with MAO inhibitors include
   A. green leafy vegetables
   B. candy and sweets
   C. wine and cheese
   D. tomatoes and fruit

Situation (Questions 168–174): Carol is a 52-year-old house-wife whose last child graduated from high school 6 months ago and moved 150 miles away. Carol comes to the mental health center because of frequent episodes of crying. She states she "has no purpose now" and "does not know what to do."

168. Factors to assess in Carol's nursing history would NOT include
    A. role perceived by client
    B. support by significant others
    C. outside interests
    D. perception of loss of youth

169. Carol is in a crisis state. As the nurse prepares to interview Carol, she would incorporate all of the following concepts EXCEPT
    A. people are capable of growth and self-control
    B. rigid external controls
    C. focusing on feelings and problem-solving
    D. work can be therapeutic

170. During crisis intervention Carol tells the nurse, "I don't know if my doctor is treating me right. I've used him for years, but he isn't helping me now." Which response is most consistent with the problem-solving model of crisis intervention?
    A. "Let's consider some things you might do about this."
    B. "Why don't you change doctors?"
    C. "Don't worry about it, he's a good man."
    D. "Did you tell your husband?"

171. Suicide is a major risk in all clients experiencing depression. A cardinal signal for potential suicide is
    A. a sudden change in mood to "better" spirits
    B. acceptance of small meals only
    C. refusal to bathe or change clothes
    D. inability to make a decision

172. Carol is in a high state of anxiety as well as being depressed. Her physician orders doxepin (Sinequan) 10 mg t.i.d. Within the first 5 days of medication therapy, the only response which is NOT expected is
    A. reduction in anxiety
    B. frequent napping
    C. reduction in depression
    D. marked sedation

173. While Carol is taking Sinequan she should be taught all of the following EXCEPT
    A. encouraging outside activities in the summer
    B. continuing the crisis intervention, problem-solving, and support
    C. encouraging physical and mental activity on a regular basis
    D. cautioning against driving her car

174. Carol has been working with the nurse for a week and is now working part-time, going to school, and making plans to travel. She and her husband do not share many common interests. What element is Carol using in overcoming her depression?
    A. Timing
    B. Accumulated wisdom
    C. Capacity for living
    D. Strong support systems

175. John Hirsch is admitted to a psychiatric unit because he is depressed and has made suicidal gestures. After several weeks of reality therapy, he continues to speak of suicide and remains aloof and dejected. Together with him, your evaluation of the situation is that John
    A. has not yet resolved problems repressed in his early development
    B. is overly dependent on others for his immediate needs
    C. is still working to fail and thus is reinforcing his failure identity
    D. is substituting defense responses for his anxieties

176. Mr. A. is receiving amitriptyline (Elavil) to treat his depression. He has been complaining of constipation. Your assessment is that Mr. A's constipation is
   A. to be expected with depression
   B. probably due to a change of diet while in the hospital
   C. an anticholinergic effect of Elavil
   D. to be expected with any antidepressant

177. Alice is a 54-year-old patient who has been hospitalized for 3 days. She refuses to eat and to leave her room. Which of the following approaches is most appropriate at this time?
   A. Forcibly take her to the dining room
   B. Feed the patient small portions of food
   C. Encourage her to ventilate her anger at being hospitalized
   D. Inform her that she will be tube fed if she does not eat

178. Angela, 47, is in her third psychiatric hospitalization for agitated depression. She cries frequently and appears apologetic and hopeless. When making rounds, the nurse finds that Angela has made superficial scratches in her wrist with a plastic knife. Which initial response is most therapeutic?
   A. "Cutting yourself is not allowed here."
   B. "Here, let me help you clean and dress your cuts."
   C. "You really must be hurting inside."
   D. "Don't worry, I won't let you hurt yourself."

179. Don is a depressed patient who has been complaining about his doctor, the food, his treatment, etc. As the day passes, he becomes increasingly resistant, refusing all milieu activities and groups. As you enter his room, Don angrily throws his book to the floor saying, "I don't want to talk today. Can't you understand that?" How might you, as Don's nurse, most therapeutically respond to his anger?
   A. "I haven't done anything to deserve this outburst."
   B. "You seem angry. How about a game of Ping-Pong?"
   C. "I set aside this time to be with you, so I'd like to stay even if you don't feel like talking."
   D. "I guess you don't feel like talking right now. I'll return in half an hour to see how you are."

180. Mrs. T. is a 63-year-old woman who is being treated in the hospital with electroconvulsive therapy (ECT) for her depression. She has had five treatments. You observe her going in and out of other patients' rooms and wandering in the corridor with a confused expression. She is unable to remember her own name or that she is in the hospital. Your evaluation of the situation would be that Mrs. T.
   A. is confused due to her treatment and is unable to locate her own room
   B. may have some brain damage and her doctor should be notified
   C. is agitated and arousing the fear of other patients
   D. is probably frightened and is seeking reassurance from other patients

181. Mrs. S. was withdrawn and seclusive when admitted 1 week ago. Which of the following behaviors best indicates that the nursing goal of establishing trust is being met?
   A. Increased eye contact during interactions
   B. Mrs. S. takes her medications readily
   C. Improvement in Mrs. S.'s appetite and intake
   D. Mrs. S. is coming to the dining room for meals

182. Andrew has been hospitalized for 2 weeks and is being treated with phenelzine sulfate (Nardil) for his depression. After breakfast he complains of a headache and goes to his room. Upon checking him a half hour later, you find Andrew diaphoretic, pale, with muscles twitching. Which nursing action is most appropriate?
   A. Check his blood pressure
   B. Alert his physician as this may be a medical emergency
   C. Ask what he ate for breakfast
   D. Check his respiration

183. Theresa has been hospitalized for 2 weeks for depression following the birth of her first child. She lacks confidence and has expressed a fear of being alone with her baby. The most important first step in discharge planning would be to
   A. meet with Theresa and her husband to facilitate sharing her fears
   B. set up regular follow-up visits at the mental health clinic
   C. refer Theresa to a public health nurse for home visits
   D. arrange for a supervised visit with Theresa and her baby

184. Norman, who is scheduled for discharge in 2 days, is still denying his depression. His doctor has ordered a daily maintenance dose of nortriptyline (Aventyl). How would the nurse best facilitate medication compliance postdischarge?
   A. Teach Norman's family about his illness and need for medication
   B. Teach Norman how the medication works
   C. Give Norman positive reinforcement for taking his medication
   D. Anticipate the side effects and instruct Norman not to discontinue his Aventyl without conferring with his therapist

185. Wilma is leaving the hospital after 6 weeks of treatment for her depression. She is a passive woman who has been very dependent upon her nurse. She expresses relief and happiness about being well enough to go home and denies having any negative feelings about leaving. How might her nurse best deal with Wilma's denial?
   A. Recognize her denial is a way of coping with the anxiety of leaving
   B. Confront her refusal to deal with her negative feelings
   C. Explain that she needs to experience her negative as well as positive feelings
   D. Share your feelings with her and invite her to explore issues of leaving

186. Mrs. Kelly, 57, was recently discharged from the psychiatric unit of a hospital in which she was treated for depression. In a follow-up visit to her home, you observe poor plumbing and cracked ceilings, no food in the refrigerator, ragged clothing, decrepit furniture, and poor ventilation and heating. In Maslow's terms, Mrs. Kelly's depression is
   A. motivated by higher-order growth needs
   B. fostered by the unrealistic and unattainable goals that she sets for herself
   C. reinforced by the unaesthetic quality of her environment
   D. motivated by deficiencies in the satisfaction of basic needs

187. Mrs. O. is admitted to the hospital for depression. She has been living alone following the death of her husband 6 months ago. One identified nursing diagnosis reads, "social isolation related to withdrawal from community activities due to grief." An appropriate short-term goal in Mrs. O.'s nursing care plan is that she will
    A. join a community group of her choice
    B. join a group activity on her psychiatric unit
    C. establish a relationship of trust with her nurse
    D. attend a group activity with her nurse after 1 week of contact with her nurse

188. Jimmy Smith, aged 15, is diagnosed with a chronic illness which necessitates a radical change in his diet. The nurse finds a letter he has written to a friend requesting the friend to bring foods into the hospital that are not allowed on his diet. The best interpretation of his behavior is that is is
    A. testing the nurse-client relationship
    B. acting out his anger about the restrictions
    C. denying the seriousness of the dietary restrictions
    D. testing his friend's commitment to their friendship

189. While Helen Jones is in the hospital for diagnostic tests, she is informed that her husband was killed in a plane crash while on a business trip. She is in a state of emotional shock and is staring off into space with very little verbal contact. The nurse best facilitates Helen's coping with this crisis by
    A. allowing her to be alone
    B. asking the physician to order a minor tranquilizer for her
    C. involving her in a conversation about a more cheerful part of her life
    D. calling in a family member

190. Mrs. Conrad has been told that her child has a terminal illness and chances for living another 6 months are unlikely. Which one of the following behaviors would the nurse expect her to exhibit initially?
  A. A vacillation between feelings; e.g., quiet, remorse, or fear
  B. A stunned numbness and inability to comprehend the situation
  C. A sense of helplessness, hopelessness, and anxiety
  D. An ability to begin to comprehend the seriousness of the situation

191. Susan, a 15-year-old, has recently been told that her mother has a terminal illness. The nurse can best help Susan understand and cope with this crisis by sharing with her that
  A. the family should take over all of the mother's responsibilities at home so that she may enjoy her final days
  B. anger expressed toward her mother at this time may be detrimental to their relationship
  C. feelings such as tightness in the throat area and loss of appetite are common for those in this situation
  D. organized and logical thinking and performance of duties both at home and at school are very important for Susan

192. Although Nancy Smith has accepted the reality of her impending (and fast–approaching) death, her husband still discusses future plans for the family as if she were going to be able to participate. How can the nurse best help Nancy plan to discuss this issue with her husband?
  A. Advise Nancy not to discuss her approaching death directly but rather use indirect comments
  B. Offer to talk with the husband privately and reinforce his wife's terminal diagnosis
  C. Explore with Nancy what she thinks will be her husband's reaction when she brings up the topic
  D. Tell Nancy that it is too stressful for her husband to handle and not to say anything

193. Mr. Grassen, a client who has lost most of his strength and is close to death, says to the nurse: "I know that I won't be around long but I'm praying that I'll last long enough to see my grandson's first piano recital." The most appropriate nursing action is to
    A. reassure Mr. Grassen that his grandson would surely understand if he was not able to attend the recital
    B. recognize that Mr. Grassen may feel guilty about not performing his expected duties
    C. inform the family that Mr. Grassen may be approaching a period of remission
    D. recognize that Mr. Grassen is in a state of partial denial of his illness

194. It is 2 years after the death of Mrs. Perry's mother and she is in the clinic for a routine examination. The nurse remembers that Mrs. Perry had a very difficult time adapting to her mother's death and decides to evaluate this as part of the interview. Which one of the following comments by Mrs. Smith would indicate that she has not successfully completed the grieving process?
    A. "On her birthday and on Thanksgiving, her favorite holiday, I still feel a lump in my throat and tears come into my eyes."
    B. "I have decided to actively work for my mother's favorite civic organization as a way to continue her work."
    C. "You know, sometimes I get so angry at her for leaving me that I can hardly keep myself from smashing her picture."
    D. "I recognize that Mom is not going to be around any more, but I still have a hard time because I want to share special moments with her."

195. Mr. Johns lost his wife Deanna 6 months ago in a skiing accident while on vacation. He is now having difficulty falling asleep which interferes with his ability to work effectively. After thorough evaluation a barbiturate is ordered for Mr. Johns. Which of the following is NOT important to include in the nurse's teaching plan for Mr. Johns?

A. Alcohol use potentiates the effect of the medication
B. Listlessness and depression often are reactions to the medication
C. Over-the-counter antihistamines should not be used
D. The medication should be taken 1 hour before the planned hour of retiring

196. According to Durkheim's sociologic theory of suicidal behavior, an individual who uses this extreme coping mechanism

A. expects society will mourn his death as a hero for behaving individualistically
B. feels powerless in a society whose norms are in a state of instability
C. feels compelled to turn his wish to destroy others in society against himself
D. wishes to experience a symbolic reunion with past heroes of society

197. According to psychodynamic theory, the unconscious conflict between self-preserving and self-destructive forces is exemplified in which of the following characteristics?

A. Blocking
B. Ambivalence
C. Isolation
D. Reaction formation

198. Which of the following profiles best describes an individual at highest risk for a successful suicide attempt?
    A. Single, elderly, Caucasian male alcoholic
    B. Caucasian female adolescent, aged 18
    C. Married Caucasian female, aged 45
    D. Black male, aged 11

199. Assessment of a suicidal client would include gathering data about
    A. violent physical outbursts
    B. symptoms of depression
    C. rigidity of boundaries
    D. sexual adjustment

200. In analyzing the data about a suicidal client, which would be associated with the greatest risk?
    A. Client's frequent comments about helplessness
    B. Unsettled family system
    C. Absence of a steady income
    D. Client's heavy alcohol intake while alone

201. Adolescents aged 15–19 are at high risk for suicidal behavior because they
    A. experience withdrawal of emotional support from their families
    B. feel anxious regarding their set expectations for achievement
    C. experience pressure from their family and society to become independent
    D. experience increased capacity for concrete thought

202. Judy, aged 16, responds to being "grounded" at home for curfew violation by threatening to overdose on a handful of aspirin while saying, "You don't understand." This behavior most likely represents a motivation to
    A. direct hostility inward
    B. live out a fantasy of reunion
    C. attain power within the family structure
    D. atone for breaking parental rules

203. In assessing a potentially suicidal client in an outpatient clinic, which of the following aspects would take priority?
    A. Age of client
    B. Presence of physical illness
    C. Degree of isolation
    D. Specificity of suicide plan

204. A delirious client may be at high risk for suicide if he is
    A. diagnosed as having a terminal illness
    B. experiencing a paradoxical drug reaction
    C. experiencing delusions of persecution
    D. a chronic alcoholic

205. You are setting up a verbal no-suicide contract with Sally, a suicidal adolescent. The primary goal of the contract is to
    A. assist the client with self-control of suicidal impulses
    B. facilitate an empathetic and genuine therapeutic relationship
    C. teach assertive verbal communication skills
    D. eliminate the need for suicidal precautions

206. A community health nurse assesses one of her depressed clients as being at high risk for suicidal behavior. Her most important initial intervention will be to
    A. maintain contact with the client until psychiatric care can be arranged
    B. refer her immediately to the crisis hot-line telephone service
    C. obtain a physician's order for an antidepressant medication
    D. arrange for immediate continuous supervision of the client by a supportive individual

207. Mr. Samuels is a 62-year-old man who lives alone and has been hospitalized three times in the past 2 years because of suicide attempts. He has been identified as chronically suicidal. Mr. Samuels would benefit most from
     A. prolonged psychiatric hospitalization
     B. being allowed to resolve his life in his own way
     C. a continuing relationship with a supportive treatment program
     D. increased antidepressant medication

208. Tom, 22, is admitted to the psychiatric unit with the diagnosis of paranoid schizophrenic disorder. He is experiencing auditory hallucinations in the form of voices telling him he is a child molester and that the only way he can escape punishment is to kill himself. Of primary importance initially is to
     A. request an order for antipsychotic medication
     B. assess for suicidal risk
     C. place him on escape precautions
     D. perform a detailed mental status examination

209. Mrs. Fenton is admitted to the psychiatric unit because of her suicidal threat. Which of the following goals would be most appropriate in the nursing care plan for the first 72 hours following admission?
     A. Medicate adequately to prevent anxiety
     B. Isolate client for close observation
     C. Provide safe environment
     D. Encourage open expression of anger

210. Mrs. Jones, aged 35, has a long history of alcoholism and drug abuse. She is brought unconscious to the emergency room after a drug overdosage precipitated by her husband's announced plans to divorce her. He shows you a note Mrs. Jones wrote which said, "Dear God, please forgive me for what I plan to do tonight. I can't go on any longer. My husband never understood me, maybe now he will." While Mrs. Jones is still unconscious, what is the most effective response the nurse can make to Mr. Jones?

   A. "I know this must be a very difficult time for you. How can I help you right now?"

   B. "Your wife's condition is very serious. Did you have any clues she might overdose before you told her you wanted a divorce?"

   C. "We have a lot of other very sick people here tonight but we'll do our best to take care of your wife."

   D. "You must feel very upset over your wife's behavior. Would you like to go for a cup of coffee?"

211. Mr. White, 75, is admitted to the psychiatric unit for severe depression. He states, "I'm so lonely since my wife died last week. We had been married 50 years. I sometimes think I'll end it all." The most effective nursing response is which of the following?

   A. "I'm concerned about your mentioning taking your own life. How would you do it?"

   B. "I hear how deeply you are affected by the loss of your wife, but we will not allow you to hurt yourself."

   C. "Your grief is very normal, Mr. White."

   D. "We can help you with your loneliness, and then these sad feelings you have won't bother you so much."

212. Mrs. Williams, 42, is being treated on an acute psychiatric unit for a major depressive disorder with suicidal ideation. She is started on amitriptyline (Elavil) today. Which approach is most important to include in her initial nursing care plan?
    A. Continue daily assessment for suicidal ideation or behavior
    B. Limit milieu group activities to maximize effects of amitriptyline
    C. Closely monitor sleep and nutritional patterns
    D. Teach the client/family about the therapeutic effect of amitriptyline

213. Mrs. Kramer is admitted to the psychiatric unit with severe depression. In talking with the nurse, she says that she has a large bottle of sedatives at home that she plans to take at the first chance. The nurse's analysis of Mrs. Kramer's suicidal risk is that
    A. it is high
    B. it is low
    C. there is no risk at all
    D. there is no need to worry while she is in the hospital

214. Mrs. Jones, 36, is experiencing a situationally induced depression with suicidal ideation. She has a high level of anxiety and is having great difficulty falling asleep at night, causing fatigue. Diazepam (Valium) has been prescribed. What does Mrs. Jones need to know about this medication?
    A. There is no potential for physical and psychologic dependence to develop
    B. Its sedative effect will promote sleep
    C. An occasional alcoholic drink at bedtime will facilitate sleep
    D. Her level of energy will be increased

215. Mrs. Monroe has been hospitalized for the past 2 weeks for treatment of suicidal ideations. In helping her regain her self-esteem, it is most important for the nurse to
    A. keep her on suicidal precautions indefinitely
    B. encourage open expression of feelings
    C. reinforce efforts at problem-solving
    D. call her by name

216. Mrs. Morgan, who has been hospitalized for several days, was immobilized by her severe depression. She has dramatically improved today and seems to have newly found energy to participate in activities on the unit. Your evaluation of this change in Mrs. Morgan is that
    A. her suicide risk is greater now
    B. she is finally responding to the medication
    C. she is improving due to effective nursing care
    D. she was merely seeking attention

217. Sally, aged 18, was hospitalized for treatment of impulsive behavior. She attempted suicide by slashing her wrists. After a therapeutic program she is ready for discharge. The nurse asks her what she will do first if she feels herself becoming suicidal before her scheduled follow-up appointment. Which client response best indicates readiness for discharge?
    A. "I'll ignore the feeling, it may be temporary."
    B. "I'll call my therapist or lifeline at once."
    C. "I'll avoid focusing on my feelings, it may reinforce them."
    D. "I'll call one of my friends to distract my morbid thoughts."

218. Which of the following approaches would be most appropriate in the nursing care plan of a suicidal client who is preparing to return home?
    A. Reestablish supportive social network
    B. Determine knowledge of lethal doses of medication
    C. Encourage client to sleep when anxious
    D. Tell client how to structure his day

219. Mr. Thomas, 45, is responding favorably to antidepressant medication and will be discharged tomorrow. You have been counseling Mrs. Thomas about the risk of suicide while Mr. Thomas continues on his antidepressant medication. Which response by his wife indicates your teaching has been effective?
   A. "I feel so relieved these pills have begun to relieve his depression. I can finally relax."
   B. "I know I still need to watch for signs of suicide because as he begins to feel stronger he might carry out his plans."
   C. "I understand the pills will stimulate his mood so he will no longer have thoughts of killing himself."
   D. "I expect he will not fully recover from his depression for a few more weeks and might try to take his own life within the next 6 months."

220. An appropriate intervention with the survivors in a family where someone has committed suicide is to
   A. encourage the family to stop thinking about the suicide
   B. help them to mourn the loss
   C. encourage acceptance of sleeping medication
   D. promote open expression of blame

221. Psychodynamic theory views manic persons as having a strong id. With this knowledge, nursing intervention would focus on assisting the client in regulating
   A. guilt
   B. impulsivity
   C. suicidal thoughts
   D. decreased confidence

222. On admission, the nurse asks a manic client what factors contributed to his hospitalization. This information could be correlated with factors related to
   A. flight-of-ideas
   B. delusions of grandeur
   C. depression
   D. inflated self-esteem

223. In an initial assessment of a manic client, it would be most important for the nurse to document his
    A. interpersonal style
    B. nutrition status
    C. physical activity level
    D. sleep pattern

224. The nurse is collecting data on the sex of those clients admitted to the psychiatric unit with manic-depressive illness. If these data are congruent with reported norms, you would expect the sex occurrence ratio to appear
    A. twice as frequently in males as in females
    B. twice as frequently in females as in males
    C. equally common in males and females
    D. in no particular pattern

225. Manic episodes usually occur in persons between the ages of
    A. 15 and 45
    B. 20 and 35
    C. 35 and 50
    D. 45 and 60

226. In assisting a manic client to plan his daily menu, the most appropriate food choices are
    A. steak, baked potato, tossed salad
    B. pork chop, greenbeans, creamed corn
    C. hot dog, potato chips, "coke"
    D. chicken salad sandwich, apple, milkshake

227. Susan, a 20-year-old college student, is in a euphoric state. She has not slept for the past 3 nights, exhibits pressure of speech, is dancing and singing, and flits about from one activity to another. In this acute phase, which goal assumes priority?
    A. Increasing group activity
    B. Increasing self-control
    C. Preventing exhaustion
    D. Counteracting denial

228. Brenda, 30, is in an acute phase of mania. This is her first night on the psychiatric unit and she is unable to sleep. She is constantly rearranging her belongings and disturbing her roommate. Which nursing intervention is appropriate in regulating Brenda's hyperactivity?
   A. Placing her in a seclusion room
   B. Helping her take her belongings to the day room
   C. Staying physically close to her
   D. Telling her she must slow down

229. Mr. Rice is an attractive middle-aged man in an elated state. The day after admission he is talking with his nurse, an attractive woman and says, "You are the first person who has understood me. I think you will really be able to help me." Mr. Rice's statement is designed to
   A. manipulate the nurse's self-esteem
   B. give appropriate and sincere flattery
   C. establish a meaningful relationship
   D. show his willingness to engage in introspection

230. In caring for Sandy, a mildly manic client, who is denying that she has any problems, it would be most important to
   A. establish a therapeutic relationship
   B. ignore her denial
   C. confront the denial
   D. let her initiate that she is denying

231. Julie, who is in an overactive state, needs to channel her excess energy in constructive activities. Which activity would be most therapeutic in the acute phase of mania?
   A. Writing
   B. Volleyball
   C. Knitting
   D. Exercising

232. When an agitated, manic client is becoming destructive on the unit, the nurse can gain his cooperation by
    A. distracting him from the situation
    B. changing him to a semiprivate room
    C. speaking in a loud tone of voice)
    D. gathering a group of friends around him

233. Peter says to his nurse, "I am God. I have powers that can help anyone. If you need any help just come to me." Which is the most appropriate response by the nurse?
    A. "How can you be God?"
    B. "What kind of powers do you have that will help others?"
    C. "You can't be God because you are in a physical body."
    D. "It sounds like it's important to you to feel powerful."

234. Jerry, a 20-year-old manic client, displays an angry outburst when the nurse enters his room. Jerry yells out, "Get out of my room and leave me alone!" The nurse leaves the room and 15 minutes later approaches Jerry. He apologizes to the nurse for his outburst. Which would be the best response by the nurse?
    A. "If you continue to yell at me, Jerry, I won't visit with you as often."
    B. "Jerry, you were acting like a child. Let's have no more of these angry outbursts."
    C. "I have other clients to care for and I cannot spend all of my time with you."
    D. "I don't like to be yelled at, but I will try to understand what you are experiencing now."

Situation (Questions 235–238): Mr. Smith is admitted to the hospital by his family. His diagnosis is manic-depressive illness, manic episode.

235. In assessing Mr. Smith, you would NOT expect to find
  A. constant movement
  B. slow, slurred speech
  C. flight-of-ideas and speech patterns
  D. 1–2 hours of sleep per night

236. Mr. Smith is placed on lithium 600 mg three times a day. His plan of care would initially include all of the following EXCEPT
  A. orders for lithium blood samples q.i.d.
  B. restriction of antacids, coffee
  C. maintaining lithium blood levels of 2.4 mEq/L
  D. avoiding thirst, fatigue, and mild muscle weakness

237. Lithium blood levels should not exceed
  A. 1.0 mEq/L
  B. 1.2 mEq/L
  C. 1.5 mEq/L
  D. 2.0 mEq/L

238. Since lithium is a lifelong regimen for the manic client, it is important for Mr. Smith to recognize its toxic symptoms, including all of the following EXCEPT
  A. nausea, vomiting, and diarrhea
  B. muscle twitching
  C. tinnitus
  D. wide mood swings

239. Roger, a 37-year-old manic client, has been receiving lithium carbonate 1500 mg/day for the past several days. He reports to the nurse that he is not feeling well. You notice he is lethargic and he complains of diarrhea. Your evaluation of the situation would be that
    A. these symptoms are not related to lithium
    B. he should be watched for signs of seizures and electrolyte imbalance
    C. his lithium dosage probably needs adjustment
    D. this response is to be expected

240. Tom is started on chlorpromazine (Thorazine) in conjunction with lithium to control his violent, agitated behavior. The nurse is teaching him the possible side effects of the medications he is taking. It is important for the client to know that the interaction of Thorazine and lithium produces
    A. no untoward side effects
    B. nausea
    C. akathisia
    D. hypertensive crisis

241. The most likely single factor that will prevent rehospitalization of Harvey, a manic client, is
    A. continuing lithium therapy
    B. emotional stressors
    C. change in life-style
    D. loss of support system

242. Joan, a 30-year-old manic client, is being discharged to return home with her husband. Joan is beginning to recognize that which family dynamics may contribute to her illness?
    A. Displaying decreasing tolerance of her manic behavior
    B. Rehospitalizing her at the onset of symptoms
    C. Not setting limits on her "crazy" behaviors
    D. Acknowledging the presence of her manic behavior

243. Steven is being discharged from the hospital after experiencing an acute manic episode. Which of the following nursing measures would be most helpful in developing compliance with continuing Steven's lithium therapy at home?
    A. Advise his wife to supervise his taking lithium as prescribed
    B. Teach him about the intended effect and side effects of lithium
    C. Tell him to call you at the hospital if he has questions about the lithium
    D. Give him a booklet describing the side effects and precautions for lithium

E. SCHIZOPHRENIC DISORDERS

244. Genetic studies have attempted to clarify the role of heredity in the development of schizophrenia. Which of the following statements about this relationship is true?
    A. Genetic factors have been explored primarily through animal and biochemical studies
    B. Genetic research indicates that heredity plays some role in developing schizophrenia
    C. Current research has identified genes that are involved in the transmission of schizophrenia
    D. Twin studies consistently indicate the occurrence of similar schizophrenic traits in twins

245. Bleuler's classic "four A's" denoting fundamental symptoms of schizophrenia are
    A. Asymmetric communication, associate looseness, affective flatness, and autism
    B. Associative looseness, affective flatness, autism, and automatic thinking
    C. Associative disturbance, affective impairment, autism, and ambivalence
    D. Associative disturbance, affective impairment, automatic thinking, and autism

246. The double-bind is a communication process which is best described as
    A. A clear, contained message from sender to receiver
    B. An unclear, contradictory message from sender to receiver, causing the receiver to feel conflict regarding the real meaning of the message
    C. A dysfunctional form of communication between mother and child
    D. A functional form of communication within the family network

247. The tendency to withdraw from involvement with reality and become preoccupied with illogical, egocentric ideas, fantasies, and distortions is called
    A. autism
    B. ambivalence
    C. inappropriate affect
    D. blocking

248. The schizophrenic individual is a social isolate but is also very dependent. This dependency occurs because the indiviudal
    A. likes people but is afraid to show any emotion
    B. has so controlled his id impulses that independence cannot develop
    C. has too much superego and feels inferior to others
    D. never differentiated from the family ego mass

249. The paranoid schizophrenic exhibits which of the following symptoms?
    A. Grandiose or persecutory delusions, hallucinations, and jealousy
    B. Psychomotor disturbance with stupor, mutism, and waxy flexibility
    C. Disorganized thinking, regressive behavior, and silly affect
    D. Apathy, indifference, and mental deterioration

250. Which of the following statements can be considered an example of a delusion of persecution?
   A. "I am a millionaire; my name is Howard Hughes."
   B. "I feel as though my heart is rotting away."
   C. "The FBI and police are out to get me."
   D. "The song on the radio is telling me what to do."

251. During your interactions with a schizophrenic individual you conclude that he has a flat affect. Which of the following behaviors is indicative of this affective disturbance?
   A. Describing an incident with no emotion
   B. Expressing an affect opposite from the one felt
   C. Displaying actions different from the thoughts expressed
   D. Presenting conflicting expressions as a result of conflicting feelings

252. Patty, an inpatient with undifferentiated schizophrenia, approaches the nurse and says, "Only carnerfwoks live here." Patty's response is an example of
   A. an hallucination
   B. an illusion
   C. a neologism
   D. a delusion

253. Tamara, a newly diagnosed schizophrenic patient, uses projection in an attempt to
   A. punish those she feels to be responsible for her hospitalization
   B. gain attention from those around her
   C. increase her level of stimulation
   D. protect herself from unacceptable impulses

254. In developing a care plan for a schizophrenic patient for whom the nurse is beginning a therapeutic relationship, initial goals should include
    A. developing techniques to respond to the patient's verbalizations
    B. collaboration between nurse and patient to identify behavioral problems
    C. providing new opportunities for the patient to try new coping behaviors
    D. formation of a working relationship with the client

255. Initiating a one-to-one nurse-patient relationship with a schizophrenic patient is most important because this patient needs one nurse
    A. to whom he can relate
    B. with whom he can identify
    C. in whom he can place trust
    D. to whom he can express emotion

256. A newly admitted patient with a medical diagnosis of catatonic schizophrenia has a disheveled appearance and displays behaviors of isolation and apathy. In addition the patient does not speak or make eye contact. On the basis of this information an appropriate nursing diagnosis would be
    A. dependence
    B. withdrawal
    C. delusional thinking
    D. regression

257. It is difficult to set mutual goals with schizophrenic patients because
    A. behavioral changes are short-lived
    B. cognitive impairments prevent patients understanding
    C. their behaviors are unpredictable
    D. their behaviors are serving as coping mechanisms

258. The schizophrenic experiences exaggerated ambivalence of an unreal nature. Nursing interventions to regulate ambivalence should focus on assisting the patient to
    A. make decisions
    B. become independent
    C. participate in activities
    D. express emotions

259. Some schizophrenic patients demonstrate regressed behaviors. An INAPPROPRIATE goal for such a patient is that he will
    A. achieve the appropriate level of functioning
    B. develop dependency upon the nurse
    C. show no further deterioration
    D. maintain his current level of functioning

260. When Mary Jane's feelings about her father were mentioned, Mary Jane, a schizophrenic adolescent, resorted to the delusional statement, "I am Cleopatra, and I command the world with my body." When such delusional thoughts are expressed the nurse should
    A. provide a rational explanation of the delusional content to the patient
    B. challenge the validity of the delusion
    C. refuse to continue the interaction
    D. respond to the theme of the delusion

Situation (Questions 261–268): Bob G., aged 39, is brought to the psychiatric intensive care unit in an agitated state by his mother. He quickly paces the emergency room, muttering to himself and laughing for no apparent reason. He is admitted to the inpatient unit and is negativistic, labile, and highly anxious. His thoughts are characterized by looseness of associations and suspiciousness, and his speech is sprinkled with neologisms. He refuses to follow the hospital's schedule. He does not wish to shower, shave, comb his hair, or change his clothes. He alternates between agitatedly pacing the hall and huddling in the corner next to his bed. He ignores the requests of others and does not participate in activities. He is noted to mutter to himself under his breath in words no one can understand. He is frequently found hiding in the laundry closet. When asked what he is doing, he responds: "Praying wasn't enough. I tried to pray—I tried! The devil is coming to get me. He says I'm a homosexual. I have to hide."

261. Bob G. is seen in intake conference on the inpatient unit. Which of the following does NOT contribute to the etiology of his illness?
    A. The biochemical processes associated with schizophrenia are not clearly understood
    B. A number of biochemical factors that rely on the neurotransmission process have been identified with the development of schizophrenia
    C. Schizophrenia is associated with overactivity in dopamine or norepinephrine tracts in the brain
    D. Biochemical studies have provided the answer to the cause of schizophrenia

262. Bob is diagnosed as having paranoid schizophrenia. In meeting with his parents and brothers for a family assessment, the nurse recognizes that
    A. a number of common feelings are generated by the family situation
    B. the family members want to change communication patterns and eagerly follow through with therapeutic plans
    C. the client is not willing to give up the sick role despite family pressure
    D. in cases of paranoid schizophrenia, family communication patterns are functional

263. Which statement best explains the effect of labeling a person as a schizophrenic upon admission to a psychiatric inpatient facility?
    A. Once a person is designated schizophrenic, all of his other behaviors and characteristics are colored by that label and he will continue to be seen as schizophrenic
    B. Diagnostic processes are accurate enough to appropriately classify psychotic behavior
    C. Sanity can be distinguished from insanity by standard diagnostic procedures identified in *DSM III*
    D. A schizophrenic patient can remove the stigma of this illness by carefully following the therapeutic plan of care

264. Bob huddles in the corner of his room without responding to or initiating communication. He speaks in a symbolic language and refuses to participate in unit activities. An appropriate initial nursing diagnosis for Bob is
    A. low self-esteem and poor reality orientation
    B. dependency related to a fused mother-child relationship
    C. lack of an adequate support system
    D. avoidance of interpersonal relatedness due to feelings of mistrust

265. When initiating a one-to-one relationship with a client identified as schizophrenic, the nurse should initially
    A. decode the client's symbolic language
    B. acknowledge feelings generated by the client
    C. ascertain that the patient has hallucinations
    D. involve the patient in goal-directed activities

266. Paranoid patients need activities that require close concentration because they
    A. need to be challenged with variety
    B. lose interest easily if not concentrating
    C. will have less time for delusional thinking
    D. will have less time to express aggression

267. An appropriate initial nursing intervention with a schizophrenic patient who is suspicious is to
    A. encourage social participation with other friendly patients
    B. be honest at all times and provide detailed explanations of routines and procedures
    C. involve the patient in competitive group therapeutic activities
    D. provide consistency in the environment and allow the patient to pace himself with others

268. Bob is experiencing paranoid delusions and states, "They are conspiring against me; they're after me day and night." Which would be a therapeutic response by the nurse?
    A. "They *are* out to get you; they *are* conspiring against you!"
    B. "Why do you feel they are pursuing you?"
    C. "I can understand how you feel, but it doesn't seem to me that this is happening."
    D. "You'll think this now because you're mentally ill. When you get well, you'll see it isn't so."

269. Mr. Crompton, admitted as a catatonic schizophrenic, demonstrates a variety of behavioral problems. In working with the hallucinations he is experiencing, the nurse recognizes that
  A. delusions are not seen in the catatonic and therefore do not complicate attempts at therapy
  B. hallucinations that occur tend to be persecutory and fraught with mysticism
  C. either agitation or immobilization may occur when he hallucinates, but not both
  D. catatonic patients remain regressed forever in personality and behavioral disorganization

270. Miss Stein's diagnosis is schizophrenia, catatonic type. The nurse finds Miss Stein in her hospital room, staring into space and not yet dressed for breakfast. Which is the nurse's most therapeutic approach to Miss Stein?
  A. "Could I bring you a tray?"
  B. "Breakfast is almost ready, Miss Stein. I'll help you get dressed."
  C. "Since you're not dressed it's better if you eat in your room."
  D. "Breakfast is almost ready, Miss Stein. You may miss it if you don't get dressed."

271. After working for 3 weeks with a schizophrenic patient who has low self-esteem, he has learned to respond to the nurse but refuses to participate in any recreational activities. The nursing action which would best assist the patient to participate is to
  A. give him a task and expect him to accomplish it
  B. go with him to the activities and participate with him
  C. take him to the activities and observe his participation
  D. indicate to him that the activities are safe and available

272. Linda Williams, a 24-year-old college graduate student, is admitted to the inpatient psychiatric unit of a general hospital. Her withdrawn behavior includes depersonalization, flat affect, hallucinations, delusions, and bizarre communication patterns. A long-term nursing goal would be to assist her to
    A. identify ways to manage anxiety
    B. allow staff members to remain with her for 15 minutes
    C. use nonverbal communication more effectively
    D. communicate in an open, direct way

273. A patient with the diagnosis of schizophrenia, paranoid type, states that he hears voices telling him what to do. The nurse understands that auditory hallucinations represent
    A. the ego's attempt to prevent unconscious feelings and thoughts from entering conscious awareness
    B. the lack of a stimulating environment to enhance the senses
    C. an overactive imagination which compensates for a dull existence
    D. a cellular pathology in the sense organs

274. The nurse is aware that a schizophrenic patient is actively experiencing auditory hallucinations. Which of the following interventions is most therapeutic?
    A. Direct the patient to include the nurse in conversations with the voices
    B. Clarify what the voices are saying and explore their dynamic meaning with the patient
    C. Acknowledge the voices exist for the patient and recognize the feeling tone in the patient's voice
    D. Direct the patient into another room so the voices will diminish

275. The prognosis for Lee, a 35-year-old schizophrenic, would be more favorable if
     A. the illness had a slow onset with obvious precipitating factors
     B. there is a prior history of schizophrenic attacks
     C. the patient's symptoms have been present for more than 6 weeks
     D. his family is interested in his treatment program

276. Susan is an undifferentiated schizophrenic patient recently transferred to the psychiatric unit of the general hospital following an episode of extremely psychotic behavior. Susan was receiving diagnostic tests for a hypertension problem when her behavior became problematic. As a nurse working with her you initially need to demonstrate
     A. acceptance
     B. warmth
     C. self-awareness
     D. limit-setting behavior

277. Joe Scott, a schizophrenic patient who has recently been started on a regimen of chlorpromazine, is experiencing tonic muscle spasms of the neck, shoulders, and eyes. This side effect is known as
     A. parkinsonian syndrome
     B. acute dystonic reaction
     C. akathisia
     D. tardive dyskinesia

278. In caring for Jason, 42, who is admitted to the psychiatric inpatient unit with undifferentiated schizophrenia, it would be most important to
     A. keep the environment full of variety
     B. provide clear directions to minimize the client's decision requirements
     C. wait until the patient asks before providing for physical needs
     D. start socializing activities immediately

279. Rosalie, 29, is in the residual phase of schizophrenia. In planning care for Rosalie, which activities would be most therapeutic during this phase?
  A. Placing her on the volleyball team
  B. Allowing her to remain in her room when desired
  C. Encouraging her to watch TV during the day
  D. Asking the occupational therapist to teach her how to crochet

280. In the initial milieu management of a schizophrenic patient, which nursing intervention is appropriate?
  A. Placing the patient in a large ward to increase social contact
  B. Minimizing contact between the patient, staff, and other patients
  C. Taking the patient off the unit to activity programs
  D. Providing thorough explanations of routines and procedures

281. Somatic therapy is based on the assumption that the psychologic condition can be influenced by nonpsychologic methods. Somatic therapy is used in the treatment of schizophrenia because
  A. somatic approaches can cure the condition by interrupting the psychotic process
  B. the effects of psychoactive drugs and electroconvulsive therapy appear to be promising in curing schizophrenia
  C. genetic and biochemical factors are known causes of schizophrenia
  D. chemical, hormonal, and physical interventions can change behavior or alter mood

282. A negativistic schizophrenic patient refuses to take his prescribed haloperidol (Haldol). The best initial nursing intervention is to
    A. inform the patient that if he refuses oral medication he will receive an injection
    B. offer the medication again a short while later
    C. omit the dose and document the reason
    D. add the medication to the beverage he drinks at meals

Situation (Questions 283–286):   Eighteen-year-old Kevin Brown is admitted with the following nursing diagnosis: auditory hallucinations related to severe anxiety and fear of possibly losing control. Chlorpromazine (Thorazine) 100 mg q.i.d., p.o. is prescribed for Kevin.

283. Which of the following statements indicates that the nurse understands the use of this medication?
    A. These symptoms are usually treated with diphenhydramine hydrochloride (Benadryl)
    B. Drowsiness often occurs when a client begins to take this medication
    C. These symptoms often occur before tardive dyskinesia develops
    D. These symptoms indicate that Kevin has dystonia

284. Chlorpromazine acts by
    A. interfering with dopamine reception or synthesis at the neural synapse
    B. causing a state of physiologic shock
    C. facilitating transmission at the neural synapse
    D. interrupting neural pathways of emotion between the frontal lobes of the cerebral cortex

285. Which of the following statements describes the use of chlorpromazine for antisocial personality disorder?
    A. It is the drug of choice
    B. It depresses the chemoreceptor trigger zone
    C. It is not prescribed for this disorder
    D. It is a cure for the antisocial personality disorder

286. Kevin says to the nurse, "Why do I have to take Thorazine anyway?" Which is the best response by the nurse?
  A. "Taking this medication will keep you from being depressed."
  B. "This medication maintains a more even mood for you."
  C. "This medication will make you feel much better."
  D. "You will feel more relaxed and be able to think more clearly."

287. Mr. Cole, 45, is receiving chlorpromazine (Thorazine) 150 mg q.i.d. during an acute schizophrenic episode. Which of the following side effects may occur?
  A. Bradycardia
  B. Decreased appetite
  C. Urinary retention
  D. Increased libido and sexual drive

288. Benztropine mesylate (Cogentin) is administered primarily to
  A. relieve mild or moderate anxiety
  B. provide adequate sedation for the agitated patient
  C. counteract extrapyramidal side effects of prescribed antipsychotic mediation
  D. normalize unacceptable psychotic behaviors such as delusions

Situation (Questions 289–294): Lorie Bear comes to the mental health clinic for a follow-up interview. She tells the nurse that she has been taking trifluoperazine (Stelazine) for the last 3 weeks when she feels like it because she had been seeing and hearing funny things.

289. Which nursing assessments are essential during the intake interview with Lorie?
    A. Evidence of angina pectoris and tachycardia
    B. Drug dosage and sedation produced; evidence of maximum therapeutic effect of the drug
    C. Antiemetic effect and interference with muscle relaxation
    D. Blurred vision and craving for sweets

290. An appropriate objective of care for Lorie is that she will
    A. cease taking medication as soon as possible
    B. independently discontinue medication during her menstrual period
    C. take the medication later in the day if she forgets the morning dosage
    D. take an antacid within 1 hour of taking her medication

291. The nurse receives Lorie's medication from the pharmacy. The medication is labeled: trifluoperazine 100 mg p.o., b.i.d. Which nursing action is appropriate?
    A. Pour the medication after checking the label three times
    B. Administer concentrated solutions directly from the bottle without mixing with juices
    C. Observe for maximum therapeutic effect 1 hour after the first dose of the drug
    D. Send medication back to the pharmacy as it is mislabeled

292. The nurse asks Lorie to return in 2 weeks to the mental
     health center. Which of the following statements by
     Lorie would indicate compliance with the planned
     therapeutic regimen?
     A. "I take my medication every night as ordered."
     B. "When I go to the beach I stop taking my medica-
        tion."
     C. "When my mouth becomes dry I stop taking my
        medication."
     D. "If I am feeling excited I take three to four addi-
        tional tablets."

293. Lorie has been taking trifluoperazine for a long time.
     Which of the following health care goals assumes the
     highest priority at this time?
     A. Providing emotional support to Lorie
     B. Observing for bizarre facial and tongue movements
     C. Monitoring daily salt intake
     D. Noting intake of foods rich in tyramine

294. A discharge teaching plan for Lorie includes the purpose
     and possible side effects of her medication, trifluoper-
     azine. Which of the following statements indicates that
     Lorie understands this teaching plan?
     A. "My perspiration will increase with this drug."
     B. "I should report excessive urination to you."
     C. "I need to be careful not to stand up quickly or
        suddenly."
     D. "I do not have to worry about drinking alcohol with
        this drug."

Situation (Questions 295-297): Susan Bristol is a patient on the adult unit of a state psychiatric hospital. She has been started on thiothixene (Navane) 5 mg p.o., q.i.d.

295. Which of the following symptoms are characteristic of extrapyramidal side effects of antipsychotic medications such as Navane?
    A. Fainting, falling, palpitations, orthopnea
    B. Dry mouth, blurred vision, constipation, vomiting
    C. Menstrual disorders, increased appetite, weight gain, anorexia
    D. Severe muscle contraction, twisted neck, eyes rolling upward

296. Susan develops symptoms of dystonia. The priority nursing action for Susan at this time is to
    A. give benztropine mesylate (Cogentin) as prescribed
    B. give Susan sugarless gum and have her rinse her mouth frequently
    C. chart bowel movements and rashes
    D. order liver function tests

297. While Susan is receiving benztropine mesylate and thiothixene her plan of care should include
    A. teaching family members to withdraw thiothixene abruptly if Susan develops side effects
    B. preparing to take Cogentin for an extended period of time
    C. preparing for short-term use of Cogentin
    D. avoiding drug "holidays" from thiothixene because they mask significant side effects

Situation (Questions 298–299):   Heather Smith exhibits agitation, disorganized thinking, auditory hallucinations and other psychotic behaviors. The physican orders haloperidol (Haldol) 5–10 mg IM q. 1 hr until client is calmer and sedated, not to exceed 60 mg in 24 hours.

298. An important nursing consideration for Heather is to
    A. observe her for hypoglycemia
    B. observe her for evidence of calm, less-disorganized behavior
    C. reduce her fluid intake
    D. keep her on complete bed rest

299. While Heather is undergoing rapid tranquilization, the nurse should plan to
    A. monitor her CPK level
    B. encourage her to participate in group activities
    C. encourage her family to visit
    D. monitor vital signs and assess for extrapyramidal symptoms

F. PERSONALITY DISORDERS

300. What percentage of Americans are characterized as having antisocial personality?
    A. 2–5%
    B. 1–2%
    C. 5–7%
    D. 7–10%

301. Peter, who has a diagnosis of antisocial personality, is admitted to a mental health unit. Which of the following aspects of his history is pertinent to his present diagnosis?
    A. Had chickenpox at aged 2
    B. Is an only child
    C. Frequently missed school
    D. Felt unwanted as a child

302. In establishing a therapeutic relationship with the antisocial client it is important for the nurse to
A. show no emotion
B. ask him what it is like to share his thoughts and feelings with you
C. be supportive of his behavior
D. help him cope with his guilt feelings

303. Chuck's diagnosis is antisocial personality. Chuck and the nurse are scheduled to talk but he leaves the unit without permission. It would be most important for the nurse to
A. assign the client to another staff member
B. act as if nothing has happened when Chuck returns
C. convey the expectation he will want to talk with her soon
D. talk with other clients about Chuck's behavior

304. Mr. Smith is an antisocial personality admitted to a mental health unit. The nurse should assess Mr. Smith for
A. signs of indifference to others
B. leadership potential in patient government
C. signs of depression
D. future goals

305. Brenda, whose diagnosis is antisocial personality, has stolen a valuable ring from another client. It would be most important to
A. document Brenda's response to being caught
B. help the victim understand the nature of Brenda's illness
C. cancel all of Brenda's privileges
D. ask Brenda's family to discuss the situation

306. Phillip's diagnosis is antisocial personality. He tells the nurse that he thinks she is cute and says in a flattering manner that he would like her to stop being a jail-keeper and let him off the unit. Which reply is most appropriate?
    A. "It depends on what you want to do."
    B. "You know the rules."
    C. "Wait until the next shift."
    D. "No."

307. Roger is a charming 25-year-old man who has had numerous conflicts with the police. His most recent admission to the mental health unit is precipitated by his threat to burn his mother's house down unless she gives him money. His mother called the police and upon arrival they find Roger crying hysterically. Based upon Freudian theory, Peter needs
    A. an outlet for his drives within enforced limits
    B. punishment
    C. classes on developing trust relationships
    D. sympathy

308. In a community meeting on a mental health unit, Tom is confronted by David, who accuses Tom of taking his lunch tray. Tom denies the action but appears somewhat anxious. After the meeting the nurse should
    A. ask group members to avoid confronting Tom
    B. allow Tom to have time to himself
    C. tell Tom she is available to talk about the situation
    D. tell Tom that feelings are difficult to cope with

309. Charles, a client on a mental health unit, whose diagnosis is an antisocial personality, expects his family to visit tonight. It would be most important for the nurse to
    A. limit the family visit to 10 minutes
    B. observe family-client interactions
    C. sympathize with the family about Charles's incorrigible behavior
    D. tell the family what Charles's needs are

310. Edna has a diagnosis of borderline personality organization. What affect is Edna likely to display?
    A. Joviality
    B. Anger
    C. Aggressiveness
    D. Arrogance

311. Karen, whose diagnosis is borderline personality, has identified her use of intellectualizing as a defense. The nurse can guide Karen in understanding this defense by sharing information about
    A. the situations that seem to provoke use of intellectualizing
    B. how to make future observations of her rigid sense of identity
    C. what causes borderline disorders
    D. how intellectualization can promote spontaneity

312. Susan Gates is admitted to the psychiatric unit with the diagnosis of a borderline personality disorder. She displays various forms of inappropriate behaviors and mood disturbances while on the unit. An appropriate nursing intervention for this behavior is to
    A. arrange care according to Susan's mood and be very flexible in approach
    B. encourage staff to make independent decisions about Susan's care
    C. recognize that her progress is rapid and these behaviors will soon disappear
    D. encourage Susan to verbally express her rage and depression

313. The nurse has been working with a borderline neurotic client on the issue of dependency and asks the client to keep a diary of important daily experiences. Which type of diary entry indicates that the client is effectively working through her dependency?
    A. Fewer instances of whining, crying, and sadness
    B. Increased ventilation of anger
    C. Decreased impulsiveness
    D. Recognition of discouragement

314. Larry, a 23-year-old borderline client, makes constant demands on the nursing staff and is being helped to label this behavioral pattern. To evaluate the effectiveness of Larry's insight, which action is most appropriate?
    A. Ask Larry to keep a log of when he requests something
    B. Observe Larry's behavior for indications he can function on his own
    C. Hold a staff meeting to discuss Larry's progress
    D. Observe Larry for evidence of increased staff manipulation

315. Sue is a 30-year-old borderline client whose request to leave the unit has been denied. Which reaction would you expect Sue to demonstrate?
    A. Forcefully asking that the decision be reconsidered
    B. Withdrawal
    C. Hallucinating
    D. Demanding her physician be notified

316. The nurse is evaluating the success of the treatment regimen to decrease hostility in Joan, a 35-year-old client with borderline personality. What response indicates the regimen is unsuccessful?
    A. Joan increases attempts to demonstrate aspects of her identity
    B. The staff increases attempts to help Joan
    C. Joan increases use of denial
    D. The staff disagrees over their treatment of Joan

317. Mr. A., 50, is being evaluated for chronic back pain. He has not worked for a long time and is unkempt in his personal appearance. He talks constantly about his health problems and readily cooperates with all procedures. In applying her knowledge of dependent patients, the nurse recognizes the client's underlying behavioral dynamic is
    A. anxiety
    B. passivity
    C. isolation
    D. lack of self-worth

318. Mr. Lyons, whose diagnosis is a narcissistic personality disorder, is talking with another client, Mrs. Smith. Mrs. Smith says, "I came into the hospital yesterday. I just can't get my husband's death out of my mind." Mr. Lyons responds by saying, "Last summer I had to give up my old apartment. You know, some apartments are. . . ." This pattern of interaction reflects Mr. Lyons's
    A. looseness of association
    B. obsession
    C. sense of omnipotence
    D. reaction formation

319. Mr. Bronson's diagnosis is a passive-aggressive personality. The dynamic underlying of this disorder is the client's need to
    A. help others
    B. intellectualize
    C. express hostility
    D. be excessively punctual

320. In working with a client with pedophilia, an appropriate goal is to
    A. increase ability to cope with anger
    B. clarify sex-role identity
    C. decrease fear of domination by others
    D. increase feelings of self-confidence

Situation (Questions 321–324): Mark Bell is a 29-year-old patient who has a definite erotic attraction toward members of the same sex. He has trouble handling feelings of depression, anger, and hostility because of the breakup of a 6-month relationship.

321. In planning care for Mark it is important to
    A. tell him to stay away from male patients on the unit
    B. provide a support system for him
    C. avoid him so he does not become dependent upon you
    D. separate him in a seclusion room

322. The nurse notices that the male staff members avoid Mark. Which of the following approaches is most useful initially in working with the staff?
    A. Transfer staff members so they are less threatened
    B. Assign male clients to the female staff members
    C. Call a staff meeting to increase awareness of the staff's own attitudes and feelings
    D. Confront the male staff with their obvious sexual biases

323. Which of the following statements indicates Mark will probably be able to deal with his homosexual feelings?
    A. "When I get home I'm going to stay by myself."
    B. "I'm so mixed up, I'll never be right."
    C. "I'll be able to meet other people now, I feel less angry."
    D. "My sexual feelings toward men will have to be kept a secret forever."

324. Which of the following statements indicates Mark has an appropriate attitude toward his homosexuality?
    A. "The nurse says I'm the only "homo" that we have on the unit now."
    B. "Because I'm different the nurses avoid me."
    C. "Homosexuals are all the same, sick and perverted."
    D. "My nurse accepts the way I am."

325. When teaching children about the possibility of sexual assault or molestation by adults it is most important to
   A. teach children to avoid their uncles and other males in the family
   B. assess how much the child already knows before discussing the topic
   C. role play dangerous scenes as a learning strategy
   D. talk about encountering dangerous situations in general

G. ORGANIC MENTAL DISORDERS

326. The diagnostic labeling of children as having "organic brain syndrome" is disputed on the grounds that
   A. children are too young to be affected
   B. all neurologic illness in children can be diagnosed
   C. ability to determine the degree of brain dysfunction in children is lacking
   D. children always outgrow the symptomatic behavior

327. The habit of pica may produce organic mental syndrome in children because
   A. eating nonfood substances can be habit forming
   B. lead may be present in paints used on toys and furniture
   C. eating nonfoods does not furnish protein
   D. manganese may be present in paints used on toys

328. A community health nurse making an initial assessment of an older patient in his home asks questions to test his orientation to time and place, and recent and remote recall of general and personal information. This test is called the
   A. Minnesota Multiphasic Personality Inventory
   B. face-hand test
   C. Rorschach test
   D. Mental Status Questionnaire

329. A commonly mistaken belief held about elderly people with organic mental syndrome is that they
   A. exhibit brand new personality traits
   B. exhibit previous personality traits
   C. behave this way because of physiologic changes
   D. are the only age group who can develop this syndrome

330. In working with psychogeriatric patients it is important for the nurse to
   A. examine her own attitudes about aging
   B. assign these patients to nursing assistants who have more time
   C. make all decisions for these patients
   D. focus on physical nursing care

331. Which symptoms are always indicative of an organic mental syndrome?
   A. Impaired memory and judgment
   B. Disturbed gait
   C. Delusions
   D. Disturbed mood

332. Mrs. White has a diagnosis of severe delirium. Which of the following is NOT characteristic of a patient with a severe, acute organic brain syndrome?
   A. Cognitive impairment
   B. Hallucinations
   C. Normal electroencephalogram
   D. Disorientation

333. Chronic infections of the central nervous system such as syphilis or brucellosis may be detected only because of
   A. classic physical signs produced
   B. gradual onset of emotional or behavioral changes
   C. wild behavioral deviations
   D. sudden onset of mental changes

334. One type of illness that can produce symptoms of acute delirium is
    A. Hypothyroidism
    B. Meningitis
    C. Concussion
    D. Barbiturate overdose

335. Ms. Brown, 45, was admitted to the hospital 3 days ago for pneumonia. The night nurse observes Ms. Brown to be restless, insomnic, and making needless picking motions at the bed clothing. She complains of insects moving across the foot of the bed. The nurse should consider the possibility that this patient is experiencing
    A. severe anxiety
    B. confusion following a nightmare
    C. actual presence of some type of insect
    D. delirium tremens

336. In caring for the patient in an acute confusional state the nurse should be calm and reassuring because the
    A. patient is frightened and anxious
    B. nurse must understand the patient's hallucinations
    C. nurse must take complete charge of the patient's care
    D. patient will identify with the nurse's mood

337. In managing a patient suffering from delirium the nurse should
    A. utilize only nonverbal behavior for communication
    B. expect medication to make the patient more comfortable
    C. speak and move slowly and deliberately
    D. order x-rays and diagnostic tests as with all neurologic patients

338. Mr. Jones, aged 25, is hospitalized with a diagnosis of lobar pneumonia accompanied by a high fever. At 10 P.M. Mr. Jones is found wandering in the hall stating he must find his clothes to go to work. Mr. Jones' behavior illustrates which organic mental disorder?
   A. Delirium
   B. Dementia
   C. Cerebral arteriosclerosis
   D. General paresis

339. Which of the following nursing interventions is effective in reducing anxiety in a delirious patient?
   A. Assigning a team of nurses to care for one patient
   B. Keeping the shades drawn and the room darkened
   C. Explaining procedures and answering questions in simple, short answers
   D. Providing the patient with solitude

340. Mr. Simms, 82-years-old, is brought to the emergency room. His daughter states he has become increasingly confused the past month, is eating poorly, and is not functioning in his "usual manner." In assessing Mr. Simms, the nurse needs to be aware of the possibility of memory loss and his subsequent "filling in the gaps" with imaginary information. This process is called
   A. reminiscing
   B. circumstantiality
   C. regression
   D. confabulation

341. Mr. Brown, aged 72, who has organic mental syndrome, was asked what he ate for lunch. In being unable to answer, Mr. Brown illustrates the most prominent characteristic of irreversible brain damage which is
   A. confabulation
   B. impaired remote memory
   C. impaired recent memory
   D. disorientation

342. A nurse caring for a patient who has had an acute myocardial infarction which has resulted in hypoxia would
observe the patient for evidence of
    A. acute anxiety
    B. la belle indifference
    C. flight-of-ideas
    D. dissociative speech pattern

343. Joan S., aged 32, is admitted to the unit for the control
of her grand mal seizures. The primary focus of nursing
care for Joan is to
    A. encourage interaction with her peers
    B. protect her from physical harm
    C. regulate her medication
    D. check her gait

Situation (Questions 344–345): Mrs. Grayson is a 62-year-old
with a diagnosis of organic brain syndrome. In interviewing
Mrs. Grayson you note that she includes excessive detail and
seems to have difficulty filtering out relevant material as she
describes events.

344. This speech behavior is known as
    A. confabulation
    B. blocking
    C. punning
    D. circumstantiality

345. Considering the implications of Mrs. Grayson's speech
pattern, which action should the nurse include in Mrs.
Grayson's care plan?
    A. Staff should avoid intervening or putting pressure on
the patient when she is talking
    B. Place Mrs. Grayson in a private room so she will not
feel pressure to talk to a roommate
    C. Encourage Mrs. Grayson not to talk any more than
necessary and try to anticipate her needs
    D. When possible, assist Mrs. Grayson by providing the
right word or words to complete her thought

Situation (Questions 346–353): Mrs. Mary P., an 82-year-old widow, is admitted to the hospital by her daughter who indicates Mrs. P. suffers occasional confusion and general slowing down but cares for herself during the day and sleeps most of the night. Her daughter thinks Mrs. P. fell at home yesterday as Mrs. P. has numerous bruises on her arms and legs. Mrs. P.'s admission diagnosis is acute brain disorder superimposed on mild senile dementia (chronic brain disorder).

346. Which of the following symptoms is NOT associated with chronic irreversible brain syndrome?
   A. Memory impairment
   B. Altered level of consciousness
   C. Lability of affect
   D. Impaired intellectual functioning

347. In assessing Mrs. P. you ask her to tell you about what happened the day before she was admitted to the hospital and other important events in her life. Mrs. P. is able to recall the date of her marriage, when her children were born, and her work as a hospital volunteer. She is unable to recall what occurred the day before admission. This impairment in ability to recall information is called
   A. attention deficit
   B. disorientation
   C. dementia
   D. dysmensia

348. Mrs. P.'s behavioral response to her cognitive impairment is LEAST affected by her
   A. personality characteristics
   B. current affective state
   C. availability of quality support systems
   D. degree of brain involvement

349. Which of the following nursing interventions would NOT be utilized in caring for Mrs. P.?
   A. Providing challenge to the patient
   B. Reinforcing reality
   C. Maintaining a familiar environment
   D. Protecting her from harm

350. Mrs. P. becomes quite agitated late in the evening. Her agitation is so severe that she requires medication to calm her and ensure adequate rest to conserve physical energy. The medication usually prescribed for this "sundown syndrome" is
   A. chlorpromazine (Thorazine)
   B. phenobarbital
   C. lithium
   D. methylphenidate (Ritalin)

351. Mr. Smith, aged 80, has been making sexual advances toward female patients and staff. To manage Mr. Smith's behavior therapeutically the nurse recognizes that Mr. Smith
   A. is just being troublesome
   B. is attempting to establish interpersonal contact
   C. is following the social expectations of an 80-year-old man
   D. must be constantly watched to prevent recurrence of this behavior

352. A 78-year-old woman is admitted to a nursing home following a brief hospitalization for a circulatory disorder accompanied by cognitive disturbance. Anticoagulants have been prescribed. In planning her care, the nurse should consider
   A. initiating seizure precautions
   B. observing for assaultive behavior
   C. her impaired communication ability
   D. possibility of hemorrhage from even a minor injury

353. A nursing goal for Mr. P., who has chronic organic brain syndrome, is for him to become more involved in social activities in the nursing home. In determining the type of activity for Mr. P., the nurse should consider that
   A. individual activities/hobbies should be progressively challenging in complexity
   B. highly structured activities provide a greater sense of security
   C. tasks requiring considerable time to complete will hold the patient's attention longer
   D. group activities can increase feelings of belonging and self-worth

354. Mrs. M., aged 76, was found wandering in the street by the police who brought her to a psychiatric hospital. Her diagnosis is chronic organic mental syndrome. A priority nursing action for Mrs. M. is to
   A. promote reality orientation
   B. allay her anxiety over being in unfamiliar surroundings
   C. initiate a sensory stimulation program
   D. encourage independent functioning to the degree possible

355. In planning the use of leisure time for an elderly client who has chronic organic brain syndrome which is most important?
   A. Watching television in her room
   B. Attending occupational therapy
   C. Napping when tired
   D. Watching television in the dayroom

356. A nursing care plan for the patient with Parkinson's disease should include
    A. reducing social contacts to avoid embarrassment about altered physical appearance
    B. moderate exercise to conserve energy and reduce tremors
    C. maintain ordinary activities of daily living as much as possible
    D. encourage solitary activities such as reading to reduce discomfort about unusual body movements

357. Ms. Brown has a moderate degree of organic brain dysfunction and is able to assist in some of her daily care. In providing care for Ms. Brown, the nurse should avoid
    A. maintaining her physical capabilities
    B. ignoring her emotional reactions
    C. promoting reality orientation
    D. encouraging independent functioning

358. Mr. Jones is admitted to the psychiatric unit with amnesia and disorientation, and Wernicke's syndrome is diagnosed. This organic brain syndrome is caused by a deficiency of
    A. ascorbic acid
    B. niacin
    C. thiamine
    D. iron

359. Improvement in the condition of a patient with Wernicke's encephalopathy is associated with the patient's increased intake of
    A. foods containing magnesium
    B. carbohydrates
    C. foods containing thiamine
    D. foods high in potassium

360. In planning for a patient who is delirious, which nursing approach is INAPPROPRIATE?
    A. Avoiding use of restraints
    B. Reality orientation
    C. Semiprivate room
    D. Constant supervision

361. Which of the following is NOT typical of hallucinations occurring in delirium tremens?
    A. Colorful
    B. Primarily visual
    C. Frightening
    D. Predominantly auditory

362. A man in his mid-40s is discharged from a psychiatric unit with a diagnosis of Huntington's chorea. He should be taught to observe for onset of involuntary movements which occur initially in the
    A. lower legs and feet
    B. face and upper extremities
    C. total body
    D. limbs only

363. Diabetes mellitus may produce changes in mental functioning such as
    A. polydipsia
    B. polyphasia
    C. fatigability
    D. polyuria

Situation (Questions 364–365): Mr. Simms has a limited degree of impaired functioning owing to chronic organic brain syndrome. Since he has improved under medical and nursing treatment, he is to be discharged to his home.

364. Because he lives alone, which approach is most reasonable to assure Mr. Simms's meal and medication routine is satisfactory?
  A. Have a home health aide prepare two daily meals and supervise him in preparing his medication
  B. Have Mr. Simms's married daughter prepare breakfast and lunch, allowing Mr. Simms to assume responsibility for his medication
  C. Teach Mr. Simms a proper medication routine and have Meals on Wheels bring one hot meal a day
  D. Allow Mr. Simms a trial period to see if he can handle his own needs

365. During a discharge planning with Mr. Simms and his daughter, the nurse learns that he takes medication for hypertension, sedatives for sleep, and a diuretic. The nurse recognizes that Mr. Simms's confusion may be due to
  A. pharmacologic agents
  B. alcohol abuse
  C. loneliness
  D. poor socialization

366. Senile dementia is generally considered to result from
  A. avitaminosis
  B. a variety of physiologic factors
  C. intracranial neoplasms
  D. frontal lobe cerebral hypertrophy

367. Senile dementia is generally accompanied by
  A. sensory and petit mal seizures
  B. retrograde amnesia and nausea
  C. headaches and fainting
  D. speech disturbances and easy fatigability

368. Cardinal symptoms of senile dementia include
- **A.** dyspnea and anxiety
- **B.** dysmnesia and disorientation
- **C.** anorexia and insomnia
- **D.** irritability and sleep disturbance

Situation (Questions 369–374): Mrs. Hernandez, a 52-year-old client, has Alzheimer's disease.

369. Mrs. Hernandez has a pattern of making up responses to questions when she cannot remember the answer. This behavior is called
- **A.** compensation
- **B.** confabulation
- **C.** depersonalization
- **D.** dissociation

370. Alzheimer's disease is characterized by
- **A.** loss of initiative
- **B.** progressive memory decline
- **C.** emotional distress and agitation
- **D.** development of extrapyramidal symptoms

371. The nurse observes Mrs. Hernandez placing soiled tissues and bread crusts in her dresser drawer. Which nursing intervention would be most therapeutic in addressing this problem?
- **A.** Confronting Mrs. Hernandez with the inappropriateness of her behavior
- **B.** Exploring Mrs. Hernandez's feelings regarding her hoarding behavior
- **C.** Assisting Mrs. Hernandez to identify articles to be discarded
- **D.** Telling Mrs. Hernandez what articles she may keep in her room

372. The nurse asks Mrs. Hernandez to join the group for dinner. Mrs. Hernandez stares blankly at the nurse, then walks away. The best initial response for the nurse to make is to
    A. repeat the statement to her
    B. tell her what time it is
    C. grasp her by the hand
    D. comment on her behavior

373. Mrs. Hernandez is becoming increasingly withdrawn, isolating herself in her room. Which activity would be most appropriate initially in resocializing Mrs. Hernandez?
    A. Playing cards in the activities room
    B. Playing Ping-Pong in recreational therapy
    C. Watching television in the lounge
    D. Baking a cake in the kitchen

374. Mrs. Hernandez becomes agitated while observing a lively volleyball game in recreational therapy. In helping to relieve Mrs. Hernandez's agitation the nurse initially
    A. explores her feelings regarding the activity
    B. offers p.r.n. medications as ordered
    C. encourages her to join in the activity
    D. removes her from the group

H. CHILDHOOD DISORDERS

Situation (Questions 375-385):   Ricky Robards, aged 3, is referred to the mental health outpatient clinic for diagnostic evaluation. Ricky has not "started to talk yet." Ricky is an only child and his parents fear he is mentally retarded. As an infant Ricky did not like to be held or rocked. The parents also report that Ricky does not play with other children and sits in the corner of his room stroking his blanket for hours. Ricky has also hit at them and screams when any unusual activity occurs.

375. Infantile autism differs from childhood schizophrenia in that children with infantile autism
    A. are usually diagnosed after the child is 10 years old
    B. have a period of normal development before developing symptoms
    C. have symptoms of withdrawal and inappropriate emotional behavior
    D. display symptoms in the first few weeks of life

376. Ricky completes a series of evaluative tests and is diagnosed as an autistic child. The staff recommends that Ricky be placed in a residential care program. On leaving the clinic, Mrs. Robards says, "I'm not sure if an institution is best for Ricky. It's such a cold, impersonal setting." Which nursing response is most appropriate?
    A. "Institutions aren't what they once were. I'm sure Ricky will be just fine."
    B. "You feel guilty about putting Ricky in a residential treatment program?"
    C. "You think Ricky won't receive the care he needs?"
    D. "You seem to feel bad about giving up your son."

377. Ricky's parents place him in the residential care center. In planning for Ricky's care, his level of growth and development will need to be assessed. According to Erikson, Ricky should be at which developmental stage?
    A. Trust vs mistrust
    B. Autonomy vs shame and doubt
    C. Identity vs role diffusion
    D. Initiative vs guilt

378. During staff conferences, a tentative plan of care is developed for Ricky. A priority nursing goal for Ricky is to
    A. help Ricky develop a sense of self-identity
    B. help Ricky form relationships with others
    C. meet Ricky's basic needs so tension and defensive behavior will decrease
    D. allow Ricky to regress and relive previous unresolved developmental stages

379. In assisting the staff to work with Ricky in a therapeutic milieu, which of the following principles is stressed?
    A. Respond only to Ricky's appropriate interactions with other children
    B. Start with where the child is
    C. Provide structure for child's daily life
    D. Isolate him from children if he hurts them

380. An early indication that milieu therapy is producing a change in Ricky's behavior would be that he
    A. plays with a group of children
    B. allows an adult to sit with him during an activity
    C. plays with one other child
    D. stops hitting other children

381. Ricky uses speech infrequently and inconsistently but not to indicate his needs or feelings. As you are sitting with Ricky, he points to a block on the floor. To help Ricky develop communication skills, which is the most appropriate response?
    A. "You would like me to give you the block?"
    B. "Go pick up the block, Ricky."
    C. "Block, say block, Ricky."
    D. "Ricky, what do you call that object?"

382. Ricky's treatment plan includes operant conditioning as a treatment modality. The basic concept of operant conditioning is
    A. response to positive or negative stimuli
    B. demonstration of desired behavior response patterns
    C. reinforcement increases the probability of behavior recurring
    D. shaping of behavior by reinforcing approximation of the desired behavior

383. Using the concept of operant conditioning to toilet train Ricky, the nurse will
    A. sensitize Ricky to use of the potty chair
    B. demonstrate use of the potty chair for Ricky
    C. punish Ricky for not using the potty chair
    D. praise Ricky each time he uses the potty chair

384. The goal of toilet training Ricky will be achieved when Ricky
    A. goes to the toilet by himself
    B. gestures to you that he has to go to the toilet
    C. looks ashamed when he wets his pants
    D. sits on the potty chair, even though he remains clothed

385. The physician orders prochlorperazine (Compazine) 2.5 mg p.o. or rectally for Ricky. An important nursing consideration is to
    A. avoid use of potent sunscreens
    B. observe for weight loss
    C. encourage adequate fluid intake
    D. give antiparkinsonian medication concurrently

386. Which one of the following responses obtained from the nursing history of a hyperkinetic child is significant as a possible causative factor?
    A. The family is of middle-class socioeconomic background
    B. The mother's pregnancy, labor, and delivery was uneventful although she experienced nausea the first trimester
    C. The child experienced a severe viral infection when he was 6 weeks old
    D. The child's two sisters exhibit moderate activity levels in school and play activities

387. Mr. and Mrs. R. are having difficulty with the behavior of their hyperkinetic son, who is the oldest of four siblings. Mr. R. blames his wife for not disciplining the child strictly enough in the home. His wife admits she has difficulty being consistent. Both parents express frustration about managing their son's behavior. Which health care goal is initially most important in working with the parents?
    A. Providing reference books on the hyperkinetic child and related problems
    B. Helping the parents enhance their effectiveness within the limitations of the home environment
    C. Enlisting their assistance in identifying their son's behavioral problems in school
    D. Increasing their opportunities to get away from home so they can become more objective

Situation (Questions 388–389):   Johnny is referred to the clinic because of complaints by his parents and teachers of "short attention span," emotional immaturity, and short temper. He is impulsive in school, has a low frustration tolerance, and is a behavioral problem.

388. A major priority in Johnny's treatment plan is
   A. initiating stimulant drug therapy
   B. placement in activity group therapy
   C. behavioral conditioning program planned for the school setting
   D. parental counseling about limit setting

389. Johnny is placed on methylphenidate (Ritalin) 10 mg/ day to help his restlessness and distractibility in school. Which observation should the school nurse or teacher be instructed to report to Johnny's physician?
   A. Falls asleep in class
   B. Continues to disrupt the class
   C. Johnny describes himself as stupid, worthless, and bad
   D. Johnny is easily distracted from class assignments

390. Jason O., 7 years old, is diagnosed as hyperkinetic. Which one of the following symptoms of brain dysfunction would you expect him to exhibit?
   A. Difficulty with attention span
   B. Highly abnormal changes in the electroencephalogram (EEG)
   C. Below-average intelligence with evidence of mental retardation
   D. Definite pathologic changes in at least one part of the central nervous system

391. Jerry, a 7-year-old, whose diagnosis is hyperkinesis, has been taking methylphenidate (Ritalin), 10 mg b.i.d. for 3 weeks, as prescribed. He is currently experiencing a lack of appetite and wakefulness during the night. The mother expresses concern about these symptoms to the nurse. Which statement accurately appraises Jerry's response to the medication?

A. "This response is to be expected in initial treatment with Ritalin."

B. "Jerry is showing signs of addiction which can be dealt with when the medication therapy is completed."

C. "It is too soon to see the therapeutic effectiveness of the medication."

D. "The medication works by decreasing the level of norepinephrine in the brain which then produces these symptoms."

392. Tom, an 11-year-old hyperkinetic child, has been in family counseling with his parents and siblings for 2 months because of recurrent conflicts within the family related to his behavioral problems. Which one of the following statements by Tom identifies a lack of progress toward goals set by the family?

A. "My parents say they won't let me go to the game, and they won't change their minds."

B. "My brothers like to do things with my parents and me."

C. "My parents never go anywhere anymore because they want to stay home with me."

D. "My parents let me go places with other kids more than they used to, as long as they know whose parents will be there."

393. Brian, a 12-year-old child with multiple symptoms of severe inattention, impulsivity, and hyperactivity, expresses a desire to be able to concentrate better. Which one of the following actions Brian suggests would you support as appropriate toward achieving his goal?

A. Constructing a model airplane from a kit during his next Scout meeting

B. Playing a game of jacks with other children during his free time at school

C. Doing his homework in his bedroom where distractions are minimal

D. Making a long list of tasks to accomplish daily so he can remember what he has to do

394. Gary's parents wish to learn more about the use of behavior modification techniques in helping him control his hyperkinetic behavior. Which of the following techniques is INAPPROPRIATE for assigning and supervising his completion of household tasks?

A. Assign responsibilities for household chores that he expresses a preference in doing

B. Reward him immediately for tasks successfully completed

C. Plan his rewards to be something he especially enjoys

D. Let him choose when he wants to perform his tasks during his daily schedule

395. Steve, a 9-year-old hyperkinetic child, is returning to school after being placed on methylphenidate (Ritalin) for 3 months during the summer. The nurse talks with his mother about conditions in the school environment that would help reduce potential behavior problems. Which one of the following situations in school would be LEAST helpful in meeting Steve's needs?
    A. School-related learning tasks that are geared to the majority of the students' learning abilities
    B. A classroom setting with a predictable environment and appropriate limitations
    C. A classroom teacher who is comfortable in setting limits with Steve despite an occasional temper tantrum
    D. Steve's placement for a part of each day with a resource teacher who is helping him develop additional skills

396. Eric, a 10-year-old hyperkinetic child, has been taking pencils and other objects from desks in his classroom. His mother asks you how to handle this situation since the teacher and students view him as a troublemaker. You suggest she talk with Eric's teacher about protecting his self-esteem while gradually assisting him to change his behavior. Which action on the mother's part would best accomplish these goals?
    A. Asking the teacher to confront Eric each time she sees him take something and making him return it immediately
    B. Suggesting the teacher replace the objects without comment when he takes them, and praising him at specified intervals for not taking others' belongings
    C. Encouraging Eric to tell people he will try not to take their things in the future
    D. Suggesting to the teacher that she make Eric sit in a corner for 15 minutes each time he takes something from a desk

397. Sara, a hyperkinetic 12-year-old, wishes to submit a project for the school science fair. The nurse has agreed to work with her on the project. Together they discuss how much time to spend on it each day. Which one of the following problematic behaviors associated with hyperkinesis did the nurse consider in arriving at a plan to spend one-half hour each day with Sara?
    A. Perceptual deficits
    B. Difficulty forming concepts and abstractions
    C. Emotional immaturity
    D. Limited attention span

398. Tom, aged 12 years, informs the nurse that he masturbates two or three times a week and lately has awakened with his bed being wet. The nurse should help the patient understand that masturbation
    A. is wrong but nocturnal emissions are normal at this age
    B. and nocturnal emissions are common at this age
    C. is normal, but nocturnal emissions are signs of being oversexed
    D. usually leads to homosexuality

Situation (Questions 399–402): Margy, 17, is a high-school senior, who comes to the school nurse because of a 50-lb weight gain over the past 4 months. She is 5'5" tall and weighs 175 lb. Margy has an IQ of 135 and states she is unpopular except when she wins horse shows.

399. Which goal is most important for Margy at this time?
    A. Nurse will instruct patient in basic four food groups
    B. Client will eat whatever she wants
    C. Client will begin professional counseling to understand cause and meaning of her eating habits
    D. Nurse and client will select a popular diet for client to follow

400. Margy also has problems at school. Which of the following is most significant as an indication of poor adjustment?

A. IQ of 135

B. Ranked second in her senior class of 405

C. States she has no close friends

D. Unsure of whether or not she should attend college

401. Margy's language includes words such as "snow," "candy," "awesome," "Teri," and "groddy," which do not fit in context with a dictionary definition of the terms. When the nurse hears these terms in assessing the patient, she should

A. apply street meanings to the words as basis for understanding

B. recognize adolescents create their own language to exclude adults and outsiders

C. prohibit the use of profanity and sexually explicit terms

D. require an adolescent to use only socially accepted words and means of expression

402. Two weeks after Margy began therapy, her day included two tests on which she made A's, followed by remarks from her peers about "being a bookworm." She was also "cold shouldered" while getting a coke. She then drank two beers, ate four pizzas and "some sleeping pills." Which of the following is Margy exhibiting?

A. Scapegoating

B. Anxiety and resistance

C. Testing limit setting

D. Helplessness and worthlessness

403. Adolescent suicide gestures and attempts include all of the following factors EXCEPT

A. lack or loss of a meaningful relationship

B. a precipitating event

C. a true desire to die

D. a bid for help

Situation (Questions 404–407):   Linda, a 14-year-old, tells the nurse she has been sexually active since aged 10 years. She thinks she might be pregnant.

404. Which of the following responses is most appropriate in talking with Linda?
   A. "You can't be pregnant, you're just a baby."
   B. "What makes you think you are pregnant?"
   C. "You probably are pregnant if you have been having sex."
   D. "The doctor will want a urine sample to determine if you are pregnant."

405. Linda is found to be 4-months pregnant. One concern is the future of the baby. Linda's decision making should be based upon awareness of all options EXCEPT
   A. adoption or foster placement
   B. special school programs for pregnant mothers
   C. work potential as a minor, including salary
   D. ambivalence about keeping the baby

406. A program for teenage pregnant girls is offered in your town and includes group therapy. Which of the following reasons is most likely to persuade Linda to join the group?
   A. Everyone wants her to join the group
   B. It would be good for her to hear other people's problems
   C. It provides a group of her age to discuss common problems
   D. The group will tell her what she should do

407. Four months later, the nurse interviews Linda to check on her progress. Which of the following statements best describes the patient's decision-making?
    A. "I am going to finish high school and give the baby up for adoption as mother wishes."
    B. "My boyfriend says that if I want to stay with him, I will keep the baby and get a job."
    C. "I want to finish school, stay with my parents, and keep the baby."
    D. "The group says I should place the baby until I get a good job."

I. DEVELOPMENTAL DISABILITIES

Situation (Questions 408–411): Jane Conrad, a 15-year-old, mentally retarded girl, is admitted to the mental health unit for evaluation.

408. The staff must determine if Jane is mentally retarded or developmentally disabled. The diagnosis of mental retardation would be confirmed by which observations?
    A. Limitations in mobility, self-care, and speech
    B. Need for a combination of special services
    C. Subaverage intellectual functioning and adaptive impairment
    D. Combination of physical and mental impairments

409. Jane uses simple communication and can read at the level of a 7-year-old; her history reflects noticeable delays in development. Which long-term goals would be most appropriate for Jane?
    A. Seeking semiskilled employment and advanced education
    B. Providing total continuous care and protection
    C. Learning self-care activities and acceptable social behavior
    D. Seeking competitive employment and marriage

410. The most helpful nursing approach for Jane would be to
    A. involve her in complex relationships
    B. obtain a detailed history from her
    C. develop a one-to-one relationship
    D. reinforce her self-perceptions

411. The nurse explains to Jane's mother that Jane has many problems with adaptive behavior. Which of the mother's statements indicates that the nurse's teaching about this concept is effective?
    A. "Jane's IQ is what is most important, nothing else counts."
    B. "Jane only has a learning disability."
    C. "Jane will always have to be institutionalized."
    D. "Jane will have problems with independence and responsibility."

Situation (Questions 412–417): Cheryl Lewis is a 4-year-old child with a protruding tongue, upward outward-slanted eyes, and hypotonic muscles. Her mother brings her to the mental health center for evaluation.

412. Cheryl's diagnosis is Down's syndrome, which results from
    A. decreased phenylalanine hydroxylase
    B. altered hexoaminodase production
    C. altered blood factor VIII due to genetic defect
    D. impairment in general material as a result of an extra chromosome

413. A behavior modification program is planned for Cheryl. Which of the following statements best describes behavior modification?
    A. Problems are unveiled on a fantasy level using dolls, toys, and clay
    B. Psychotherapeutic goals are achieved by using dramatic techniques
    C. A therapy based on the concept that behavior is determined by its consequences
    D. Insight therapy that uses techniques of free association

414. For Cheryl's behavior modification plan to be successful, it is most important to
    A. deprive Cheryl of things that are pleasurable
    B. assess what is rewarding to Cheryl
    C. reward undesirable behaviors
    D. apply punishment frequently

415. Cheryl's father says to her, "You dummy! Can't you get dressed by yourself?" This statement contradicts principles of care for the mentally retarded because it
    A. will prevent Cheryl from becoming independent
    B. fails to build Cheryl's self-confidence and respect
    C. makes Cheryl feel worthy despite her defects
    D. treats Cheryl's inability to dress herself as an understandable mistake

416. One objective in Cheryl's plan of care is that Cheryl's father will assist her with dressing procedures by the end of 1 week. Which of the father's statements indicates that this goal has been achieved?
    A. "Cheryl will never learn how to dress."
    B. "Cheryl is very slow, she'll just have to have help."
    C. "I'll just button her shirt this one time."
    D. "I'm so pleased, I only had to help Cheryl with one button."

417. Cheryl's parents plan to have more children but ask what they should do to have a normal child. Which of the following statements should form the basis of the nurse's response?
   A. Genetic counseling referral would benefit this family
   B. Most mental retardation is caused during the post-natal period
   C. Errors in metabolism cause most mental retardation
   D. This family should be discouraged from having children

Situation (Questions 418–422): Sharon Cooper is a 35-year-old retarded client living in a supportive-living home.

418. To develop a realistic nursing care plan for Sharon, which of the following assessment should be made initially by the nurse?
   A. Socioadaptive capacity, maturity, and self-help skills
   B. Sexual impulses, psychotic behavior patterns, and ambivalent feelings
   C. Organic factors, neurologic causes, and motor abilities
   D. Flexibility of environment, toxic factors, and medical diagnosis

419. Sharon sometimes has emotional outbursts, is inflexible, passive, and dependent. An appropriate short-term goal for Sharon is that at the end of 1 week, she will
   A. go shopping unassisted
   B. make simple decisions without help
   C. control all angry outbursts
   D. lead the residents in their house meeting

420. The doctor orders chlorpromazine hydrochloride (Thorazine) to control Sharon's occasional hyperactive episodes. Sharon develops extrapyramidal side effects. The drug prescribed to combat these side effects is
    A. thiothixene (Navane)
    B. diazepam (Valium)
    C. benztropine mesylate (Cogentin)
    D. imipramine (Tofranil)

421. The nurse teaches Sharon to report to the staff if she has a sore throat while taking chlorpromazine (Thorazine) because a sore throat
    A. is a sign of liver complications
    B. accompanies extrapyramidal symptoms
    C. can forewarn of a hypotensive episode
    D. can mean her white blood cell count is depressed

422. Which behaviors indicate that Sharon is ready to have more advanced nurse-client goals?
    A. Short attention span, autism, and restlessness
    B. Emotional vulnerability, irritability, and hypersensitivity
    C. Dependency, ambivalence, and worthlessness
    D. Unassisted dressing, improved decision-making skills, and control of emotional outbursts

J. PERSON ABUSE

Situation (Questions 423–432): Mrs. Jane Smith, aged 34, has been married for 10 years and has four children, ages 10, 8, 6, and 4. Her husband Richard, aged 30, works in a steel mill and maintains a steady job, but drinks excessively on weekends and occasionally during the week. Jane and Richard have frequent fights when Richard drinks. It takes little or no provocation from Jane or the children to set Richard off into a rage, throwing and breaking furniture and occasionally hitting Jane and the older children.

423. Using the developmental approach in family assessment, at what stage of family development is the Smith family?
   A. Beginning
   B. School age
   C. Launching center
   D. Empty nest

424. Richard's abusive behavior is most likely related to
   A. effective coping with stress
   B. threats of rejection
   C. realistic expectations about marriage
   D. excessive drinking

425. Jane comes to a health clinic requesting help for Richard's drinking problem and his "bad temper." Your assessment of Jane should include
   A. relationship to her parents
   B. her mannerisms and style of clothing
   C. presence of multiple bruises
   D. her loyalty to her husband

426. Jane should be encouraged to
   A. talk about her family problems
   B. look for a job
   C. leave Richard
   D. report her experiences to the police

427. Richard's family background probably reflects
    A. inadequate sex education
    B. being abused as a child
    C. a strong male self-image
    D. a warm family relationship

428. A week later Jane Smith comes into the clinic with her four-year-old daughter, Margaret, in her arms. She claims that her daughter fell off a bike. Knowing the Smith's family history, your initial nursing action is to
    A. separate the mother from her child
    B. examine the child for bruises and old scars
    C. tell the physician about the Smith's family history
    D. tell Jane your doubts about the cause of the child's injury

429. Margaret is diagnosed as being an abused child. Since either Richard or Jane could potentially be the abuser, what data would support your belief that Jane is the abuser?
    A. Jane's unrealistic expectations of her daughter
    B. Jane's ineffective use of defense mechanisms
    C. The age difference between Jane and Richard
    D. The Smith family's low educational, social, and economic background

430. Violent behavior is associated with all of the following factors EXCEPT
    A. ethnicity
    B. psychosis
    C. drug use
    D. delirium

431. The sexually abused child is exploited in all of the following ways EXCEPT
    A. physically
    B. socially
    C. educationally
    D. emotionally

432. Strategies for primary prevention of child abuse include
    A. hospitalizing the abused child
    B. criminal punishment of abusers
    C. courses in parenting
    D. separating the abused child from parental abusers

Situation (Questions 433–440): Ann, a 28-year-old graduate student, returns to her apartment around 11:30 P.M. She is greeted by a man who says: "Hi Ann, remember me?" Ann recalls dating him once but before she can say or do anything, the man pushes her to the floor and forces intercourse. As the man leaves he says, "You deserved what you got tonight." Ann calls the local rape victims' clinic.

433. Ann calls the clinic saying, "I have to talk to someone or I'll go crazy. I should not have dated him." Before you can effectively respond to Ann, it is essential to
    A. recognize any bias you hold about rape
    B. call for assistance
    C. tape the conversation
    D. know some of the myths about rape

434. Ann arrives at the clinic alone, crying, but generally calm. In assessing Ann's condition it is important to first identify
    A. her support network and social relationships
    B. your legal responsibilities
    C. signs and symptoms of physical and emotional trauma
    D. her need to be alone

435. A complete physical and gynecologic examination is set up for Ann over her protest. Your role as the nurse is to
    A. convince Ann that this examination is essential
    B. contact Ann's parents
    C. inform the local police department of the incident
    D. inform Ann about her rights and support her decisions

436. Ann decides to undergo physical and gynecologic examinations. The nurse's initial action is to
    A. ask Ann what she wants to know about the examination
    B. provide Ann with a written explanation of each test
    C. request Ann to write down what she can remember about the incident
    D. assure Ann that the examining physician is an expert in rape victimization

437. Ann decides to prosecute the assailant. Evidentiary material should be gathered by the examining physician in the presence of a witness and the examining physician must
    A. personally do the laboratory analysis
    B. sign all laboratory results
    C. report all his findings to the police
    D. personally hand all specimens to a laboratory technician or a pathologist

438. Half of all rapes occur in a private residence and a third to a half of all sexual assaults are committed in
    A. a park
    B. the victim's residence
    C. a car
    D. the rapist's residence

439. Supporting the concept that rape is a violent nonimpulsive attack using sex as a weapon, what percentage of rapes are planned in advance by the rapist?
    A. 38%
    B. 50%
    C. 68%
    D. 98%

440. One of the myths of rape is that
     A. rapists choose victims without regard for age, race, or socioeconomic class
     B. rape is provoked by the victim
     C. rape is the fastest rising violent crime in the United States
     D. most rapes are intraracial

441. When a battered woman recognizes that her husband will not, or cannot, stop his violent behavior and she will no longer submit to it, she is in which stage of the battered woman syndrome?
     A. Denial
     B. Guilt
     C. Enlightenment
     D. Responsibility

442. Family dynamics in abusive families are characterized by
     A. tight social networks
     B. dominance of emotionality
     C. dependence upon cognitive processes
     D. dependence upon fundamentalist religious beliefs

K. SUBSTANCE ABUSE

443. Which of the following factors indicate a client is at high risk for the development of alcoholism?
     A. Being a middle child
     B. Having an alcoholic father
     C. Being the wife of a business executive
     D. Being the son of a Jewish banker

444. The nurse bases her assessment of the alcoholic client on the knowledge that, chemically, alcohol is a
     A. stimulant
     B. hallucinogen
     C. depressant
     D. phenothiazine

445. Coping mechanisms used by the alcoholic include
   A. repression and regression
   B. rationalization and denial
   C. reaction formation and undoing
   D. substitution and sublimation

446. A nursing care plan for a female alcoholic client would contain strategies for
   A. confronting her irresponsible parenting
   B. encouraging a divorce to lessen stress
   C. strengthening her self-concept
   D. teaching breast self-examination

447. In communicating with an alcoholic client, the most effective nursing approach is to
   A. be nonjudgmental and listen to his feelings
   B. encourage him to return to work
   C. give him pamphlets to read about alcoholism
   D. help him realize how unfair he has been

448. In working with alcoholic clients, the nurse encounters many situations that can lead to a stall in the therapeutic process. Among the common stall situations the nurse may experience is
   A. recognizing alcoholism as a disease
   B. judgmental attitudes toward drinking
   C. working toward prevention of alcoholism
   D. general optimism about selected treatment plan

449. A client in the emergency room tells you that she has had four drinks in the past hour; her blood alcohol level is 0.15%. Your analysis of this data is that she
   A. has developed tolerance to alcohol
   B. has a serious alcohol problem
   C. is at the level of legal intoxication
   D. must be feeling depressed

450. Acute alcoholic intoxication causes delirium in individuals by
   A. altering neurochemical responses in the brain
   B. decreasing the supply of oxygen or other nutrients to the brain
   C. increasing cerebral demand for oxygen
   D. increasing cerebral demand for metabolites

451. In assessing an alcoholic client for evidence of mild withdrawal symptoms, the nurse would be alert for the presence of
   A. diaphoresis and restlessness
   B. disorientation to time and place
   C. visual and auditory hallucinations
   D. highly disorganized agitation

452. Nursing assessment of the alcoholic during detoxification would include data related to
   A. ability to tolerate job-related stress
   B. ability to express emotions
   C. response to major tranquilizers given
   D. seizure potential

453. The priority nursing action during the detoxification phase of alcoholism treatment is
   A. teaching relaxation to control stress
   B. education about alcohol-related liver disease
   C. managing physiologic or psychologic instability
   D. uncovering of maladaptive defenses

454. Mr. Smith, a patient on the alcoholism detoxification unit for 24 hours, is now displaying elevated vital signs and marked disorientation. Your evaluation of this situation would be that Mr. Smith is
   A. oversedated
   B. progressing toward delirium tremens
   C. drinking on the unit
   D. developing renal failure

455. John, 17, is admitted for alcoholism. He is the youngest client in the unit and seems to be alone much of the time. When he attempts to kiss his nurse, she responds in a matter-of-fact way, telling him that such behavior is not necessary to maintain her interest in his therapy and welfare. The nurse indicates that John has shown a capacity for communicating his feelings, which is important in his treatment. In terms of Maslow's hierarchy, the nurse recognizes that John

    A. is out of control and should be restrained
    B. is really attempting to establish a meaningful relationship
    C. has fallen in love with her
    D. has a deep-seated sexual problem

456. One of the clients on the alcoholism treatment unit says, "They say I drink too much, but my real problem is my family doesn't appreciate me." Your analysis of this comment is that the client is

    A. using alcohol to maintain emotional distance in family relationships
    B. displaying insight into his alcoholism
    C. being too harsh on his family
    D. expressing feelings of depression that precede suicide

Situation (Questions 457–463): Mr. Pierce has frequent automobile accidents, outbursts of rage, and suicidal gestures when drinking. He also has a decreased tolerance to alcohol.

457. Which interpretation of Mr. Pierce's behavior is correct?

    A. His behavior is characteristic of the late stage of alcoholism
    B. His behavior is characteristic of early stage alcoholism
    C. His behavior is indicative of a long period of abstinence from alcohol
    D. His behavior is characteristic of an antisocial personality

458. Mr. Pierce frequently denies that he abuses alcohol. Which approach would be most appropriate in dealing with Mr. Pierce's denial?
   A. Confront him when he uses denial
   B. Teach the staff that denial can occur when the client does not always experience all effects from drinking
   C. Teach him the consequences of alcohol abuse
   D. Ignore his use of denial

459. Mr. Pierce needs to be observed for signs of delirium tremens (DTs). An early sign of DTs is
   A. vascular enlargement of the face
   B. coma
   C. hyperglycemia
   D. tremulousness

460. Mr. Pierce has lost many friends because of his inconsistent behavior while drinking. Which nursing action would facilitate achievement of the goal of increasing Mr. Pierce's socialization on the unit?
   A. Give Mr. Pierce plenty of time alone during the day
   B. Have Mr. Pierce join his group of "drinking buddies" in the evenings
   C. Appoint Mr. Pierce the president of the alcoholism unit
   D. Help Mr. Pierce learn to relate to others through a therapeutic relationship with the nurse

461. Which of the statements below indicates that Mr. Pierce has achieved the goal of increased socialization?
   A. "I prefer to drink by myself after work."
   B. "I don't need anybody."
   C. "When I can't find someone to drink with, I get a supply of beer."
   D. "I have twice as many friends now that I don't drink."

462. The nurse considers referring Mr. Pierce to Alcoholics Anonymous (AA). Which service does AA provide?
    A. Support to alcoholics and their families
    B. Job referral
    C. Physician referral
    D. Help to the alcoholic only

463. Mr. Pierce attents AA for a year by himself and has been assigned to another AA client. This is an indication that he is
    A. seeking a cohort for companionship while drinking
    B. is unable to stay away from alcohol
    C. recovering
    D. not showing improvement

Situation (Questions 464-465): Ms. Barnes has agreed to lead a therapy group of recently admitted alcoholic clients.

464. The nurse's role during the first session of this group is to
    A. function as a psychodynamic therapist
    B. be nondirective
    C. leave the group after members start talking
    D. provide information about the unit and program

465. Ms. Barnes and a group of female clients engage in a "rap" session. The role of the nurse at this time is to
    A. frequently interject her opinion during the session
    B. act as a listener and clarifier
    C. allow the clients to manipulate her as a way to build trust
    D. control the group to prevent expression of feelings

Situation (Questions 466–471):   Mr. Range is admitted to the alcohol detoxification unit.

466. Which nursing assessment of Mr. Range assumes priority?
   A. Skin turgor, nutrition, anxiety
   B. Respiratory or cardiac embarrassment, excessive bleeding
   C. Hyperreflexia, fever, diaphoresis
   D. Diarrhea, nausea, and vomiting

467. During the acute care phase of Mr. Range's withdrawal from alcohol, which goal is most appropriate?
   A. Verbalizing increased feelings of self-worth
   B. Exploring alternatives to drinking
   C. Identifying his drinking problem
   D. Stabilizing his overall physical condition

468. Mr. Range's vital signs are: T, 102°F; P, 90; R, 30; BP, 140/90. Which nursing action is most appropriate?
   A. Providing a calm supportive environment
   B. Giving client the ordered hypnotic
   C. Increasing fluid intake
   D. Socialize with others on the unit

469. Which observations by the nurse indicate that Mr. Range is out of the acute withdrawal phase?
   A. He says he will only drink beer from now on
   B. He is semiobtunded with petechiae and icteric scelera
   C. His vital signs are normal with no signs of agitation
   D. He continues to have seizures

470. Chlordiazepoxide (Librium) 100 mg IM q6hr is ordered for Mr. Range depending upon the severity of his symptoms. The purpose of this medication is to
   A. help the client's nutritional status
   B. interfere with alcohol consumption
   C. act as an aversive agent
   D. temporarily duplicate the depressant action of alcohol on the central nervous system

471. Disulfiram (Antabuse) is prescribed for Mr. Range. Which statement indicates that he understands the effects of this medication?

   A. "I can eat a gourmet dinner now."
   B. "A small drink can make me very ill."
   C. "This drug will cure my alcoholism."
   D. "If I stop taking disulfiram I can have a drink in 3 hours."

472. An alcoholic client tells you he has been taking disulfiram and has just had several drinks. Your immediate care plan would focus on relief of the resulting

   A. paralytic ileus
   B. profuse bleeding
   C. leg cramping
   D. severe hypotension

Situation (Questions 473–477): Ms. Lewis is admitted to the detoxification unit. She is obviously intoxicated, talkative, and belligerent.

473. Which nursing assessment assumes priority?

   A. The client's perceptual ability
   B. Degree of psychomotor hyperactivity
   C. Client's degree of self-esteem
   D. Client's hygiene

474. The goal of care assuming priority for Ms. Lewis at this time is to

   A. promote personal hygiene
   B. detect changes in vital signs
   C. motivate client for treatment
   D. protect client from self-inflicted injury

475. While caring for Ms. Lewis it would be most important to

   A. give her a backrub
   B. determine the nature of her work
   C. talk with her about alcoholism
   D. provide for safety factors

476. Ms. Lewis's blood alcohol level is 0.13%. How should this result be interpreted by the nurse?
    A. This is a low level; it should produce no problems
    B. This is a dangerously high blood alcohol level
    C. Ms. Lewis should be observed for ketoacidosis
    D. Ms. Lewis probably is not following her prescribed diet

477. During a termination interview with Ms. Lewis, which statement indicates the highest degree of client insight?
    A. "I will never be cured of my alcoholism."
    B. "If I wait 3 weeks I'll be able to have another drink."
    C. "It's my mother's fault that I drink."
    D. "I just want to stay here and not leave."

478. As you counsel an alcoholic who is about to be discharged, you encourage him to seek continuing health supervision of common health problems associated with chronic alcohol abuse such as
    A. malnutrition
    B. fear and anxiety
    C. insomnia
    D. susceptibility to respiratory infections

479. Mr. Smith is to be discharged from the alcoholism treatment unit today. He tells you that the most important part of his treatment was learning to communicate more openly with his family. Your evaluation of his progress is that he is successfully learning to
    A. become independent and self-sufficient
    B. give up all association with drinkers
    C. face the grief he has caused others
    D. rely more on people than alcohol

Situation (Questions 480–482): Mr. Green comes to the emergency room sweating profusely, trembling, and showing signs of agitation. He is disoriented as to time and place, and believes he has hives from a mosquito bite.

480. Which nursing action assumes priority at this time?
   A. Requesting an order for an antihistamine
   B. Taking a nursing history to document possible causes of presenting symptoms
   C. Isolating the client to protect others
   D. Restricting oral fluid intake

481. Mrs. Green is worried her husband will have a convulsion. The nursing assessment should focus on Mr. Green's
   A. history of seizures
   B. medication history
   C. nutritional status
   D. psychologic history

482. A diagnosis of alcohol withdrawal syndrome is made and Mrs. Green's physician orders chlorpromazine to control his withdrawal symptoms. Which aspect of the patient's nursing history is important to report to his physician?
   A. History of insomnia
   B. Liver disease
   C. Consumes 8–10 cups of coffee per day
   D. Takes multivitamins daily

483. The feature distinguishing hallucinogenic drugs from other drugs of abuse is their capacity to
   A. induce states of altered perception
   B. produce severe respiratory depression
   C. provide both stimulation and depression
   D. produce rapid physical dependence

484. The nursing care plan for a drug abuser would include strategies for helping the addict deal with his
    A. dependency needs
    B. hostility
    C. regression
    D. displacement

485. Mrs. Smith tells you that she has been taking pills to calm her nerves and pills to help her sleep. She adds that she finds herself using more of the pills lately to get the same relaxation. Your analysis of this data is that Mrs. Smith is displaying
    A. blackouts
    B. physical illness
    C. tolerance
    D. withdrawal symptoms

486. Mr. Johnson is admitted for heroin detoxification. Your assessment is based on the knowledge that psychologic dependence is characterized by the
    A. presence of withdrawal symptoms
    B. need for continually larger doses
    C. drive to continue the drug
    D. use of several types of drugs

487. Tony is a 15-year-old who is hospitalized for an orthopedic problem. As you are making rounds you detect the odor of marijuana at his doorway and you observe him smoking in his room. An appropriate nursing action is to
    A. call the security guard to handle the situation
    B. ignore Tony's behavior as he is seeking attention
    C. accept Tony's behavior as he is not disturbing anyone
    D. confront Tony and tell him this behavior is unacceptable there

488. In assessing a client who has suddenly stopped taking amphetamines, it is most important for the nurse to note the presence of
    A. suicidal ideation
    B. muscle cramping and pain
    C. respiratory distress
    D. euphoria

489. Mr. Anderson is admitted with a diagnosis of narcotic withdrawal. Symptoms of narcotic withdrawal include
    A. lack of coordination
    B. rhinorrhea and sore throat
    C. combativeness and dizziness
    D. slurred speech and confusion

490. In caring for a client with a sedative overdose, which nursing action assumes priority?
    A. Administering the appropriate antagonist
    B. Ensuring an adequate airway
    C. Starting an IV
    D. Obtaining an accurate drug history '

491. Nursing actions assuming priority during barbiturate detoxification include
    A. preventing seizure activity
    B. preventing psychiatric complications
    C. developing client insight
    D. developing client identity

492. The chief goal of nursing intervention in heroin overdose is the maintenance of
    A. contact with reality
    B. adequate fluid intake
    C. a safe environment
    D. adequate respiration

493. Which nursing intervention is most appropriate for the client who overdoses with hallucinogens?
   A. Assisting with goal-directed activities
   B. Preventing flashbacks
   C. Administering IV fluids for stabilization of cardio-vascular system
   D. Maintaining a safe environment while client sleeps off drug effects

494. A client experiencing a cocaine overdose can develop which complication?
   A. Circulatory collapse
   B. Gangrene
   C. Septicemia
   D. Vascular rupture

495. In caring for Mr. Nelson, aged 61, who is admitted for treatment of severe, chronic low-back pain, it is most important to determine his
   A. financial status
   B. family support
   C. level of consciousness
   D. potential drug dependence

496. You have developed a teaching plan to help female clients who have been abusing sedatives and tranquilizers. Which of the following would be important to include?
   A. That tranquilizers are safe to take during pregnancy
   B. That prescription drugs are safe if taken as directed
   C. Strategies for ensuring adequate nutrition are essential
   D. Diazepam (Valium) and alcohol can be a lethal combination

497. Mr. Johnson has been sentenced by a criminal court judge to your facility for treatment of his narcotic addiction. You recognize that his motivation for treatment is
    A. internal and receptive
    B. dependent on his physical discomfort
    C. external but promising
    D. reality-based and strong

498. Rehabilitation of the drug addict involves helping the client to alter his life-style. Which of the following nursing measures would be most helpful?
    A. Demanding total abstinence from all drugs
    B. Imposing restrictions when client is inappropriate
    C. Positive reinforcement of non–drug-oriented problem solving
    D. Using street jargon when talking with client

499. Mrs. Samuels has been making satisfactory progress in the drug rehabilitation program and is about to be discharged. Which of the following would indicate control of drug use at a recreational level?
    A. Having a daily after-dinner glass of wine
    B. Restricting coffee to 2 cups a day
    C. Smoking no more than one pack a day
    D. Smoking two joints a day

500. The client most likely to suffer relapse following drug abuse treatment, because of the powerful primary reinforcement of the substance, is the client who has used
    A. cocaine and heroin
    B. LSD and PCP
    C. marijuana
    D. sleeping pills

501. Mr. Adams is being discharged following detoxification from heroin. He is going to be attending the methadone clinic. After considering his comments about looking forward to getting back into circulation with his old friends, your evaluation is that he
   A. greatly needs the support of others
   B. does not feel stigmatized by society
   C. continues to need assistance in altering his life-style
   D. may not benefit from continued administration of methadone

502. Mr. Jonnson is being discharged following narcotic detoxification. He tells you that he will be attending a day-treatment center for addicted clients. You reinforce his decision because
   A. he needs confidence in his decision making
   B. such programs provide needed structure
   C. his family is unable to help him
   D. he has successfully manipulated you

4

Answers and Rationales

For each question the nursing behavior (NB) and locus of decision making (LDM) has been identified following the rationale.

A. BASIC CONCEPTS OF NURSING PRACTICE IN MENTAL HEALTH

1. Theories of Personality and Psychosocial Development and Their Application

1. **B.** In Sullivan's theory the three modes of perception are syntaxic, prototoxic, and parataxic. He believed human beings must be socialized into people able to live in a social organization. Emphasis is on interpersonal growth and development, and the motivation for behavior is the avoidance of anxiety and satisfaction of needs. *(NB, analyzing; LDM, nurse centered)*

Haber et al., p. 51

2. **D.** In this situation the mother's anxiety is communicated to her infant, leading to uncertainty and a sense of mistrust in the infant. The infant's anxious behavior may generate further inadequate or inconsistent nurturing patterns, perpetuating a cycle of anxiety. Options A, B, and C are

explanations sometimes used by lay persons to allay parental concerns. *(NB, analyzing; LDM, shared)*

Haber et al., pp. 52, 151

3. B. Late adolescence, the last stage in Sullivan's theory, is concerned with developing an enduring intimate relationship with one member of the opposite sex and occurs by about 21 years of age. Maturity is the last stage in Erikson's theory of social growth and development, occurring between 45 years and death. Self-actualization is the highest level of Maslow's hierarchy of needs. Civilized identity is the fourth stage of societal development postulated by Glasser. *(NB, evaluating; LDM, client centered)*

Haber et al., pp. 50–52

4. D. According to Sullivan's theory of anxiety, hysteria is the result of an unresolved conflict with a significant person. Option A describes Freud's explanation for neurosis and neurotic behavior, and option B, Engel's theory of the cause of anxiety. Option C describes Bateson's theory of the cause of schizophrenia. *(NB, analyzing; LDM, nurse centered)*

Burgess, pp. 236–237, 275; Pasquali et al., p. 143

5. A. Freud theorized that sexual growth and development was the basis of many unconscious conflicts, and he developed a scheme to clarify the stages and emerging conflict. The oral state is the initial one, followed by the anal, phallic, latency, and genital stages. Option B describes the stages which Erikson describes in his theory of social growth and development. Option C describes developmental tools which are a part of Sullivan's theory of interpersonal growth and development. Option D describes Freud's aspects of consciousness. *(NB, assessing; LDM, nurse centered)*

Haber et al., pp. 48–52

6. A. According to Freudian theory, anxiety is the response of the ego to unconscious material that threatens to emerge into conciousness. Because anxiety is such an unpleasant experience, people have several built in mechanisms to defend themselves from it. Defense mechanisms are abilities the ego calls into play to protect against anxiety; they operate outside awareness. *(NB, assessing; LDM, nurse centered)*

Haber et al., p. 48

7. **D.** The id, one of three aspects of personality described by Freud, includes the instinctual forces and is primarily unconscious, expressed as thoughts and feelings. The ego assesses reality. The id is unable to delay gratification. *(NB, analyzing, LDM, nurse centered)*

Haber et al., p. 48

8. **B.** The ego appraises environment, assesses reality, stays in touch with bodily and environmental changes, and directs the motor activity of the body. The ego substitutes reality for pleasure. Conscience is analagous to the superego, and the ego is reality oriented, maintaining the balance between id and superego. *(NB, analyzing, LDM, nurse centered)*

Haber et al., p. 48

9. **C.** The superego contains the rigid, absolute rules that direct a person's thoughts, feelings, and actions; it is analagous to conscience except that the superego contains conscious and unconscious material. The superego often directly opposes the forces of the id. *(NB, analyzing, LDM, nurse centered)*

Haber et al., p. 48

10. **B.** In the developmental task of trust-vs-mistrust, experiences with the nurturing person are the foundations of the level of trust a person will develop. In this situation the girl wants lasting relationships but is afraid to trust people, expressing her discomfort in sarcasm, hostile behavior, and overprotection of her possessions. She has not mastered the

task of trust-vs-mistrust, the first in Erikson's scheme, so cannot be in the successive stages of initiative-vs-guilt, industry-vs-inferiority, and intimacy-vs-role diffusion. Chronologically the girl should be mastering industry-vs-inferiority but her behaviors are directed toward trust relationships, not work situations.(*NB, analyzing; LDM, shared*)

Haber et al., p. 50

11. D. Ego integrity is an affirmation of meaning in one's life, and lack of ego integrity is manifested by fear of death and despair. Relations to self and others are negotiated earlier in life. Behavior as a conditioned response is emphasized in the behavioral model, not in Erikson's framework. Irrational thinking is seen as the primary cause of maladaptive behavior by the cognitive school. *(NB, analyzing; LDM, nurse centered)*

Haber et al., pp. 50, 54, 60–61

12. D. Jung believed that a person is predisposed to certain deep expectations, longings, and terrors rooted in his history and above his experiences as an individual. Dream interpretations should be used in a goal-focused way rather than in seeking causative sources. Freud used dreams to explain sources of psychic problems. Jung's approach does not deal with belief systems or thinking nor with external stimuli and reinforcers. *(NB, assessing; LDM, shared)*

Burgess, pp. 389–391

13. B. In the psychologic model, therapy consists of clarifying the psychologic meaning of events, feelings, and behaviors. Forgotten events may be remembered, reexperienced, and put into perspective so the patient can be freed to see current situations as they really are. In the social model the focus is on the way the individual functions in the social system. The behavioral model emphasizes that behavior is learned and maintained because it leads to positive results. The biologic model views psychiatric illness as a disease like others. *(NB, analyzing; LDM, shared)*

Burgess, pp. 110, 119, 126, 128

14. D. In the interpersonal model anxiety is experienced interpersonally and symptoms occur when security operations are unable to protect the self from anxiety. The crux of the therapeutic process is corrective interpersonal experience. The nurse-patient relationship builds patient security. In the social model social resources are used to work toward resolution of the patient's problem. The psychoanalytic model uses the patient's thoughts and dreams which the therapist interprets. In the behavioral model the patient practices behavioral techniques and develops behavioral hierarchies. *(NB, planning; LDM, shared)*

Stuart and Sundeen (1979), pp. 22, 37–39

15. C. In client-centered therapy groups the respect for and confidence in a client's capacity to direct his or her life makes them responsible for the course, direction, and speed of therapy; the locus of evaluation of change always lies with the client. Social interaction occurs in a client-centered group but not for the purpose of control. Identification and support of existing coping patterns reflect didactic therapy. Etiology, diagnosis, and prognosis are not components of client-centered therapy. *(NB, analyzing; LDM, client centered)*

Haber et al., pp. 58–59

16. C. Reinforcement schedules are basically operant-conditioning techniques based on Skinnerian principles. Dreams, past experiences, and free association are key concepts in psychoanalytic theory in which all behavior is considered meaningful. *(NB, assessing; LDM, shared)*

Haber et al., pp. 47, 54

17. B. Behavioral therapists believe all behavior is learned, and since it is learned, can be unlearned and replaced by more adequate, appropriate behavior. Self-understanding or insight are not components of behavior therapy, which begins with the client's maladaptive behavior; past life is not extensively reviewed as the maladaptive behavior is the focus of attention. Deconditioning uses external stimuli to shape behavior. *(NB, analyzing; LDM, nurse centered)*

Haber et al., pp. 54–55

18. **A.** A planned response pattern to extinguish inappropriate modes of behavior is a component of behavior therapy, as part of the deconditioning process. Verbalization is not a major component of behavior therapy. "Support" is non-specific and not a behavioral principle. Intellectual understanding of symptoms is more psychodynamic than behavioral in orientation. *(NB, planning; LDM, shared)*

Haber et al., pp. 54–55

19. **A.** Systematic desensitization is a step-by-step use of a counteracting emotion to overcome an undesirable emotional habit; it involves training in deep muscle relaxation, use of a scale of subjective anxiety, construction of anxiety hierarchies, and use of relaxation techniques. Sharing of perceptions, meaning, and values; self-exploration and self-assessment; and developmental history are not components of the behavioral model of care. *(NB, planning; LDM, shared)*

Haber et al., pp. 54–55

20. **B.** Rogers views people as able to direct their lives in healthy ways. In a climate of unconditional acceptance people are able to become aware of unconscious material that is controlling their lives. The locus of therapy lies with the client. Rogers states that current needs are the only ones the person endeavors to satisfy. Focus on distracting topics diverts the client from thinking about current feelings. Prognosis is future oriented, and the focus is on current needs. *(NB, planning; LDM, client centered)*

Haber et al., pp. 58–59

21. **C.** Reality therapy focuses on what one is doing rather than on what one is feeling. After clients become more aware of their behavior, they are helped to look at it critically to

judge its effectiveness and social acceptability. In reality therapy, talking about the patient's specific problems is not emphasized because it is thought that talking too much about problems increases feelings of failure. Reality therapy emphasizes two major psychologic needs: to love and be loved and to feel worthwhile to oneself and others. People who cannot satisfy these needs without harming others are irresponsible. *(NB, evaluating; LDM, client centered)*

Wilson and Kneisl (1979), pp. 670–671

22. C. In rational-emotive therapy both emotions and behavior depend upon cognitive mediation occurring in relation to every experience. Rational beliefs help the individual accept reality and live in intimate relationships with others, while irrationality is synonymous with self-destructive behavior. Healthy functioning is possible only when the values in which one believes are rational ones. In this situation the husband's values are irrational. Since there was a harmonious marital relationship before the wife's surgery, the husband was capable of such a relationship. Rational-emotive therapy does not try to evaluate past conflicts and repressed feelings. Illogical thinking, not overdependence on others for gratification, is the root of maladaptive behavior. *(NB, evaluating; LDM, shared)*

Wilson and Kneisl (1979), p. 671

23. A. Rational-emotive therapy helps people dispel their disturbing beliefs by explaining what irrational beliefs are and how they cause emotional difficulty. After logical analysis, one sees that irrational beliefs are unnecessary and eliminates them. There is no way the daughter could know her father would need care while she was away. She can participate in her father's convalescence once she corrects her irrational beliefs. There are no data concerning the father's perceptions. *(NB, analyzing; LDM, shared)*

Wilson and Kneisl (1979), p. 671

24. C. Adler emphasized the social aspects of human involvement and the role of education as an essential means to foster and expand social interest. Differentiating feelings and behaviors would be used in a psychodynamic approach, while prescribing behavior changes and desensitization are components of the behavioral model. *(NB, implementing; LDM, shared)*

Burgess, p. 391

25. B. The center of Horney's theory is the self, viewed in terms of actual self, real self, and idealized self. Goals of therapy are self-realization and self-actualization and dealing with here-and-now issues. Challenging the patient to a game of table tennis allows her to resolve the immediate conflict and cope effectively with the situation. The patient is probably unable to deal immediately with her behavior, especially in front of others. Limit setting would probably make the patient more angry and increase her acting out. *(NB, implementing; LDM, nurse centered)*

Burgess, p. 393;
Wilson and Kneisl (1979), p. 539

26. C. Anticipatory guidance such as explaining the meaning of negativistic behavior in a 2-year-old helps the mother understand and deal more effectively with the behavior. Option A describes intervention after an event occurs, not preventing its occurrence. Option B describes a secondary prevention approach rather than anticipatory guidance. Establishing a trust relationship, while important, is not part of anticipatory guidance. *(NB, analyzing; LDM, shared)*

Taylor, p. 147

27. C. An overemphasis on safety is considered a general characteristic of neurotic behavior. Vivid recall of past life events is not indicative of any psychiatric disorder. A loss may precipitate a crisis but is not the only cause for neurotic behavior. Disrespect for the law is characteristic of an individual with an antisocial personality disorder. *(NB, assessing; LDM, nurse centered)*

Grace and Camilleri, pp. 152–153

28. **C.** The psychotic patient experiences gross distortion of external reality (i.e., hallucinations, delusions, illusions). Therefore control of distorted thought perceptions would be appropriate for a psychotic patient. Options A, B, and D reflect goals pertinent for neurotic patients. *(NB, analyzing; LDM, shared)*

Burgess, p. 235

2. Coping/Defense Mechanisms

29. **C.** Ego defense mechanisms protect the ego from being overwhelmed with anxiety. Everyone uses them in coping with mild to moderate levels of anxiety; they operate on relatively unconscious levels. No person can be consistently free of anxiety and the mechanisms do not always work. *(NB, analyzing; LDM, nurse centered)*

Burgess, pp. 26–27;
Stuart and Sundeen (1979), pp. 82–83

30. **B.** Isolation is the exclusion from awareness of the feelings connected to a thought, memory, or experience. The person remembering the experience or thought does not reexperience the emotion that originally accompanied it. Regression is a return to an earlier stage of development. In repression, painful thoughts are barred from conscious recognition. Rationalization is an attempt to make one's behavior appear to be the result of rational thinking rather than of unconscious origin. *(NB, analyzing; LDM, nurse centered)*

Haber et al., p. 46

31. **A.** Regression is the ego's return to an earlier stage of development in thought, feeling, or behavior. It appears transiently during times of stress when it is used as a retreat from anxiety and conflict. This girl's behavior is typical of that of a 2-year-old. Repression is the barring from consciousness of painful experiences or unacceptable thoughts. Denial is the total failure to acknowledge the existence of an affect, experience, idea, or memory. Isolation is the exclusion of awareness of the feelings connected to a thought, memory, or experience. *(NB, analyzing; LDM, client centered)*

Haber et al., pp. 46–47

32. C. The new graduate is using rationalization as a coping mechanism. She is attempting to make her behavior appear to be the result of logical thinking rather than of unconscious impulses or desires. Rationalization is used when a person has a sense of guilt or uncertainty, a face-saving device that may or may not deal with the truth. The supervisor's approach indicated interest in the new graduate and offers opportunity to explore the meaning of her behavior. Options A, B, and D all pass judgment without attempting to clarify the meaning of the nurse's behavior. *(NB, planning; LDM, shared)*

Haber et al., p. 47

33. C. This physician perceives his stature negatively and is trying to overcome this by being aggressive, forceful, and controlling in his interactions with the staff. The head nurse's approach acknowledges the physician's behavior and could provide an opportunity to discuss staff concerns with him. Options A, B, and D all emphasize the physician's poor self-concept and closed communication channels. *(NB, implementing; LDM, shared)*

Stuart and Sundeen (1979), p. 84

34. A. Sublimation is the acceptance of a socially approved substitute goal for a drive whose normal channel of expression is blocked. In this situation the woman wants children but has been unable to have any as yet; her desires find natural expression in working with babies as a hospital volunteer. Compensation is the process of making up for a deficiency in self-image by emphasizing another feature regarded as an asset. Regression is return to an earlier developmental level. Repression is the exclusion of a painful thought or impulse from awareness. *(NB, analyzing; LDM, client centered)*

Stuart and Sundeen (1979), pp. 83–84

35. B. In projection, one's feelings, thoughts, or wishes are attributed to others in an effort to deny their existence in the self. This nurse is projecting her insecurities on the head nurse. Option A is an example of rationalization of anxiety. Option C is a mature, reality-oriented statement, not a defense mechanism. Option D is an example of denial. *(NB, evaluating; LDM, shared)*

Haber et al., pp. 46–47

36. A. Condensation involves concentrating several thoughts and feelings into a relatively simple verbal or nonverbal message. In this situation, the "old bat" hit the boy or inflicted some other type of punishment on him. Identification is the unconscious modeling of self after some admired figure. In projection characteristics or thoughts are attributed to another. Displacement is the shift of emotion from a person or object toward which it was originally directed to a neutral or less dangerous person or object. *(NB, analyzing; LDM, client centered)*

Stuart and Sundeen (1979), pp. 84, 151

37. C. In a conversion reaction symptoms of some physical illness appear without an underlying organic pathologic condition, relieving anxiety. The organic symptom usually symbolizes the conflict; in this instance, the man hitting his father. Suppression is the intentional exclusion of material from consciousness. Displacement is the shift of emotion from the original person or object to a neutral or less dangerous person or object. Undoing is the act or communication that partially negates a previous one. *(NB, analyzing; LDM, shared)*

Stuart and Sundeen (1979), pp. 83–86

38. A. Denial is the avoidance of disagreeable realities by ignoring or refusing to recognizing them. This patient is avoiding the reality of his diagnosis by saying he is going home. Repression is the involuntary excluding thoughts or feelings from consciousness, and suppression is the intentional, conscious exclusion of thoughts or feelings. Compensation is a process of making up a deficiency in self-image by overemphasizing another. *(NB, analyzing; LDM, client centered)*

Stuart and Sundeen, pp. 215–216

39. A. In reaction formation the patient develops conscious attitudes and behavior patterns that are the opposite of what one really feels or would like to do. This patient's anger toward the male staff is opposite to her feelings. Reaction formation is voluntary, whereas repression is involuntary exclusion of feelings from conscious awareness. The patient has not incorporated another person's values, and her behavior does not suggest return to a previous developmental level. *(NB, analyzing; LDM, client centerd)*

Stuart and Sundeen, pp. 215–216

40. A. This patient appears to be displacing her own feelings of unworthiness, guilt, and being "dirty" to the coffee cups and does not want anyone else to use them. Suppression is the intentional exclusion of material from consciousness. Regression is the return to an earlier developmental level. Denial is the avoidance of painful realities by refusing to recognize that they have occurred. *(NB, analyzing; LDM, client centered)*

Stuart and Sundeen (1983), pp. 215–216

41. A. This patient is displacing her feelings of anger from a more powerful figure, her husband, to a less powerful figure, the nurse. In denial, painful or anxiety-producing aspects of reality are blocked out. Projection involves attributing one's own unacceptable attitudes to another person.

Rationalization is an attempt to make one's behavior appear to be the result of logical thinking rather than of unconscious origin. *(NB, analyzing; LDM, client centered)*

Haber et al., pp. 46–47

42. C. The nurse understands that this patient is displacing her guilt by excessive handwashing in an attempt to allay her anxiety. The patient's anxiety cannot be controlled until her anxiety level is reduced, and shaming will only increase her anxiety. The patient may or may not be aware that her behavior is irrational, but she cannot control it, so asking if her hands are dirty is irrelevant. *(NB, implementing; LDM, shared)*

Stuart and Sundeen (1983), pp. 215–216

43. B. By profusely apologizing about his outburst the previous day, the patient is undoing, attempting to cancel its significance. Rationalization is the offering of a logical explanation for behavior resulting from unconscious impulses. In repression, painful thoughts or feelings are involuntarily excluded from conscious awareness. Blaming others for one's own actions is projection. *(NB, analyzing; LDM, client centered)*

Haber et al., p. 46

44. B. This patient is explaining away his apparent lack of friends by saying he is not appreciated; he is rationalizing, attempting to make his personal situation the result of logical thinking rather than unconscous impulses or desires. Fantasy is a retreat into daydreaming where the individual can fashion his own world. Sublimination is the substitution of socially acceptable pursuits for unwanted sexual or aggressive drives. Compensation is overcoming a deficiency in one area by excelling in another. *(NB, analyzing; LDM, client centered)*

Haber et al., pp. 46–47

45. A. In introjection the feelings, attitudes, and values of a most significant other are incorporated into one's own ego, becoming a part of oneself without which one cannot psychologically survive. Projection is the process of attributing one's unacceptable attributes to another. In displacement dangerous thoughts and feelings are transferred from a more powerful to a less powerful figure. Undoing is the negation of prior behavior by subsequent behavior. *(NB, analyzing; LDM, client centered)*

Stuart and Sundeen (1983), pp. 215–216

46. C. This patient is retreating to behavior appropriate at an earlier developmental level, i.e., regressing. Option A describes an aggressive response. Option B suggests projection, and option D, rationalization. *(NB, analyzing; LDM, client centered)*

Stuart and Sundeen (1983), pp. 215–216

47. A. Patients with phobias have persistent fears of some object or situation that presents no actual danger to the patient. The phobic object often symbolizes the original object or situation, and the dynamics of this reaction include the exaggerated use of displacement to obtain relief from anxiety. Projection involves attributing one's own thoughts and feelings to another. Suppression is the intentional exclusion of material from consciousness, and repression, the involuntary exclusion of such material. *(NB, assessing; LDM, client centered)*

Stuart and Sundeen (1979), pp. 83–84

48. C. The patient who is experiencing a conversion reaction needs to have the sick role minimized because it becomes the source of meeting his needs. Positive interactions with other patients is a means of verbalizing anxieties rather than somaticizing them. Focusing on the patient's impairment serves to reinforce the importance of the disability to him. Insisting the patient attend physical therapy calls additional attention to the disability. Telling the patient to "grow up" will only increase his anxiety. *(NB, planning; LDM, shared)*

Haber et al., p. 465

3. Communication Skills

49. C. From the data presented, it appears that there is a discrepancy between the patient's verbal and nonverbal messages which the nurse needs to explore. Nonverbal communication is often unconscious, and whether the patient is lying or is simply unaware of how upset she is must be validated by the nurse. While the patient's verbal communication must be taken seriously, she may be unaware of her nonverbal messages. *(NB, analyzing; LDM, shared)*

Burgess, p. 70

50. B. The patient's verbal and nonverbal behavior is blocking the interview process and the patient may or may not be aware that she seems to be demonstrating resistance. For this reason the patient's behavior should be explored to determine if the behavior is indeed resistance or if the patient is simply anxious. Ignoring the patient's behavior will not remove the apparent communication barrier, and telling her that you find her behavior annoying will probably increase her defensiveness. It is premature to terminate the interview without exploring the meaning of the patient's behavior. *(NB, implementing; LDM, shared)*

Wilson and Kneisl (1979), p. 146

51. B. From the data presented, all that can be said is that the nurse is expressing the anger the patient has not, or cannot, express. The presence of a depressed patient tends to evoke feelings of sadness, irritability, hostility, and helplessness in the nurse. The depressed person may not know the source or object of his anger and avoids confronting these feelings. To assess a countertransference response, data concerning whether or not the nurse's response to the patient is similar to her response to an earlier significant figure in her life must be presented, and they are not. Although the nurse may feel anger toward a patient who allows himself to be misused, it is more likely she is picking up his unconscious anger at being misused. Even if the nurse is depressed and overidentifying, the crucial issue is still how the patient experiences being misused by others. *(NB, analyzing; LDM, nurse centered)*

Haber et al., pp. 541–544, 548

52. C. The theme of loss is evident from the patient's statements concerning loss of his father, loss of his leg, and the anticipated loss of his girl friend. Guilt and dependence are not mentioned. While it might be inferred that the patient's losses cause grief, the only data explicitly stated concern loss. *(NB, analyzing; LDM, shared)*

Haber et al., p. 262

53. A. Nonuseful responses occur as a spontaneous reaction to increased anxiety and when we do not know what to say. A cliche such as, "How are you today?" is not useful because it does not provide opportunity for greater verbal exchange. A statement of recognition, observation, or a broad opening would be more useful. We have insufficient data to know whether or not the patient is depressed. Questions that begin with "how" or "why" are often viewed as threatening by the patient. Even though this interaction begins with a probing word, "how," the content is not meaningful and should not provoke patient anxiety. Direct questions are often useful in clarifying and extending nurse-patient communication. *(NB, evaluating; LDM, nurse centered)*

Burgess, pp. 65–69

54. D. In challenging, the nurse feels that if the patient is challenged to prove unrealistic ideas or perceptions, the client will realize there is no proof to support such ideas and will be forced to acknowledge what is true. The nurse forgets that unrealistic thoughts, perceptions, and feelings serve a purpose for the client. When challenged, the client feels threatened and tends to cling to and expand the misinterpretation because they support his point of view. Giving reassurance is an effort to soothe and avoid rather than explore the patient's painful feelings. Changing the subject diverts the focus of interaction at a crucial time to something less threatening. Being judgmental is responding to a patient with value-laden judgments which come from the nurse's value system. *(NB, evaluating; LDM, nurse centered)*

Haber et al., pp. 244–245

55. B. Only when the nurse's feelings, thoughts, and behavior are identified through self-assessment and are synchronized through self-awareness can the nurse perceive how these dimensions of self influence client behavior and care. Awareness that the client in this situation reminds the nurse of significant others and recognizing the feelings which the client's behavior generates will help the nurse better understand the dynamics of the relationship. Both objective and subjective data about the patient are important to the care plan. Even with the patient who has a history of substance abuse there are areas of trust that can be established. Asking another nurse to care for this patient is unnecessary and only delays the nurse's thorough self-assessment. *(NB, planning; LDM, nurse centered)*

Haber et al., pp. 197–198

56. A. At the end of an interview there should always be a feeling of satisfaction that something of significance was accomplished. There should be a definite closing with both nurse and patient acknowledging that both understood what was said. Planning may be a more appropriate component of a subsequent session. The quality of the nursing diagnosis has nothing to do with the therapeutic benefit of an interview nor does the amount of historical data obtained. *(NB, evaluating; LDM, shared)*

Burgess, pp. 64–65

57. A. At termination the patient often tries to convert the therapeutic relationship into a social one, requesting personal information, etc. This situation gives the nurse the opportunity to help the patient talk about other times when he has had to terminate relationships and how he has dealt with saying goodbye to other individuals. Accepting the patient's invitation would fulfill the patient's wish to avoid the pain of losing a significant relationship. Hospital policy and joking are both ways of the nurse hiding from her own feelings. *(NB, implementing; LDM, shared)*

Burgess, pp. 64–65

4. Group and Family Therapy

58. C. Suggesting that the former therapist be involved in making a decision about group therapy for this client is a way of redirecting him back to the therapist for help since the client is delusional. Delusional patients are not candidates for group therapy. The client's written or verbal permission is necessary to properly obtain medical records. Contacting the patient's wife should be considered but is not a priority. *(NB, implementing; LDM, shared)*

Stuart and Sundeen (1979), pp. 324–325, 328–329

59. C. Group therapy is useful in treating emotional stress and disorder through group process. However, individuals may be frightened and feel more vulnerable because of the self-disclosure expected. The group leader probably did not ignore the client but was waiting for her to determine her role in the group. Orientation to the group is essential to determine suitability for participation in the group. After two sessions the client did not have sufficient information about the other members to make a realistic assessment of mutual compatibility. *(NB, evaluating; LDM, shared)*

Stuart and Sundeen (1979), pp. 324, 328–329

60. B. Effectiveness of group therapy is often contingent upon the ability and willingness of group members to be open and disclose information about themselves. Self-disclosure is usually viewed as being more difficult in a group setting, but the group can help people become more aware of their interaction and coping patterns. If the patient feels blocked with his individual therapist, he must work this out with the therapist. Meeting a mate is not a group therapy goal, and fear of consensual validation may contraindicate the group therapy approach as such validation is one advantage of the group. *(NB, planning; LDM, shared)*

Burgess, p. 417;
Stuart and Sundeen (1979), pp. 324–325

61. D. Selection of group members is an important task since the composition of the group will greatly influence its outcome. The leader develops selection criteria on the basis of purposes of the group, and interviews prospective members to determine their appropriateness for the group based on these criteria, which are shared with the prospective members. Ability to give time to the group, willingness to attend regularly, and ability to verbalize feelings are all important but secondary to meeting stated criteria for membership. *(NB, assessing; LDM, nurse centered)*

Stuart and Sundeen (1979), pp. 328–329

62. A. Factors fostering group cohesion and therapeutic problem solving are important in selecting group members. Homogeneous variables such as age, education level, and individual adaptation style will increase attractiveness to the group. The effectiveness of group therapy is often contingent upon the members' ability and willingness to disclose information about themselves, and conflicted feelings about intimacy may lead to withdrawal. When the potential group member is very satisfied with himself he may profit less from group experience. The patient with ability to relate symptoms, give advice, and have definite opinions may use those abilities to avoid discussing feelings. *(NB, analyzing; LDM, nurse centered)*

Burgess, p. 417;
Stuart and Sundeen (1979), pp. 328–329

63. **B**. The group leader does not know at this point why the client wishes to withdraw from the group. A face-to-face interview to explore the client's concerns and feelings is preferable to a generalization about the stress of group participation communicated by phone. Forcing the client to attend another session for proper termination is usually unsuccessful. Referral to another group may be appropriate when the reasons for the client's withdrawal from the present group are explored. *(NB, implementing; LDM, shared)*

Burgess, pp. 417–419;
Stuart and Sundeen (1979), pp. 328–333

64. **A**. The task of encouraging group interaction may necessitate the leader's assuming a less verbal role. The timing of remarks and responses to the group are important leadership skills; stalls can occur if the nurse responds too quickly or offers premature interpretations. Reflecting on observation seems appropriate here. Sharing personal feelings is not usually advisable because the focus should be on members' feelings. Confrontation may be premature; for example, more information about the phase of group development is needed. Choosing a topic may provide conversation but may move the group away from the process issues. *(NB, planning; LDM, nurse centered)*

Burgess, pp. 418–419

65. **D**. Data suggest the group is beginning its working phase. At the resolution of the cohesive stage, the final stage in the initial phase of group development, members learn self-discovery, and differences should not be feared. At the end of this stage, the group loses its false sense of happiness and gains ability to work together. During the working

phase the group directs its energies mainly toward task completion. The initial phase consists of the orientation and conflict stages which precede the cohesive phase; the group moves through the working phase before the termination phase occurs. *(NB, evaluating; LDM, shared)*

Stuart and Sundeen (1979), pp. 332–333

66. **C.** In a group that is relatively passive it is important for the leader to note covert feelings and ask group members if they are aware of any raising issues that no one in the group would feel comfortable doing. Group members should be treated fairly, but the issue of "special treatment" needs to be confronted. When the group is active, the group will raise the question of a member's behavior as an issue. Dealing with the member's behavior outside the group does not help the group deal with his behavior. *(NB, implementing; LDM, shared)*

Haber et al., pp. 370–371

67. **C.** It is important to encourage and allow the group to deal with each member's issues. Excusing the patient from the group or allowing him to observe only are autocratic leadership decisions, reducing the group's decision-making power. Making a disclaimer about the expectations concerning the group task will not allow the individual to deal with an issue important for him. *(NB, planning; LDM, shared)*

Grace and Camillari, p. 501

68. **D.** It is important to review the sequence of events with the group and to have members work together to better understand the silent member's behavior. Asking the silent member to speak may increase her resistance and exempt the group from analyzing their process. A group member who expresses feelings by silence will tend to remain entrenched in silence if left to his own devices for too long. Silence is itself a powerful nonverbal cue, and other observations of nonverbal behavior are probably limited. *(NB, analyzing; LDM, shared)*

Haber et al., p. 370

69. A. When a group is discussing how difficult life is outside the group, members are collectively using the defense mechanisms of deflection and avoidance and are unconsciously speaking of their experience within the group. Supporting the group's expressed feelings supports their avoidance of dealing with these feelings. When the leader either supports or refutes expressed group feelings, discussion remains at the content level and helps avoid process issues. The leader's behavior is not necessarily in question, but the leader must be able to sustain group criticism. *(NB, planning; LDM, shared)*

Haber et al., p. 372

70. D. Only when the group process is interfering with completion of its tasks is it appropriate for the leader of an activity group to raise a process issue. When scapegoating occurs, it is critical to the life of the group to raise the issue and deal with it in the group. Options A, B, and C all take the issue outside the realm of the group and place it in the realm of leader-patient; the process issue needs to be explored within the group. *(NB, planning; LDM, shared)*

Haber et al., p. 373

71. D. Termination generally occurs when the patient is able to relate to others in a nondefensive way and exhibits other signs of healthy self-esteem. Ability to make a decision to terminate is not the only or best indicator of readiness for it. Progress over time and expressed reasons for leaving are important but less crucial than the ability to relate to others. *(NB, evaluating; LDM, client centered.)*

Haber et al., p. 376

72. A. Denial and repression are the most common defenses a group collectively uses to protect against the sadness and loss of termination. There are no data to support option B, and there is no evidence of reaction formation by the group. If a group member could clearly express process issues during termination, the leader should be delighted as this indicates an effective group and effective leadership. *(NB, analyzing; LDM, shared)*

Grace and Camilleri, pp. 508–509

73. A. The process of goal clarification is essential in family therapy, and clarification of each member's view of the problem is essential before intervention can be planned. Specifically focusing on the son's problem negates the concept of the holism of the family system, where the action of one member impacts on others within the system. If there is documented conflict within this family, the family as a unit must be the therapeutic focus. Subsequent group therapy for the son may be appropriate but only after family system problems are resolved. *(NB, implementing; LDM, shared)*

Burgess, pp. 493;
Haber et al., pp. 322–323

74. C. There are many roles in a family system and expectations and norms of role behavior will differ in each family group. In this situation where communication is dysfunctional, it would be important to document roles assumed, role reversal, etc. Since the situation reflects dysfunctional, nonfocused communication, it is unlikely that there is any family secret protected by guarded communication. This situation also reflects that no one is dominant. Provision for physical survival, socialization, regulation, and support are all basic family functions that are not necessarily in question at this point. *(NB, assessing; LDM, shared)*

Burgess, pp. 434, 440–441

75. B. Overadequate-inadequate reciprocity is the process that occurs when one partner in a marriage functions well when the other spouse is dysfunctional. Wives of alcoholics often appear dominant, but since this husband is no longer drinking, this pattern is dysfunctional. There are insufficient data about personality characteristics of either spouse, and in family therapy the focus is on relationship and communication patterns, not individual characteristics. *(NB, analyzing; LDM, shared)*

Haber et al., p. 326

76. D. Triangles are predictable dysfunctional patterns of interactions among three persons. Triangulation is dysfunctional because it offers emotional stabilization through diversion rather than through resolution of issues within a dyad. Emotional cutoff is the process of separating, isolating, withdrawing, or denying the importance of the parental family. In this case, the daughter's pregnancy has increased her emotional involvement with her parents. The double-bind is a communication process in which the verbal message is contradictory to the nonverbal one, but the receiver must obey both; it is characteristic of schizophrenic families. Withdrawal is one form of emotional cutoff. *(NB, evaluating; LDM, client centered)*

Burgess, p. 437;
Haber et al., pp. 327–328, 330–331

77. B. Paradoxical injunction is prescribing the symptom or reversal of the symptom; it results in behavior changes because consciously controlled behavior cannot serve unconscious purposes. In freezing, a family member pantomimes a situation that is problematic, then freezes at that point. Role playing involves family members acting parts of other members. In sculpting a family member arranges others as he or she perceives them relationally. *(NB, analyzing; LDM, nurse centered)*

Haber et al., p. 332

5. Psychosocial and Mental Status Assessment

78. D. Physical malfunctions, including metabolic, nutritional, and endocrinologic, can all produce aberrant behavior. Physiologic malfunctions include biochemical factors. Some genetic factors appear to be related to development of schizo-phrenia and manic-depression. *(NB, analyzing; LDM, nurse centered)*

Wilson and Kneisl (1979), pp. 358–359

79. A. Symptoms such as those described in the statements of family members do not occur in isolation but generally reflect lack of communication within the family system. While perceptual differences are involved here, the larger issue is the family disequilibrium that is represented, not simply an individual problem. One or two family members using drugs to escape tension is not a normal family situation. However, there are no data indicating either mother or daughter have serious drug problems. *(NB, analyzing; LDM, shared)*

Lancaster, p. 171

80. B. By assessing the client's communication patterns you can determine a great deal about how he thinks. General appearance and family support systems cannot provide information about thought processes, and attitudes reflect more than thought processes, including such things as cul-ture, beliefs, and family influences. *(NB, assessing; LDM, nurse centered)*

Lancaster, p. 171

81. A. The son may be sharing his feelings of neglect and wishes that his mother was as attentive to him as to non-family members. The father's feelings are less important than the son's feelings at this point. The mother's educational preparation is unrelated to the son's feelings. Whether or not the mother avoids her family by doing for others is a secondary concern to the son's feelings. *(NB, analyzing; LDM, shared)*

Stuart and Sundeen (1979), p. 296

82. A. By asking the client about his level of education and employment, the nurse can determine if his answers reflect whether or not his vocabulary is consistent with his educational achievement, status, and role. Strange speech patterns may reflect limited education. Rapport is established by the nurse's approach, not necessarily by asking direct questions. Client interests may be useful at a later point. Determining the need for vocational rehabilitation would be done upon completion of the examination and after all data are analyzed. *(NB, analyzing; LDM, shared)*

Stuart and Sundeen (1979), p. 303

83. C. Repeating digits both forward and backward is a means of evaluating the client's immediate recall of what was just said. Recent memory deals with information or events occurring in the recent past, while remote recall deals with recollection of past events. *(NB, assessing; LDM, shared)*

Stuart and Sundeen (1979), p. 304

84. C. Echolalia is the purposeless repetition of a word or phrase. In word salad ordinary words or phrases are linked in a way that seems meaningless and illogical. Flight-of-ideas is the sudden rapid shift from one idea to another before the preceding one has been concluded. Neologism is a privately coined word or group of words having meaning only for the speaker. *(NB, analyzing; LDM, nurse centered)*

Haber et al., pp. 605–606

85. C. Once the data base has been established during the assessment phase, planning begins with the development of goals. Client and family history are part of the assessment phase. Establishing rapport is usually done in the assessment phase and continued throughout the nursing process. *(NB, planning; LDM, nurse centered)*

Haber et al., p. 222

6. Social, Legal and Ethical Aspects of Mental Health Nursing

86. C. Primary prevention of depression emphasizes promotion of healthy personality development so that the incidence of depression is reduced. Helping the client to become involved in an activity that is meaningful is one primary prevention approach. From data provided, this client is not clinically depressed. Group therapy is a secondary preventive approach. The client needs to establish a feeling of belonging and a vacation may further isolate her. *(NB, planning; LDM, client centered)*

Haber et al., pp. 549–550

87. A. Secondary prevention involves the early identification of emotional disorders that require prompt treatment. Encouraging an apparently depressed person to see a counselor is an example of a secondary preventive approach. Taking the apparently depressed person to a mental health facility or having her committed may be unnecessary until the diagnosis is established. Medication is only one approach to treating depression. *(NB, implementing; LDM, shared)*

Burgess, p. 190

88. A. Tertiary prevention is the attempt to reduce the residual effects of mental illness. In this situation the client is functioning in sheltered work and living environments; she is productive, not disabled, and thus would meet the goal of tertiary prevention. Home care programs and halfway houses are part of the rehabilitative efforts of tertiary prevention. While specific data and individual goals are not identified, the sense of the situation is that the goals of tertiary prevention have been met. *(NB, evaluating; LDM, shared)*

Burgess, p. 190

89. B. The catchment area concept divides a population into small enough segments so that collaborative working relationships may be established between community agencies and the mental health center. The client's age, length of time symptoms have been present, and support systems are unrelated to catchment, which is determined by where the person lives. *(NB, planning; LDM, shared)*

Burgess, p. 189

90. B. Community assessment should focus on consumers' special needs rather than the perceptions of health care providers as to what the consumer ought to have. It is unrealistic for one person to collect all data needed for a thorough community assessment. The key to a successful assessment lies in where to gather data more than in what data to gather. Current recipients of services form only one part of the comprehensive assessment. *(NB, planning; LDM, nurse centered)*

Stuart and Sundeen (1979), pp. 540–541

91. A. Because sufficient mental health services and financial assistance are not available, many outpatients' needs are unmet; basic changes in policies and programs are needed in how mental health care is planned, coordinated, and financed. Using the energies of a community leader to form and lead a group to lobby for such changes is appropriate and likely to be effective. Explaining the impact of limited resources is explaining the obvious to this community leader. Emphasizing the positive things being done could be perceived as defensive. While asking the leader for neighborhood program suggestions is possible, impact would be more limited and the potential for using her energies to benefit a larger community seems most appropriate. *(NB, implementing; LDM, client centered)*

Burgess, p. 193

92. B. Confidentiality relates to the responsibility of the agency and professionals to keep all information, records, and correspondence confidential. Access to this information is allowed only under specifically defined circumstances. No information should be given to the client's employer by either nurses or physicians. *(NB, implementing; LDM, nurse centered)*

Burgess, p. 210

93. D. All family members provide input to the crisis and should be included in dealing with the situation. Option A does not provide sufficient explanation as to why the family needs to become involved in counseling. Ignoring the daughter's behavior is not appropriate. While anxiety is present, family involvement is most important. *(NB, analyzing; LDM, client centered)*

Taylor, p. 149

94. C. Emergency involuntary admission may be used for patients who are acutely ill; time is limited for a specified period. Voluntary admission is not an option for this client as she has refused to consider hospitalization. Formal commitment is not required, and foster home placement is not a form of admission. *(NB, analyzing; LDM, shared)*

Stuart and Sundeen (1979), pp. 285–286

95. B. Since it is unlikely that the manic client will recognize his need for hospitalization, his wife should be informed about her role as guardian and how to begin emergency commitment procedure. Mental health centers located nearer to the family residence are preferable to state hospitals which are often located at some distance. The client's manic episode is likely to be accelerated if his wife tried hiding his money and credit cards. *(NB, implementing; LDM, client centered)*

Taylor, p. 625

96. C. By allowing the client to call, he retains some independence while careful monitoring may prevent him from compromising his business status because a poor sense of judgment is often associated with mania. Denying the client any calls will increase his anger and agitation, and it is inappropriate for his wife to phone for him. Monitoring calls is preferable to taking over for the client. *(NB, implementing; LDM, shared)*

Taylor p. 626

97. C. Mutual goal setting is often helpful to patients in helping them clarify their own thinking, and these goals become more useful since they have been determined in part by the person responsible for their implementation. To avoid intervention in what you think are poorly conceived goals may set the client up for failure. People rarely carry out goals to which they are opposed for whatever reason. Unless the client's goals are detrimental to her recovery or she is unable to renegotiate them in a mutual process, it is inappropriate to confront her physician about her lack of readiness for discharge. *(NB, planning; LDM, shared)*

Burgess, p. 114

B. PYSCHOPHYSIOLOGIC DISORDERS

98. D. The client using reaction formation displays attitudes or feelings that are the opposite of those operating unconsciously. Anger is the normal response associated with hostility. Appearing aloof represents withdrawal, and depression is associated with introjection. *(NB, assessing; LDM, shared)*

Burgess, pp. 27, 223–224;
Haber et al., p. 779

99. C. The social model of care considers social environment as it impacts on the person and his life experience. Culture is considered instrumental in defining mental illness, prescribing the nature of therapy and determining the individual's prognosis. Option A describes the basic premise of the interpersonal model of care, and option B the existential model. Option D describes the major premise of the communication model. *(NB analyzing: LDM, shared)*

Stuart and Sundeen (1979) pp. 20–28

100. D. According to Selye, stress is the nonspecific response of the body to any demand made upon it. The statements in options A, B, and C are all part of Selye's model of stress. Only option D is inaccurate and inconsistent in terms of Selye's model. *(NB, analyzing; LDM, nurse centered)*

Burgess, p. 218

101. A. The multicausal model is based on the premise that illness results from a variety of stressors: psychologic, physiologic, and sociologic. The specificity model asserts that specific types of emotional conflict produce certain types of personalities which have a propensity for certain disease conditions. The nonspecific stress model postulates that the physiologic response to stress is the same for everyone and that the disease developed is determined by organ sensitivity. The individual response specificity model proposes that there is a tendency toward specific, consistent, physiologic response to stress. *(NB, analyzing; LDM, nurse centered)*

Wilson and Kneisl (1979), pp. 615–617

102. D. In the behavioral model the nurse would help the client identify habits that are maladaptive and need to be changed. Option A represents a nursing approach consistent with the psychologic model of care, and option B, the social model of care. Option C represents an approach consistent with the biologic model of care. *(NB, planning; LDM, shared)*

Burgess, pp. 110–130

103. B. Dependent persons need to have others make decisions for them, thus beginning to make individual decisions would indicate progress toward resolving dependency needs. Options A, B, and D are all behaviors typical of the dependent patient. *(NB, evaluating; LDM, client centered)*

Stuart and Sundeen (1979), p. 183

104. D. A nursing model approaches illness as resulting from a combination of biopsychosocial stressors; this entry is consistent with a nursing model approach. The entry in option A reflects the communication model; option B the behavior model; and option C, the medical model. *(NB, evaluating, LDM, client centered)*

Stuart and Sundeen (1979), p. 38

105. B. In asthma the difficulty is in expiration as the bronchioles tend to narrow during expiration under normal conditions. Assessments in Options A, C, and D are all commonly associated with asthma. *(NB, assessing; LDM, nurse centered)*

Pasquali et al. p. 297

106. D. Providing for the client's oxygen needs will decrease hypoxemia, and this will help in reducing the client's restlessness; as a consequence, both anxiety and discomfort are reduced. Anxiety reduction and relief of discomfort are best met initially by oxygen therapy. The type of asthma is not an essential early determinant of therapy but could be explored later. *(NB, planning; LDM, nurse centered)*

Robinson, pp. 461–462

107. A. Sedatives are contraindicated in severe asthmatic attacks because they may produce respiratory depression and increase hypoxemia. Phenobarbital is used to promote relaxation and prevent asthmatic attacks. Epinephrine and aminophylline are used to treat severe attacks as well as in their prevention. Beclomethasone is used as an inhalant for chronic asthma. *(NB, analyzing; LDM, shared)*

Luckmann and Sorensen, pp. 1318–1321

108. D. The autonomic nervous system is overstimulated in asthma. Allergic sensitivity, genetic predisposition, and dependency needs are all associated with development of asthma. *(NB, assessing; LDM, shared)*

Haber et al., p. 708

109. D. Patient teaching is essential so that the patient understands the disease process, accepts it, and can help prevent future crisis states and the development of chronic disease. Option A reflects a physiologic source of illness and options B and C psychologic sources of illness. Option D incorporates all of these aspects into improving the client's understanding the nature of the disease process. *(NB, evaluating; LDM, client centered)*

Burgess, p. 229

110. C. Persons developing psychophysiologic conditions typically suffer from dependency conflicts, making it difficult for them to establish warm personal relationships. They characteristically lack the motivation for self-awareness, focus on the physical rather than the emotional aspects of the illness, and their impatience makes them poor candidates for psychotherapy. *(NB, analyzing; LDM, nurse centered)*

Robinson, p. 461;
Wilson and Kneisl (1979), p. 392

111. D. The patient with a peptic ulcer has strong dependency needs. Options A, B, and C are all characteristic of the person with peptic ulcer. *(NB, planning; LDM, shared)*

Pasquali et al., p. 296

112. B. The type A personality frequently feels pressured by time, and this statement reflects this pressure. He is unable to relax, and free time is anxiety producing, so a vacation would not be a desired choice. The type A personality puts work before family, characteristically working late and bringing work home. *(NB, analyzing; LDM, client centered)*

Pasquali et al., p. 443

113. **A.** Unless the client with a peptic ulcer recognizes he is under stress and needs help, only the biologic aspects of his illness can be treated. Options B, C, and D are all pertinent goals, but less significant than the stress component for this client. *(NB, analyzing; LDM, shared)*

Burgess, p. 228;
Luckmann and Sorensen, p. 1435

114. **B.** The patient with a peptic ulcer needs to develop warm, safe relationships and to be encouraged to overcome his tendency toward social isolation. Options A, C, and D reflect appropriate goals for this client. *(NB, analyzing; LDM, shared)*

Robinson, p. 461

115. **C.** The client with a peptic ulcer needs to recognize his need for love and attention, recognizing that it is acceptable to have feelings and share them with others. This client has dependency needs which need to be gratified, at least in part, without eliminating the possibility of developing greater independence. Power and authority connote independence, and the need to achieve precludes rest and recreation. *(NB, analyzing; LDM, shared)*

Robinson, p. 461;
Wilson and Kneisl (1979), pp. 395–396

116. **A.** Since restlessness is a common sign in type A personalities, decreased feelings of restlessness would indicate positive response to the care plan. Options B, C, and D all represent characteristics of the type A personality. *(NB, evaluating; LDM, client centered)*

Pasquali et al., p. 443

117. **B.** Cimetidine (Tagamet) is classified as a histamine antagonist. *(NB, analyzing; LDM, nurse centered)*

Luckmann and Sorensen, pp. 1434–1435

118. **A.** In anorexia nervosa the person is obsessed with the idea of being thin and is preoccupied with avoiding food. Excessive exercise routines do not occur in all instances of anorexia nervosa nor is tomboyish behavior associated with this disorder. Ambivalence toward parents is a characteristic of adolescents. *(NB, assessing; LDM, shared)*

Haber et al., p. 723–724

119. **B.** The anorexic client needs close, one-to-one supervision for at least 30 minutes following meals to prevent attempts to induce vomiting. The client also needs to be supervised by the staff in the bathroom during this period. Options A and D are punitive; bed rest will not provide the supervision needed, and forcing her to eat again will not make food more desirable. Restricting bathroom privileges immediately after meals provides no supervision and assumes the client will vomit only in the bathroom. *(NB, planning; LDM, shared)*

Wilson and Kneisl (1979), p. 548

120. **C.** Amenorrhea, which is characteristic of anorexia nervosa, occurs in 50% of all women before weight loss. Listlessness and diarrhea are not associated with this condition, and increased oral intake is not seen unless as a component of the related condition, bulimia. *(NB, assessing; LDM, shared)*

Haber et al., p. 724

121. **D.** This option allows the anorexic client some decision in food selection while being supervised by staff and provides her with some feeling of control. Option A is an authoritative response with little evidence of consideration for the client's feelings. Option B is also authoritative with

punitive implications. Option C implies distrust of the client and is not conducive to building a therapeutic relationship. *(NB, implementing; LDM, shared)*

Haber et al., p. 747

122. B. Once the behavior modification regimen is established in which bringing in food is not allowed, the regimen must be strictly adhered to or the client will have the opportunity to manipulate the regimen and the staff. Options A and D would be counterproductive, and option C implies the nurse is not capable or willing to make a decision based upon the clearly defined treatment regimen. *(NB, implementing, LDM, nurse centered)*

Haber et al., p. 747

123. C. Behavior therapy would indicate that an undesirable behavior should not be reinforced; thus only appropriate statements would be responded to by the staff. Focusing on food should be avoided and the staff should not encourage her to eat. Having the client eat alone removes her from the normal social environment when she needs to learn appropriate behavior. Monitoring conversation is authoritarian and not conducive to increasing self-esteem. *(NB, analyzing; LDM, nurse centered)*

Wilson and Kneisl (1979), p. 547

124. C. Examining the reasonableness of the client's request can assist her to develop responsibility for her behavior and positively reinforce desired behavior. Option A is punitive and does not provide reward for desirable behavior. Option B implies distrust of the client and can be destructive in a therapeutic relationship. Option D is a way for the nurse to avoid appropriate decision making. *(NB, implementing; LDM, shared)*

Haber et al., pp. 724, 747

125. B. Diminished interest in, and preoccupation with, food and weight is a positive indicator that the client is progressing toward recovery. Option A reflects lack of insight on the client's part as to the nature of the problem and denies a problem existed. Option C denies that in reality she did not have the self-control she felt existed. Option D reflects some continued preoccupation with food in a more acceptable, selective manner. *(NB, evaluating; LDM, client centered)*

Haber et al., pp. 747–748

126. B. Returning to school and developing peer involvement will help her continue to develop personal strength. Quitting school is really not an option, and being around food will not insure her ability to cope with it. Moving back with her family and being tutored at home can tax the client's coping ability. Beginning a comprehensive fitness program again emphasizes her body. *(NB, evaluating; LDM, client centered)*

Haber et al., pp. 747–748

127. A. This option indicates insight into the parental dynamics contributing to the development and maintenance of anorexia and the client's awareness that she should not get caught up in the argumentative process. Option B implies anger and lack of insight into the real issue. Option C uses the therapist as a substitute parent, and option D ignores the obvious existing problems. *(NB, evaluating; LDM, client centered)*

Haber et al., pp. 725–726, 747–748

C. ANXIETY REACTIONS

128. D. Physiologic responses associated with anxiety are primarily mediated through the autonomic nervous system. A variety of physiologic symptoms can be observed in the anxious patient, including elevated blood pressure, difficulty breathing, dilated pupils, and vasoconstriction. *(NB, assessing; LDM, nurse centered)*

Stuart and Sundeen (1979), p. 81

129. B. Since this patient's symptoms are those that can also occur in physical illness, the possibility of any organic illness should be ruled out. Monitoring vital signs will indicate changes in physiologic responses but will not aid in the patient's diagnosis and treatment. The ability to answer questions or follow directions is limited during an anxiety reaction. Isolation increases anxiety and may increase the patient's symptoms and overwhelming fear. *(NB, planning; LDM, shared)*

Pasquali et al., p. 339

130. A. According to Freudian theory, amnesia results from a basic conflict between the desire to express and the desire to prevent expression of unconscious fantasies. Option B describes Leighton and Murphy's sociocultural theory of amnesia, and Horney's theory is described in option D. *(NB, analyzing, LDM, nurse centered)*

Pasquali et al., pp. 327–332

131. C. Requesting diet counseling is an active behavior which will help the client achieve the goal of better health. Eliminating or reducing intake of fats, salt, and sugar will improve his diet. Setting goals and working until they are achieved continues the client's pressured, time-oriented lifestyle. Allowing others to make decisions is helpful but probably insufficient to change the client's life-style. Making a list of needed life-style changes does not necessarily mean the client will put them into effect. *(NB, evaluating, LDM, client centered)*

Blattner, pp. 186–196

132. A. Keeping the client's environment calm and approaching her quietly will facilitate the client's adjustment to the unit and developing a trust relationship. Interrupting the client's ritual may cause a panic attack. Obsessive-compulsive clients need purposeful activities since pleasurable activities bring discomfort. They know their rituals are absurd and discussing them increases their anxiety. *(NB, planning; LDM, shared)*

Haber et al., pp. 462–467

133. B. Anxious clients may display demanding behavior and being with an anxious client tends to increase one's own anxiety because anxiety is highly communicable. The nurse must resolve her own feelings of anxiety before she can intervene effectively with the client. The anxiety is probably related to her family's impending visit; there is no need for her to be placed in seclusion. Leaving the client alone is a dysfunctional method of escaping one's own anxiety. There are insufficient data to determine if the patient's medication needs to be increased or what medication she is taking. *(NB, analyzing; LDM, nurse centered)*

Haber et al., pp. 445–447

134. C. The underlying cause of a conversion reaction is a fixation in early psychosexual development leading to anxiety. The repressed tension is converted into a physical symptom representative of the conflict. Repetitious comments such as suggested in option A increase the patient's anxiety contributing to the need for the symptom, belittle the client's feelings, and prevent development of trust. Family dynamics can contribute to initiating, reinforcing, and perpetuating the conversion reaction behavior pattern. People with a conversion reaction enjoy being the center of attention and will use their symptoms as a way of meeting this need. *(NB, planning; LDM, shared)*

Haber et al., p. 465

135. C. An important way to build self-esteem is to provide opportunities for the client to succeed through incremental structuring of activities and expectations. Helping people become more effective parents is a means of primary prevention of somatoform disorders, since early childrearing patterns along with stressful life events are significant etiologic factors in their development. Assigning this patient a group leadership role may only increase her anxiety. The patient with a conversion reaction is attempting to relieve stress and anxiety in a socially acceptable way; symptoms are real to the client, and the nurse needs to help the client deal with his feelings more effectively. *(NB, planning; LDM, shared)*

Haber et al., pp. 475–477

136. B. The defense mechanisms involved in amnesia are repression and denial. Amnesia is a response to an extreme anxiety-provoking situation. Repression is the primary forgetting of material not subject to conscious recall, while suppression is conscious forgetting of material. In reaction formation an individual assumes attitudes or needs which are directly opposite to consciously disowned ones. In undoing, an individual symbolically erases a previous consciously intolerable action or experience. *(NB, analyzing; LDM, client centered)*

Pasquali et al., pp. 345–346

137. B. Most clients with somatoform disorders do not understand or know why they behave as they do. By nurses labeling the emotion they sense clients are expressing through their behavior, the client is forced to become consciously aware of what is being experienced by considering a specific feeling, which can then be expressed. If clients who use somatoform behavior as a defense against anxiety are asked to approach that which they fear or are forced to relinquish their symptoms, their anxiety levels will rise. Focusing on topics outside the patient increases the secondary gain of attention. *(NB, planning; LDM, shared)*

Haber et al., pp. 460–462, 475

138. D. Desensitization is the gradual systematic exposure of the client to a feared situation under controlled conditions. Presented in a gradual way from least to more frightening, the client becomes desensitized to each stimulus and what was most anxiety-producing is no longer capable of eliciting that anxious response. Option D reflects such an outcome. Muscle relaxation alone does not mean the phobia has been overcome. Option B only states conditions, not outcomes, and Option C does not measure effectiveness of the desensitization program. *(NB, evaluating; LDM, client centered)*

Haber et al., p. 478

139. D. To prevent recurrence of a conversion reaction the client must begin to recognize feelings of anxiety and use effective coping mechanisms. Option A is helpful in developing such coping mechanisms but presumes the client can identify her own anxiety. Option B is a part of the current plan of care as is option C. *(NB, planning; LDM, shared)*

Stuart and Sundeen, pp. 228–233

140. C. Obsessive-compulsive behaviors are an unconscious attempt by the client to reduce an intolerable level of anxiety. The greater the anxiety, the more attention is devoted to a rigid routine. The ritualistic behavior represents a return to earlier methods of dealing with anxiety. Conversion reactions are evident through physical symptoms. Hysteric reactions are now referred to as somatoform disorders. In phobic reactions there is an object, but it is maladaptive. *(NB, analyzing; LDM, client centered)*

Haber et al., pp. 460–463

141. A. The repetitive actions of the obsessive-compulsive client's rituals relieve anxiety but only temporarily; therefore the action must be repeated at intervals as anxiety increases. Contemplation does not remove the client's anxiety, and the physical action must be repeated over and over to reduce this anxiety. Energy may be transferred to the environment through rituals, but this is not the source of reducing anxiety. *(NB, planning; LDM, nurse centered)*

Pasquali et al., pp. 340–345

142. B. Engaging the client in constructive activities which leave less time for compulsive behavior is an effective means of reducing dependence upon the ritual. Requesting that the client change his routine is ineffective because ritualistic clients have a low tolerance for change. Accepting the patient is important but may not reduce dependence on rituals. The client needs to be helped to set limits on his own behavior rather than the nurse doing it alone. *(NB, implementing; LDM, shared)*

Haber et al., p. 476

143. B. Behavior modification has been an encouraging approach to patients' compulsive overeating. Desensitization is not usually employed for treatment of obesity. Typical psychotherapy has been relatively unsuccessful with overeating patients unless their behavior is stress related. Gestalt therapy is one type of psychotherapy. *(NB, analyzing; LDM, shared)*

Wilson and Kneisl (1979), pp. 399–400

144. D. A strict behavior modification program is used with anorectics to alter their eating behavior. Such programs impose severe limits on nurse-client interactions so that relationship time with the client can be used as a reward; therefore, restrictions may be frustrating to the nurse who values such therapeutic relationships. Family dynamics may have helped create the anorectic behavior, but the behavior itself must be reversed since it can be life-threatening. Weighing the patient is reinforcing her need to restrict eating. *(NB, analyzing; LDM, shared)*

Haber et al., pp. 723–726, 730–731

145. C. The therapeutic dose and antianxiety effect of benzodiazepines such as chlordiazepoxide (Librium) are experienced when the client experiences relief without being oversedated. Sedation is an expected side effect. Peak blood levels of Librium are reached in 2–4 hours, and it will enhance sleep by reducing anxiety. This client is probably experiencing situational anxiety; if her fears are underscored by factors such as low self-esteem, other approaches such as psychotherapy may be beneficial. *(NB, implementing; LDM, shared)*

Burgess, pp. 383–385;
Haber et al., pp. 402–404

146. D. When the client can state the reasons for which his prescribed medication should be taken, he understands the use of the medication. Options A, B, and C are all aspects about the prescribed medication but do not indicate when the medication is to be used. *(NB, evaluating; LDM, client centered)*

Grace and Camilleri, p. 365

147. B. Benzodiazepines such as diazepam (Valium) can produce physical and psychologic dependence and tolerance to the sedative and euphoric side effects. Assessing the client's drug dependence is an essential priority so that the drug can be withdrawn safely as indicated. Assessing the client's coping mechanisms would be important after possible drug dependence is determined. The client's feelings about the operation should have been explored at the time of surgery, and while current feelings should be considered, this action is of secondary importance. Antianxiety agents are useful for a short-term situation such as that experienced by the client originally; continuing their use is unwarranted now. *(NB, planning; LDM, shared)*

Haber et al., pp. 402–404

D. AFFECTIVE DISORDERS/DEPRESSION/ GRIEF/SUICIDE

148. C. Early morning awakening is one of the primary characteristics of severe depression, and weight loss (or gain) is an indicator of moderate to severe depression. Grief often leads to depression and anhedonia (lack of pleasure in previously pleasurable activities) and can reflect a normal mourning process. Sadness and crying spells are seen more often with mild depression. Lack of concentration and feelings of fatigue are symptoms of anxiety as well as depression, and more data are needed to determine if a psychiatric evaluation is warranted. *(NB, analyzing; LDM, shared)*

Pasquali et al., pp. 384–387

149. C. Adolescent males between 15 and 19 are at a high risk for suicide; therefore assessing and documenting suicidal ideation would be a priority. Options A, B, and D are all components of the mental status examination but are less significant in light of his history. *(NB, assessing; LDM, shared)*

Haber et al., p. 578

150. D. Sleep disturbances are common in depressed clients; sleep is desired but not satisfying. Anxious patients may have difficulty falling asleep but awaken more refreshed. Discussing client problems is helpful to both the depressed and the anxious client. The depressed client feels worse as the day progresses. The anxious patient enjoys activities but the depressed client has little energy for them. *(NB, assessing; LDM, shared)*

Haber et al., pp. 535–536

151. A. The psychologic model of care of the depressed patient deals with establishing a nurse-patient relationship, helping the patient bear and resolve painful feelings, and responding to the dynamic issue. The biologic model involves use of somatic therapy. The behavioral model helps provide controls for the patient, and the social model involves the therapeutic milieu of the unit environment. *(NB, analyzing; LDM, nurse centered)*

Burgess, pp. 256–259

152. **A.** A history of previous suicide attempts would place this client at high risk for suicide since it is a serious problem among the elderly. Options B, C, and D are all necessary assessments but potential for suicide would assume priority. *(NB, assessing; LDM, shared)*

Haber et al., pp. 579–580

153. **C.** Delusional thinking may be present in the depressed client. The delusions confirm the person's feelings of worthlessness, guilt, and powerlessness. Delusions of grandeur are uncommon in depression, and thought broadcasting is more commonly experienced by persons with schizophrenia. Hearing voices is an auditory hallucination and more commonly occurs in schizophrenia. *(NB, analyzing; LDM, nurse centered)*

Haber et al., p. 537

154. **A.** The response that the depressed person tends to evoke in the nurse can influence clinical management unless the nurse is aware of her own feelings. Reassurance tends to discount the person's feelings. Options C and D are appropriate nursing actions after the nurse has explored her own feelings. *(NB, implementing; LDM, shared)*

Haber et al., pp. 541–543

155. **D.** There is sufficient evidence that one biochemical cause of depression is due to neuropharmacologic dysfunction resulting in reduced norepinephrine. Decreased catecholamines, and sodium and potassium are associated with

depression, but no single hormone has been related to depression. *(NB, analyzing; LDM, nurse centered)*

Burgess, p. 247;
Stuart and Sundeen (1983), p. 296

156. A. The mood state of depression may be described as one of despair, gloom, a sense of foreboding, a feeling of emptiness, or a feeling of numbness. Options B and C refer to cognitive functioning which is not affected in depression. Delusions and hallucinations are not associated with depression. *(NB, analyzing; LDM, shared)*

Burgess, p. 246

157. B. In a short hospital stay there is insufficient time for planned therapy with the client. Options A, B, and C all describe relevant components of a care plan for a short hospital stay. *(NB, planning; LDM, shared)*

Wilson and Kneisl (1983), pp. 324–326

158. A. Chlordiazepoxide (Librium) produces a calming effect, relieving nervousness and anxiety in small dosages and in larger dosages, produces drowsiness and sedation. Syncope, vertigo, urticaria, and menstrual irregularities are all potential adverse side effects. *(NB, evaluating; LDM, shared)*

Haber et al., pp. 403–404

159. B. Hypotension or drop in blood pressure from the baseline is a common side effect of antipsychotic drugs such as chlorpromazine (Thorazine); Thorazine is the most potent drug when considering hypotensive reactions of clinical significance. Isolation may be contraindicated in involutional psychosis because depressive features, suicidal ideation, and delusions often accompany this psychosis. Antipsychotic drugs do not cause physiologic dependency and are not physically addicting. Forcing fluids is unnecessary with Thorazine. *(NB, planning; LDM, nurse centered)*

Haber et al., pp. 398–399

160. B. Tricyclic drugs such as imipramine (Tofranil) are often used in treating depression and have little potential for causing hypertensive crisis. Benzodiazepines such as chlordiazepoxide (Librium) are used primarily to treat anxiety. Monoamine oxidase inhibitors such as phenelzine sulfate (Nardil) are used to treat depression but can produce hypertensive crisis. Phenothiazides such as chlorpromazine (Thorazine) are used primarily to treat psychotic behavior. *(NB, analyzing; LDM, nurse centered)*

Pasquali et al., pp. 410–411

161. D. Setting realistic goals that the patient can achieve increases the probability that he will achieve some success, which will raise his self-esteem. Options A, B, and D are valid components of a plan for a depressed client but will not necessarily raise his self-esteem. *(NB, planning; LDM, shared)*

Haber et al., pp. 551–552

162. D. Normal grieving may take days, weeks, or months; depression is delayed grievance. Both depression and grief convey the feeling of loss, although the quality may vary. The feeling of helplessness is characteristic of both grief and depression, and while both result in inability to function, grief is more limited in this respect. *(NB, analyzing; LDM, nurse centered)*

Stuart and Sundeen (1983), pp. 287–288

163. D. Widespread use of tranquilizers may suppress grief. Option A suppresses grieving when significant others inhibit mourning and attempt to orient the bereaved too quickly to the future. The circumstances of the death may contribute to failure to resolve grief, including the nature of the relationship and perception of ability to prevent the death. Option C reflects the mourner's perception that the death was preventable. *(NB, analyzing; LDM, shared)*

Stuart and Sundeen (1983), pp. 290–291

164. C. This option reflects the nurse's support of and respect for the client. Option A ignores the patient's feelings by communicating that the nurse is too busy. Option B tells the client how and what to do, and option D substitutes another activity for exploring the client's feelings. *(NB, implementing; LDM, shared)*

Burgess, pp. 248–249

165. D. Following electroconvulsive therapy (ECT) orientation may need to be repeated several times, and confusion may occur with each treatment. Postural hypotension may occur following ECT. There may be amnesia before ECT, and on occasion the patient may become agitated. *(NB, evaluating; LDM, nurse centered)*

Stuart and Sundeen (1983), pp. 491–492

166. B. Tranylcypromine (Parnate), a monoamine oxidase (MAO) inhibitor can produce orthostatic hypotension. Toxic effects and drug interaction with MAO inhibitors may occur up to several weeks following termination of therapy. Hot showers and baths may cause a fall in blood pressure, especially with MAO inhibitors. The MAO inhibitors may mask signs of ischemic attacks so patients should begin exercise programs cautiously. *(NB, planning; LDM, client centered)*

Haber et al., pp. 404–405, 407–408

167. C. Hypertensive crisis is the most serious adverse effect of MAO inhibitors and is produced when the medication is taken in combination with tyramine- rich foods such as wine and cheese. No adverse reaction has been noted with green leafy vegetables, sweets, tomatoes, or fruits. *(NB, analyzing; LDM, client centered)*

Haber et al., pp. 407–408

168. D. The midlife crisis of loss of youth generally occurs in the early 40s. If a woman perceives herself only as a homemaker and mother, she will experience the depression of "empty nest syndrome." The need to move from "us-ness" to "me-ness" requires independence and growth. Hobbies and secondary interests can blossom into new energies. *(NB, assessing; LDM, shared)*

Wilson and Kneisl (1983), pp. 263–265

169. B. People in crisis need to have psychologic equilibrium restored; focus of the intervention is on the immediate problem the person is facing through exploring feelings using a problem-solving approach. The person in crisis does not need rigid external controls but rather to experience growth in problem solving. Work is necessary to existence for physical and social reasons. *(NB, planning; LDM, shared)*

Burgess, p. 461;
Wilson and Kneisl (1983), p. 272

170. A. The problem-solving model emphasizes thorough assessment of the client's problem, then shifting to a plan for implementation; this option reflects moving toward possible solutions. Options B and D tell the client what to do, and option C negates the existence of a problem. *(NB, implementing; LDM, shared)*

Burgess, p. 461

171. A. Suicidal risk increases for severely depressed clients as they begin to feel better. Options B, C, and D all indicate characteristics of the depressed person. *(NB, assessing; LDM, client centered)*

Wilson and Kneisl (1983), pp. 292, 372–375

172. C. Maximum antidepressant effect from doxepin (Sinequan) occurs in 14–21 days, but antianxiety effects occur within several days. Marked sedation may occur during early treatment, and the patient may need frequent naps. *(NB, evaluating; LDM, shared)*

Burgess, pp. 378–379;
Haber et al., pp. 405–406

173. A. Tricyclic antidepressants such as doxepin (Sinequan) may cause photosensitivity. Antidepressants may be indicated when anxiety is present although not encouraged during crisis intervention. Regular activity is encouraged, and driving may be dangerous because of the sedative effect of Sinequan. *(NB, planning; LDM, client centered)*

Burgess, pp. 379–380;
Haber et al., p. 406

174. C. This client is exploring her capacity for living with independence and "me-ness." Timing is not involved, and her husband does not serve as a strong support at this time. While the client has wisdom, it did not prevent the crisis; having negotiated this crisis, she will be more prepared for the next. *(NB, analyzing; LDM, client centered)*

Wilson and Kneisl (1983) pp. 264, 277

175. C. The most crucial element in finding an identity, according to Glasser's reality therapy, is a genuine, loving relationship with another person. Therapy focuses on what one is doing rather than on what one is feeling; if this patient focuses on feelings of failure, he cannot move on because the past cannot be altered. Unresolved developmental conflicts, psychosexual maturity, and defense mechanisms are not components of reality therapy. *(NB, evaluating; LDM, shared)*

Wilson and Kneisl (1979), pp. 670–671

176. C. Constipation is an anticholinergic effect of tricyclics such as amitriptyline (Elavil). While constipation can be a symptom of depression, its severity would be increased because of the medication's side effect. There are no data concerning diet in this situation, and there are antidepressants which can be less constipating than others. *(NB, analyzing; LDM, shared)*

Haber et al., pp. 406–407

177. B. Clients who will not eat or drink may be in danger of dehydration, electrolyte imbalance, and starvation. In these situations the nurse must intervene and do for the client until she can carry out the activity independently. Forcibly removing the client is not likely to make her eat. No data about the client's feelings are provided, and while such exploration is desirable, it would be secondary to her inadequate nutritional intake. Tube feeding may be used but only as a last resort. Use of threat is nontherapeutic. *(NB, planning; LDM, nurse centered)*

Haber et al., p. 551;
Robinson, pp. 347–350

178. A. The nurse needs to communicate that the patient's life is worth saving, that she means to protect the patient by setting limits while she feels so bad about herself. The patient needs to develop feelings of self-worth and clearly communicating to the patient that she is perceived as being worthwhile will help her to participate in the therapeutic process. Options B and D reinforce and perpetuate the patient's helplessness and lack of responsibility. Option C is the response appropriate after the initial expression of limit setting. *(NB, implementing; LDM, nurse centered)*

Robinson, pp. 344–345

179. B. Acknowledging the client's emotion and arranging for a physical activity that allows expression of the emotion without harming anyone is most therapeutic. Option A reflects the nurse's anger at the client's behavior, which can inhibit communication. Option C does not recognize the client's anger or acknowledge his right to refuse. Option D accepts the client's refusal to communicate but does not offer assistance or alternative ways for him to express his anger. *(NB, implementing; LDM, shared)*

Haber et al., p. 551

180. A. Loss of memory and confusion are the two most common side effects of electroconvulsive therapy and would account for her behavior; this reaction would be considered normal, not an indication of brain damage. Other patients are likely to understand and help the client. Her wandering is more suggestive of being lost rather than of being frightened. *(NB, evaluating; LDM; shared)*

Haber et al., pp. 388–389

181. A. Eye contact usually takes place more often when one person is comfortable with another. Such nonverbal messages are important indicators of change and of response to the relationship. Options B and C are inappropriate because there is no indication that the client was not eating or taking her medications. Option D indicates that the client is relating better to others, but it is not a specific measure of establishing trust. *(NB, evaluating; LDM, shared)*

Stuart and Sundeen (1979), p. 185

182. B. Phenelzine sulfate (Nardil) is a monoamine oxidase (MAO) inhibitor and can produce hypertensive crisis. Since hypertensive crisis is a medical emergency because it may lead to intracranial hemorrhage, the physician must be notified immediately. Once the physician is notified, the patient's blood pressure should be checked. What the patient ate is important to determine but secondary to the crisis. Checking respirations is not a major concern in hypertensive crisis. *(NB, implementing; LDM, nurse centered)*

Haber et al., pp. 407–408

183. D. The safety of the baby and the mother-child relationship may be at risk and needs to be assessed before making discharge plans. It would be more appropriate to schedule a meeting with the couple, during which the nurse could offer opportunities for the patient to express her fears, after an assessment of the client's ability to handle the baby. Options B and C are logical components of a discharge plan but would be more effective and specific following assessment of mother-child interaction. *(NB, planning; LDM, shared)*

Haber et al., pp. 981–982

184. B. Compliance with a medication regimen is dependent upon the client's understanding of the medication. While the client's family needs to be informed, this measure would not necessarily increase client compliance. Providing positive reinforcement for taking medication while hospitalized may increase compliance during hospitalization but not necessarily at home; with the nurse providing the reinforcement, the patient is not becoming more independent. Teaching about side effects will not ensure compliance. *(NB, planning; LDM, shared)*

Haber et al., p. 397

185. D. It is especially important for the nurse to be genuine during the termination phase of a relationship. The nurse is teaching communication by role modeling when she shares her own feelings; inviting exploration of issues related to leaving also demonstrates alternative coping skills. By allowing the patient's denial the nurse misses an opportunity to share feelings and to teaching alternative coping skills. Confrontation will increase the patient's anxiety and might lead to further withdrawal. Telling the patient what she needs to experience reinforces her dependency and passivity. *(NB, planning; LDM, shared)*

Haber et al., p. 270

186. D. The patient in this situation is concerned about physiologic necessities and safety; these basic needs must be satisfied before she can move on to others, according to Maslow. There are no data to suggest the patient has set unattainable goals. Satisfaction of this patient's physiologic and safety needs are the motivators of her present behavior. *(NB, analyzing; LDM, nurse centered)*

Haber et al., pp. 8–9

187. D. The goal of attending a group activity after a week of contact with her nurse is a specific, short-term goal relating to the stated nursing diagnosis. Achieving this goal would be an initial step in increasing the client's socialization. Option A is a long-term goal which should be preceded by more realistic short-term goals. Option B, while desirable, would follow the patient's trust and safety in the environment. Option C is general and does not relate to the identified nursing diagnosis. *(NB, analyzing; LDM, shared)*

Stuart and Sundeen (1979), pp. 178–179

188. C. Requesting foods known to be restricted is a clear behavioral indication that the patient is denying his illness. There is no evidence that the patient wanted the nurse to see the letter, and testing would be evidenced by more active behaviors. There are also no data to indicate that the patient is angry or testing his friend. *(NB, evaluating; LDM, shared)*

Haber et al., p. 860

189. D. Sharing grief with others who are also affected is a healthy way to resolve their loss. Isolation increases feelings of helplessness and hopelessness. Ordering a tranquilizer postpones the patient's realization of the crisis. Talking with the patient about more cheerful subjects belittles the patient's feelings. *(NB, implementing; LDM, shared)*

Haber et al., pp. 869–872

190. B. The initial reactions in the normal process of grief are shock and disbelief. Vascillating between feelings and comprehending the situation occurs in the stage of restitution. A sense of helplessness is characteristic of the developing awareness of grief. *(NB, analyzing; LDM, client centered)*

Burgess, pp. 262–263

191. C. Tightness in the throat and loss of appetite are characteristic symptoms of somatic distress related to the grieving process. The client needs to maintain her independence as long as possible. The daughter's anger toward the anticipated loss of her mother is to be expected and may be shared with her mother. During the grieving process individuals are usually unable to maintain patterns of organization. *(NB, planning; LDM, shared)*

Pasquali et al., pp. 380–381

192. C. Exploration of problems with the client supports her and gives realistic, sensible encouragement with rational planning and preparation. Advising indirect comments blocks communication and adds stress. The nurse should not interfere by talking privately with the husband, but rather should support the client's healthy coping. Avoiding discussion belittles the situation for the client and reinforces the husband's denial. *(NB, planning; LDM, shared)*

Haber et al., pp. 423, 862–865

193. B. Feelings of guilt are common in the bargaining stage of death and dying, according to Kubler-Ross. Option A belittles the client's feelings, and options C and D are both inaccurate and inappropriate. *(NB, implementing; LDM, shared)*

Haber et al., pp. 862–863

194. C. Angry comments about a client's mother years after her death indicate unresolved feelings. Option A indicates intense feeling of loss precipitated by anniversary dates. Healthy resolution involves the incorporation of some aspects of the dead person into the bereaved person's ego structure. Ability to remember pleasures is a sign of healthy adaptation. *(NB, evaluating; LDM, client centered)*

Pasquali et al., p. 382

195. D. It is unnecessary to take a barbiturate an hour before desired hour of retiring because barbiturates are readily absorbed; they should be taken at bedtime. Options

A, B, and C are all accurate statements about the use of barbiturates. *(NB, planning; LDM, client centered)*

Haber et al., pp. 162–171

196. B. According to Durkheim the anomic suicide occurs when the individual feels alienated from a society that is in a state of changing structures and values. Altruistic suicide would be demanded by society, not the individual. Egoistic suicide is brought about by lack of relatedness to others in society. Option D represents a Freudian dynamic, being reunited with another person in death. *(NB, analyzing; LDM, nurse centered)*

Haber et al., p. 581;
Pasquali et al., pp. 396–397

197. B. A common feature of suicidal people is their ambivalence; within these people is a struggle between self-preserving forces and self-destructive forces. Blocking is an interruption in flow of thoughts of both life and death instincts. The emotion associated with suicidal thought is dissociated from consciousness. In reaction formation the individual expresses an attitude that is directly opposite the unconscious feelings and wishes. *(NB, analyzing; LDM, nurse centered)*

Haber et al., p. 583

198. A. Each variable in this profile is associated with high risk for suicide, making it the profile of highest risk. Adolescents have a high rate of suicide, but male adolescents are at greater risk than female. Being married and female puts this individual at lower risk. A black preadolescent is at higher risk for homicide. *(NB, assessing; LDM, nurse centered)*

Wilson and Kneisl (1979), pp. 254–255

199. B. Suicidal clients display a variety of behaviors but among the most common are depression, psychosis, and extreme irritability and agitation. Many suicidal clients have slowed motor activity as a result of their depression and violent physical outbursts would be unusual. There are no data to suggest any relationship between suicidal thoughts and rigid boundaries, or that sexual adjustment is related to suicide. *(NB, assessing; LDM, shared)*

Haber et al., pp. 589–591

200. D. Alcoholism and lack of relatedness are among the most clearly identified high-risk factors associated with suicide. Helplessness and an unsettled family system are not high-risk factors by themselves, and while absence of regular income is stressful, it is not a high-risk factor for suicide. *(NB, analyzing; LDM, nurse centered)*

Haber et al., pp. 578–583

201. C. Adolescents are bombarded with pressures from family and society to make their way as adults, yet life goals are not yet formed. In developing their own goals, adolescents may find these goals in conflict with those of family and society, increasing their vulnerability to suicide as a solution to stress. Healthy families can provide a balance of emotional support while encouraging the adolescent's individualization. Mastery over concrete thought occurs between 7 and 12 years; adolescents develop abstract-thinking capacity which is essential to their developing life goals. *(NB, analyzing; LDM, shared)*

Haber et al., pp. 578–579

202. C. The adolescent in this situation is attempting to manipulate her parents and punish them for punishing her. Her hostility is directed toward her family rather than herself. There are insufficient data to support the adolescent's wish to rejoin a significant other in death. *(NB, analyzing; LDM, client centered)*

Haber et al., pp. 584–586;
Wilson and Kneisl (1979), pp. 554–555

203. D. The suicide plan is an important area to assess because it is an index of danger and may also suggest something about the client's mental state. Age, history of physical illness, and degree of isolation are insufficient in themselves to determine the lethality of suicide. *(NB, assessing; LDM, shared)*

Haber et al., p. 591

204. C. People who are psychotic are vulnerable to suicide because of their impaired ability in reality testing and problem solving. The psychotic person may hallucinate self-destructive messages which are acted upon. The delirious patient's awareness of his terminal illness will be blunted and thus is not a relevant dynamic. Experiencing a paradoxical drug reaction would not necessarily place the patient at risk for suicide. The alcoholic client's mood disturbance will be secondary to his clouded consciousness and impaired orientation while in a delerious state. *(NB, assessing; LDM, nurse centered)*

Haber et al., p. 581

205. A. In planning care for the suicidal patient the nurse must help the patient learn to control self-destructive impulses; a contract implies the patient accepts this responsibility. Facilitating a therapeutic relationship is not specifically related to this goal, nor is teaching assertiveness. The nurse is responsible for supervising the suicidal client until he is no longer suicidal. *(NB, analyzing; LDM, shared)*

Burgess, pp. 495–496

206. D. Continuous human contact by a caring individual decreases the client's feeling of hopelessness and provides the best prevention against suicide. Maintaining intermittent contact is an insufficient deterrent to preventing suicide in the high-risk client; the hot-line by itself also will not deter this client. Antidepressant medication may be indicated but is a secondary concern. *(NB, planning; LDM, shared)*

Burgess, p. 494

207. C. People who make suicide attempts are usually outside of a caring system, and those who are successful are generally not actively engaged in treatment. A continuing relationship with a treatment program helps those high-risk suicidal persons who have had poor personal relationships. Prolonged hospitalization can increase client dependency and decrease his self-esteem and control. Allowing the client to solve problems in his own way can result in another suicide attempt. Increasing medication will not alleviate this client's loneliness. *(NB, planning; LDM, client centered)*

   Burgess, pp. 493–494

208. B. Acutely psychotic clients with persecutory hallucinations are at high risk for suicide because of impaired reality testing. Requesting an order for antipsychotic medication can be pursued after suicidal risk is ascertained. Escape precautions are probably less significant than suicidal precautions because of the impact of hallucinations on client behavior. Assessment of suicidal risk is part of the mental status examination and takes priority over other aspects of the examination for this patient. *(NB, implementing; LDM, shared)*

   Haber et al., p. 581

209. C. The first priority in intervening with suicidal clients is to protect them from themselves. Medication may be an adjunct to other therapy and nursing care but can be dangerous if the client hoards them; medication may also mask the severity of symptoms. Isolating the client is contraindicated because it will further decrease the client's self-esteem and control. Open anger may frighten the client and increase guilt if encouraged too soon. *(NB, analyzing; LDM, shared)*

   Wilson and Kneisl (1983), p. 291

210. A. This response conveys regard for the husband's feelings but is nonjudgmental; it provides a means of helping him identify adaptive coping mechanisms. Option B conveys guilt to the husband for causing his wife's suicide attempt. Option C reflects a negative response to the husband and the client based on her feelings about suicidal attempts. Option D cuts off communication with the client's husband. *(NB, implementing; LDM, shared)*

Haber et al., pp. 586–588

211. B. This client needs protection from self-harm because of his loneliness; his interpersonal resources are eroding and he needs care and nurturing. Before exploring the client's suicide plan the nurse needs to provide a safe environment for the client and to build a trusting relationship. The client's expression is more than normal grief; offering false reassurance is inappropriate. Option D denies the client's true feelings while offering vague reassurance. *(NB, implementing; LDM, shared)*

Haber et al., pp. 579–580, 582–584

212. A. The maximum effect of amitripyline occurs in 14–21 days after onset of administration, so assessment for suicidal ideation or behavior must be continued until risk is decreased. Therapeutic interpersonal contact helps build self-esteem, an important component of treating depression. The effectiveness of amitripyline is independent of group activity. Monitoring sleep and nutrition patterns are less reliable indicators of suicidal risk than suicidal ideation. Teaching about amitriptyline is not a priority but needs to be included in the care plan. *(NB, planning; LDM, shared)*

Haber et al., pp. 405, 552, 554

213. A. This client has a specific plan and an available method with high lethality; these factors place her at high risk for suicide. Options B and C are inaccurate and option D is a conclusion of comfort to the nurse, since the client is indicating a crisis state needing resolution. *(NB, analyzing; LDM, shared)*

Wilson and Kneisl (1983), p. 290

214. B. Diazepam produces sedative and hypnotic effects in large dosages. It can also produce physical and psychologic dependence, and it potentiates the effects of alcohol. The client's energy level will probably be decreased as a result of the drug's sedative effect. *(NB, planning; LDM, shared)*

Haber et al., p. 403

215. C. Activities that are appropriate with a suicidal client include positively teaching and reinforcing problem-solving skills so that the client feels in better control and is better able to cope with life stresses. Suicidal precautions convey the message that the client cannot care for himself, decreasing self-esteem. Encouraging expression of feelings is helpful but must be followed by problem-solving action or little progress is made. Calling the client by name offers recognition but little else. *(NB, implementing; LDM, shared)*

Haber et al., pp. 593–594

216. A. Making a suicide plan and following through requires energy. For this reason, severely depressed people are at greater risk when their drive and energy begin to return. Antidepressant medication does not produce maximum therapeutic effectiveness for several weeks and would not account for the change in client behavior. Dramatic changes in client behavior are significant and should not be taken lightly or used to make the nurse feel better. Assuming the client was seeking attention denies the seriousness of the client's illness. *(NB, evaluating; LDM, shared)*

Wilson and Kneisl, p. 292

217. B. Interpersonal contact with a professionally trained health care provider is necessary to determine the lethality of a suicidal risk and the type of crisis intervention required. Options A and C reflect avoidance and denial of feelings. Calling a friend may provide support but is not the priority action. *(NB, evaluating; LDM, client centered)*

Aguilera and Messick, pp. 118–125

218. A. A long-term goal for the suicidal client being discharged is to provide the client with a support system at home. Determining knowledge of lethal doses of medication will not decrease client isolation. Encouraging the client to sleep when anxious supports the client's denial of problems. Telling the client how to structure his day is appropriate when he is in a state of panic or disorganization, but after treatment it should not be necessary and may make the client more dependent. *(NB, planning, LDM, client centered)*

Wilson and Kneisl (1983), p. 292

219. B. As the client's depression lifts, he will experience an increased energy level and may be able to carry out his suicide plan. Option A reflects denial or lack of understanding about the client's risk of suicide at this time. Full therapeutic effect of antidepressant medication occurs in about 3 weeks; thus risk of suicide remains if the wish to die strongly persists. Within 6 months the client will have either recovered or been successful in his suicide attempt. *(NB, evaluating; LDM, client centered)*

Haber et al., pp. 404–409

220. B. Family members or significant others who are left behind feel guilt and anger. They need to be helped to mourn their loss in a healthy manner. Encouraging the family to stop thinking about the suicide enforces denial of an event which they need to talk about. Encouraging acceptance of sleeping medication promotes maladaptive coping. Expressing blame only increases the family's guilt feelings. *(NB, implementing; LDM, shared)*

Wilson and Kneisl (1983), p. 292

221. B. A strong id in the manic person leads to uncontrollable impulsive behavior. Manic clients lack feelings of guilt, and suicidal thoughts are more common in depressed individuals because of a punitive superego. Manic clients are extremely self-confident. *(NB, planning; LDM, nurse centered)*

Pasquali et al., p. 392;
Stuart and Sundeen, p. 306

222. C. Manic behavior is viewed as the mirror of depression, and the person may go from a cycle of depression to a manic phase. Options A, B, and D are all characterisitcs of mania. *(NB, analyzing; LDM, nurse centered)*

Burgess, pp. 250–251;
Haber et al., pp. 559, 562, 567

223. C. Hyperactivity in a manic client requires decisive nursing intervention because the consequences of continued activity can be life threatening. Interpersonal style is significant but not life threatening. Nutrition and ability to sleep are problematic in the manic client but will resolve as the hyperactivity decreases. *(NB, assessing; LDM, nurse centered)*

Haber et al., pp. 567–568

224. B. Manic-depressive illness appears twice as frequently in females as in males. *(NB, assessing; LDM, nurse centered)*

Haber et al., p. 558;
Robinson, p. 341:
Wilson and Kneisl (1983), p. 764

225. B. Manic episodes usually occur in persons between 20 and 35 years of age. Schizophrenia usually occurs between the ages of 15 and 45. Depressive episodes usually occur in persons 35–50 years of age. *(NB, assessing; LDM, nurse centered)*

Pasquali et al., pp. 393, 448, 521

226. D. High-caloric finger foods and drinks that can be consumed easily while standing or moving are suggested for the manic patient, thus this menu is desirable for its nutritional value and calories. In the manic phase the patient is not likely to take time to sit down and eat complete meals such as those in options A and B. Foods in option C, while finger foods, do not provide as much nutritional value as those in D. *(NB, planning; LDM, shared)*

Haber et al., p. 569

227. C. This manic client can exhaust herself from constant physical and verbal exertion, and the most important goal is to provide opportunities for rest to prevent exhaustion. Decreasing environmental stimuli is imperative, so group activities are contraindicated. Increasing self-control is a long-term goal. Counteracting denial is an appropriate goal when hyperactivity has decreased and the client no longer needs denial for conservation. *(NB, analyzing; LDM, shared)*

Burgess, pp. 250–251;
Haber et al., pp. 569–570;
Stuart and Sundeen (1983), p. 319

228. B. Moving the manic client's belongings to the dayroom will allow her to rearrange them without disturbing other patients. Seclusion would probably increase her agitation and while the client needs to be observed, the nurse must remove herself to decrease stimuli to the client. Telling the client to slow down is ineffective as the client is unable to stop her activities. *(NB, implementing; LDM, shared)*

Wilson and Kneisl (1983), p. 445

229. A. Manic clients are adept at manipulating the self-esteem of others. The good reality orientation of this client makes the flattery seem sincere and appropriate. Manic clients often use manipulation to resist rather than establish involvement in interpersonal relationships. They usually show little evidence of introspection. *(NB, analyzing; LDM, shared)*

Haber et al., pp. 559, 564;
Stuart and Sundeen (1983), p. 319

230. A. The first step in assisting a client to counteract denial is to establish an open relationship where thought and feelings can be discussed. If this client is to modify denial behavior, she needs to face her inner feelings. Confrontation can be utilized after a nurse-client relationship has been established. The manic client has the ability to maintain the flow of information on a superficial level when information about self is offered. *(NB, planning; LDM, shared)*

Haber et al., pp. 570–571

231. D. Physical activities for the client in the acute manic stage should require large sweeping movements. Writing is an excellent outlet for the mildly elated person, and volleyball is too competitive and causes the elated client to become overly stimulated. Overactive clients will lose interest in activities such as knitting, which require fine, discriminative skills. *(NB, planning; LDM, shared)*

Taylor, p. 287

232. A. The nurse can make use of the elated individual's inability to maintain sustained attention by directing his thoughts elsewhere. Because other people irritate the manic client and provoke him to talk excessively, the manic client should be in a single room. A firm, kind, low-pitched voice is most effective with the manic client, and the nurse should reduce environmental stimuli, including people. *(NB, implementing; LDM, shared)*

Taylor, pp. 285–286

233. D. The nurse should respond to the theme that underlies the verbal content of the client's delusion. The delusion should not be attacked or challenged, and communication should avoid supporting or reinforcing the delusion. Rational explanations will only make the client adhere more firmly to his delusion. *(NB, implementing; LDM, shared)*

Haber et al., p. 643

234. D. It is most appropriate for the nurse to tell clients in a matter-of-fact way when she is angry with them. Option A deprives clients of nursing care when they display unacceptable behaviors. In option B the nurse assumes an attitude of superiority and discounts the client's concern. Option C reflects the nurse's retaliation to anger by asserting herself as one with authority. *(NB, implementing; LDM, shared)*

Stuart and Sundeen (1983), pp. 418–419;
Wilson and Kneisl (1983), pp. 438–439

235. B. The manic client is very talkative and his speech is not slow or slurred. Constant activity, flight-of-ideas, and decreased need for sleep are all characteristic of manic clients. *(NB, assessing; LDM, client centered)*

Wilson and Kneisl (1983), p. 422

236. C. Therapeutic serum lithium levels range from 1.0–1.5 mEq/L, and at no time should serum levels exceed 2.0 mEq/L. Routine blood serum levels are done to regulate dosage, and the effects of lithium may be decreased by alkalizing agents. Thirst, fatigue, and mild muscle weakness are common side effects. *(NB, planning; LDM, shared)*

Haber et al., pp. 409–410

237. C. Significant side effects of lithium therapy are correlated with lithium blood levels above 1.5 mEq/L; 1.0 and 1.2 mEq/L are therapeutic serum levels, and 2.0 is correlated with severe toxicity. *(NB, analyzing; LDM, nurse centered)*

Haber et al., p. 409;
Wilson and Kneisl (1983), pp. 685–687

238. D. Lithium is used to prevent recurrence of cyclic attacks of mania, stabilizing mood swings. Lithium toxicity is characterized by blurred vision, diarrhea, tinnitus, fine muscle tremors, and increased urination. *(NB, analyzing; LDM, client centered)*

Haber et al., pp. 409–410

239. C. Lethargy and diarrhea are early signs of lithium toxicity, not common side effects. Seizures and electrolyte imbalance should be prevented by dosage adjustment. *(NB, evaluating; LDM, shared)*

Wilson and Kneisl (1983), pp. 685, 687

240. A. Antipsychotic drugs such as chlorpromazine (Thorazine) act more quickly than lithium to bring exaggerated manic behavior under control; antipsychotics are useful in the first week of a manic episode. There are few interaction problems in use of lithium with antipsychotic or antidepressant drugs. Nausea, a side effect of lithium, may be masked by the antiemetic action of Thorazine. Akathisia, the extreme inability to sit still, is an extrapyramidal side effect of antipsychotics such as Thorazine but resembles the client's manic behavior that will be controlled by Thorazine and lithium. Hypertensive crisis is a severe side effect of monoamine oxidase inhibitors. *(NB, analyzing; LDM, shared)*

Burgess, pp. 371, 381–382;
Wilson and Kneisl (1983), pp. 670, 682

241. A. People suffering from manic-depression will probably reenter the health care system in an acute episode when they stop taking lithium. Although environmental dynamics such as emotional stressors, change in life-style, and loss of support systems can contribute to the onset of manic symptoms, discontinuing lithium therapy is the most significant factor. *(NB, analyzing; LDM, client centered)*

Haber et al., p. 563;
Wilson and Kneisl (1983), p. 429

242. C. The family may participate in the escalation of manic behavior when members do not consistently set limits on "crazy" client behaviors. The family often participates in maintaining the client's manic behavior when they deny its presence, display increasing tolerance for it, and do not act on the need to rehospitalize the family member until the situation has reached crisis proportions. *(NB, evaluating; LDM, client centered)*

Haber et al., p. 573

243. B. Recent studies indicate that the intended effect and side effect of drugs are common concerns of clients who refuse to take medication as prescribed. A client who does not assume responsibility for taking his medication suffers a blow to his self-image of being an autonomous, capable person. The nurse's ethical obligation is to inform the client, within his ability to understand, about prescribed medications; this should be done before discharge. Written instructions are helpful but insufficient without individualized teaching. *(NB, planning; LDM, client centered)*

Haber et al., p. 412;
Wilson and Kneisl (1983), p. 667

E. SCHIZOPHRENIC DISORDERS

244. B. Research indicates that heredity is a component in developing schizophrenia, but does not indicate how or the precise nature of the genes involved in transmission of schizophrenia. Genetic factors have been explored primarily through twin and family studies. Concordance rates (occurrence of similar traits in twins) of schizophrenia vary widely. *(NB, analyzing; LDM, nurse centered)*

Haber et al., p. 614;
Wilson and Kneisl (1979), p. 358–359

245. C. Bleuler's classic four "A's" denoting fundamental symptoms of schizophrenia are ambivalence, associative disturbance, autism, and affective impairment. Automatic thinking and asymmetric communication are not among the classic symptoms. *(NB, analyzing; LDM, nurse centered)*

Burgess, p. 278

246. B. The double-bind is a communication process wherein the verbal message is contradictory to the nonverbal one, but the receiver of the message must obey both. Since the message sent is contradictory, it is unclear. The double-bind is a dysfunctional form of communication occurring between any individuals or groups, not just within a family or between mother and child. *(NB, analyzing; LDM, nurse centered)*

Haber et al., p. 331

247. A. Autism is an extreme retreat into fantasy in which the person is continually preoccupied with daydreams, fantasies, or psychotic thoughts. Ambivalence is an unstable blending of love and hate, with sudden unaccountable shifts in affection and hostility. In inappropriate affect, emotional expression is urelated to reality. Blocking involves disconnecting thought associations. *(NB, assessing; LDM, nurse centered)*

Burgess, p. 280

248. D. The schizophrenic's ego strength is fragile, largely because he has never differentiated from the family ego mass and developed self-confidence in relationship to personal capabilities or a separate identity, resulting in dependency. Option A deals with the patient's affect or emotion, not dependence. Id is not related to dependence and feeling inferior to others results in low self-esteem. *(NB, analyzing; LDM, nurse centered)*

Haber et al., pp. 613–614

249. A. Paranoid schizophrenia is associated with persecutory or grandiose delusions or hallucinations with persecutory or grandiose content. Suspiciousness, jealousy, and mistrust of others are other characteristics of this type of schizophrenia. Option B describes characteristics of catatonic schizophrenia, while option C indicates characteristics of disorganized schizophrenia. Apathy, indifference, and mental deterioration are nonspecific symptoms not indicative of any type of schizophrenia. *(NB, assessing; LDM, nurse centered)*

Haber et al., pp. 600–601

250. C. Delusions of persecution reflect a person's belief that he or she is being harassed, threatened, or persecuted under the influence of some powerful force. Option A is an example of a delusion of grandeur, an exaggerated sense of importance that has no basis in reality. Option B represents a somatic delusion, reflecting the belief that the person's body is changing in a way that has no basis in reality. Option D is an example of an idea of reference in which the person believes certain events or interactions are directly related to himself. *(NB, assessing; LDM, nurse centered)*

Haber et al., p. 606

251. A. Flat affect is one in which there is absence of feeling tone. Expressing an affect opposite from the one felt is not an affective disturbance. Affect involves feelings or emotions, not thoughts or actions. Presenting conflicting expressions as a result of conflicting feelings is displaying one's felt emotions. *(NB, analyzing; LDM, shared)*

Haber et al., p. 610

252. C. Neologisms are words coined by the schizophrenic that have personal meaning but are not understood by others. Hallucinations are spontaneous, unwilled sense perceptions for which there is no reality basis. An illusion is a misinterpretation of an actual sensory experience. A delusion is a false, fixed belief that cannot be corrected by logic. *(NB, analyzing; LDM, shared)*

Burgess, pp. 280–282

253. D. Coping mechanisms are used to excess in schizophrenia but become inadequate in reducing anxiety to tolerable levels. The person who is intensely anxious about some impulses perceived as unacceptable may project these impulses onto others in the environment. By this projection the self rids itself of the anxiety-probing impulses and enables them to reside in others. Coping mechanisms would not punish others but relieve the individual's internal anxiety; their use is not related to gaining attention from others. Coping mechanisms tend to reduce stimulation by relieving anxiety. *(NB, analyzing; LDM, nurse centered)*

Haber et al., p. 600

254. D. The primary objective of the beginning phase of a therapeutic relationship is establishing contact, the formation of a working relationship with the client. The working relationship in this phase is the framework on which the client constructs behavioral change. Developing techniques for responding to the patient's verbalizations would be more appropriate in the working phase of the relationship, as would be nurse-patient collaboration to identify behavioral problems. Providing opportunities for the patient to try new coping behaviors is also a component of the middle or working phase of the relationship. *(NB, analyzing; LDM, shared)*

Wilson and Kneisl (1979), pp. 137–142

255. C. The goal of nursing intervention with the schizophrenic patient is establishment of trust in the nurse. As a result of this trust relationship the patient can hopefully learn to trust others. Relating and identifying will occur after trust is firmly established. Trust must be present before feelings and emotions can be expressed. *(NB, planning; LDM, shared)*

Haber et al., pp. 637–639

256. B. Isolation, apathy, mutism, and lack of eye contact all reflect withdrawal. On the basis of the data presented, there is insufficient information to support a nursing diagnosis of dependence, delusional thinking, or regression. *(NB, analyzing, LDM, nurse centered)*

Stuart and Sundeen (1983), pp. 368–375

257. D. The behavioral disruptions of schizophrenic patients serve as coping mechanisms and are therefore resistant to change; this makes mutual goal setting difficult. While behavioral changes may take a long time to develop, these changes can be lasting. Schizophrenia does not affect the patient's cognitive understanding, and schizophrenic behaviors are predictable, meaningful, and fulfill patient needs. *(NB, analyzing; LDM, client centered)*

Stuart and Sundeen (1983), pp. 385–386

258. A. The ambivalent patient is unable to make decisions. The nurse initially makes decisions for the patient and helps the patient to gradually progress toward independent decision making thus decreasing his ambivalent behavior. The ambivalent schizophrenic could not tolerate independence or function adequately without supervision. Participating in activities does not directly relate to decreasing ambivalence. Expressing the contradictory feelings of ambivalence may or may not be helpful in changing behavior. *(NB, planning; LDM, client centered)*

Wilson and Kneisl (1983), p. 442

259. B. Dependency of the client upon the nurse should be avoided because it fosters regression; the goal of independence is to promote the client's return to a higher level of functioning. Attaining an appropriate level of functioning is a long-term goal. Further client regression should be prevented, and maintaining the current level of functioning is a short-term goal that will help prevent further regression. *(NB, analyzing; LDM, shared)*

Burgess, pp. 292–293

260. D. Responding to the theme of the delusion shifts the focus to the client's real feelings that underlie the delusion, encouraging the client to explore the purpose for which the delusion serves. Rational explanations will make the patient adhere more firmly to the delusion. Challenging the validity of the delusion strips the client of her defense against over-whelming anxiety and may precipitate an outburst of assaultive behavior. Refusing to continue talking with the client indicates nonacceptance of the client by the nurse. *(NB, planning; LDM, shared)*

Haber et al., pp. 642–643

261. D. Biochemical studies have thus far proved inconclusive regarding a specific biochemical basis for schizophrenia. Information in all of the other options is accurate regarding what is known about the biochemical processes associated with schizophremia. *(NB, analyzing; LDM, nurse centered)*

Haber et al., pp. 614–615

262. A. Families of schizophrenic clients may generate a variety of feelings in the nurse; these feelings may range from empathy regarding the difficulties the family may face to anger about the client's lack of progress. Families often express desire to restructure family relationships and communication patterns, but then do not follow through with these plans. The nurse may perceive the client as a helpless victim, unable to overcome family forces which operate to keep the client "sick." Family communication patterns are often dysfunctional. *(NB, analyzing; LDM, nurse centered)*

Haber et al., p. 620

263. A. Labels such as schizophrenia frequently determine what care clients receive based upon interpretation of client behavior in light of the label. The label often creates expectations and interpretation of behavior associated with diagnosis whether or not the label is valid; significant symptoms or behavior may be negated because of the label.

While there is movement toward unifying psychiatric diagnoses, there is still lack of precision in these diagnoses. The initial diagnostic label remains beyond the immediate illness. Sanity cannot be distinguished from insanity on the basis of a classification system such as the *Diagnostic and Statistical Manual of Mental Disorders (DSM III)*. Since the diagnostic label can become a self-fulfilling prophecy for patient, family, and mental health professional, its potential stigma cannot be removed. *(NB, analyzing; LDM, shared)*

Haber et al., pp. 24–26

264. D. Schizophrenic clients display profound mistrust of self and others, arising from early interpersonal relationships experienced as threatening and rejecting. These clients develop and use defense strategies such as avoidance and ambivalence for self-protection in current relationships. Dependency is a common problem among schizophrenic clients, but this diagnosis is established after more data are gathered. The full extent of low self-esteem may become apparent only after the nurse spends time interacting with the client. There are insufficient data to determine if the client indeed lacks an adequate support system. *(NB, analyzing; LDM, shared)*

Haber et al., pp. 625–626, 634–635, 637–639

265. B. In a one-to-one relationship with a schizophrenic client it is especially important to acknowledge feelings generated by the client because the client is acutely sensitive to the feelings of others. Feelings in the nurse that can go unrecognized and unacknowledged can create barriers in the nurse-client relationship. Decoding the client's symbolic language, assessing the client's hallucinations, and involving the patient in goal-directed activities are all interventions that would be initiated after the relationship was established. *(NB, planning; LDM, nurse centered)*

Haber et al., pp. 618–619

266. C. Because delusions occupy much of the paranoid patient's thinking, structured activities will decrease time spent in this process. Too much variety and stimulation will be ineffective because of the patient's intense, narrowly focused attention span. The paranoid patient rarely has interest in concentrating on an activity. When the patient becomes aggressive, he cannot concentrate on activities. *(NB, analyzing; LDM, shared)*

Wilson and Kneisl (1979), pp. 336–337

267. D. The nurse needs to be consistent in working with the suspicious client. The patient must know what is expected from him and what to expect from the staff; the sameness provides security for the client. The suspicious client is intimidated by an overbearing, friendly attitude of others, and clear, concise explanations are preferable. Contact with others and competition is frightening to this client. *(NB, implementing; LDM, shared)*

Burgess, pp. 288–289

268. C. In communicating with the delusional patient, the nurse should avoid supporting and reinforcing the client's delusion without attacking or challenging the delusion. The client needs to be helped to relinquish his delusion without losing face. Option A is an example of supporting the client's delusional system. In option B the nurse questions the delusion which confuses the client who is unable to test external reality. Option D belittles the client and may provoke violent behavior on the client's part. *(NB, implementing; LDM, shared)*

Haber et al., pp. 641–643

269. B. Both hallucinations and delusions occur in the catatonic schizophrenic with identified themes of persecution and fear-inducing mysticism. Delusions are frequently part of the catatonic patient's disturbed thought process. Both agitation and mute immobilization can be seen in the same catatonic patient. The catatonic patient regresses to a primitive level of functioning during the acute phase of illness but may return to reality and be symptom-free from time to time. *(NB, analyzing; LDM, nurse centered)*

Lancaster, pp. 364–366

270. B. This option demonstrates awareness of this withdrawn patient's inability to care for herself and displays acceptance of her as an individual. Option A is inappropriate because the patient is withdrawn, preoccupied, and unable to make a decision in response to the question. Option C does not facilitate decreasing the client's withdrawn behavior and may be perceived as punitive by the client, further decreasing self-esteem. Option D is also threatening to the patient who is already immobilized. *(NB, implementing; LDM, shared)*

Stuart and Sundeen (1983), pp. 386–388

271. B. Going to the activity with the client and participating with him uses the established trusting relationship as a means of expanding his participation in other activities in which he can experience success. Option A will only serve to increase the patient's anxiety and option C will not serve to encourage patient participation. Reassurance is nontherapeutic for the patient with low-esteem and feelings of worthlessness. *(NB, implementing; LDM, shared)*

Haber et al., p. 635

272. D. Goals for the schizophrenic client should be realistic to avoid discouragement for both nurse and client. The goal of open, direct communication, for instance, may take months to achieve. Option A is an intermediate goal, while option B reflects a short-term goal. The client's nonverbal communication should be congruent with her verbal communication, and this may also be a long-term goal; using only nonverbal communication is not therapeutic. *(NB, analyzing; LDM, shared)*

Haber et al., pp. 625–629

273. A. Auditory hallucinations represent a high level of interpersonal anxiety and a projection of repressed ideation to objects outside of the self. Projection permits the ego to deal with unconscious feelings and impulses as external threats, thus reducing anxiety. Hallucinations are unconscious in nature and unrelated to environmental stimuli. Biologic theorists believe that hallucinations result from a metabolic response to stress, not cellular pathology. *(NB, assessing; LDM, nurse centered)*

Stuart and Sundeen (1983), p. 369

274. C. Acknowledging the reality to him of the client's hallucination reflects an accepting, nonjudgmental attitude on the nurse's part that is essential in decreasing client anxiety. The nurse also needs to clearly indicate that these sensory perceptions are not shared by others. Option A would reinforce the client's hallucinatory world. The psychotic client is unable to explore the meaning of the hallucination; he is not capable of dynamic insight at this time. Option D is another nontherapeutic response that would serve to reinforce the hallucination. *(NB, analyzing; LDM, shared)*

Haber et al., pp. 641–642

275. D. Researchers have concluded that the current status of the patient's life provides the most valid prognostic clues. Strengths within the social environment, such as family interest and participation in treatment, are positively related to patient improvement. Prognosis is poor when onset is slow, there is a prior history of schizophrenic symptoms, and the symptoms have been present more than 6 weeks. *(NB, analyzing; LDM, shared)*

Burgess, pp. 297–298

276. C. Feelings that the schizophrenic client generates in the nurse may reflect unresolved issues in the nurse's own life and interfere with accurately synthesizing cognitive and affective experiences. Therefore self-assessment will help the nurse develop self-awareness, self-understanding, and understanding of clients. Acceptance of the client occurs after the nurse's self-assessment. Warmth may be a useful intervention in some clients but may intensify problems in others. Limit setting may be initiated in response to testing behavior on the client's part. *(NB, implementing; LDM, nurse centered)*

Haber et al., pp. 620–621, 639

277. B. Acute dystonic reactions involve bizarre and severe muscle contractions that can be physically painful and frightening to the client; these reactions occur early in treatment with phenothiazides. Parkinsonian syndrome includes symptoms such as masklike facies, resting tremor, and postural rigidity. Akathisia is a motor restlessness experienced as an urge to pace. Tardive dyskinesia is a disorder characterized by involuntary movements of the face, jaw, and tongue. *(NB, assessing; LDM, nurse centered)*

Wilson and Kneisl (1979), pp. 592–593

278. B. The nurse needs to provide directions to the schizophrenic client that enable him to follow daily routines with a minimum of decision-making requirements. The environment needs to be consistent and predictable, with environmental stimuli kept to a minimum to prevent sensory overload. Immediate involvement in stimulating activities may initially be too anxiety producing for the client. The client may have difficulty communicating and may not initiate requests for needed care, hence the nurse needs to assess and intervene on his behalf. *(NB, planning; LDM, shared)*

Haber et al., p. 630

279. A. In residual schizophrenia the patient is without overt psychotic features but has other clinical signs such as social withdrawal, eccentric behavior, emotional flatness, illogical thinking, and loose association. Volleyball would be an appropriate activity because it involves working with others, decreasing social isolation. Remaining in her room, encouraging TV watching, and learning to crochet are all solitary activities which reinforce her social isolation. *(NB, planning; LDM, shared)*

Haber et al., p. 601

280. B. Initially, contact between the schizophrenic patient and the staff and other patients should be kept to a minimum because the patient tends to be distrustful and suspicious. The patient needs a small unit, preferably a private room, to overcome his feelings of intimidation by the staff or other patients. The environment should be limited for this patient to enhance his sense of security, thus taking the patient off the unit should occur only when he feels comfortable with the unit environment and himself. Providing long verbal explanations will anger the client but no explanation whatsoever will decrease his trust of the staff; concise explanations are appropriate. *(NB, implementing; LDM, shared)*

Burgess, pp. 288–291

281. D. Chemical, hormonal, and physical interventions influence the brain either directly or indirectly, changing behavior, altering mood, or both. Somatic approaches cannot cure the condition but do interrupt the psychotic process and alleviate symptoms. Somatic therapy can be used even if the cause of the psychosis is not organic. Psychoactive drug therapy and electroconculsive therapy have been established as effective measures in alleviating symptoms of schizophrenia. *(NB, analyzing; LDM, nurse centered)*

Wilson and Kneisl (1979), p. 363

282. B. Negativism is common in schizophrenics, and the patient should be given another opportunity to take the medication. Threats cause the patient to become increasingly anxious. Omitting the medication without notifying the physician is inappropriate and irresponsible, as is concealing medication in food, tricking the patient into taking medication. *(NB, implementing; LDM, shared)*

Taylor, pp. 247–248

283. B. When clients first take antipsychotic drugs they often feel oversedated, but this effect decreases after taking the medication for a few weeks. Diphenhydramine hydrochloride (Benadryl) is used to treat extrapyramidal side effects of antipsychotic medication. Oversedation is not a symptom of dystonia and is unrelated to tardive dyskinesia. *(NB, analyzing; LDM, nurse centered)*

Stuart and Sundeen (1983), p. 502

284. A. While the exact mechanism of the action of chlorpromazine is unknown, it is theorized that it interferes with dopamine reception or synthesis at the neural synapse. Insulin shock therapy produces a state of physiologic shock. Antidepressant drugs appear to facilitate transmission at the neural synapse. Psychosurgery interrupts the neuropathways of emotion between the frontal lobes of the cerebral cortex. *(NB, analyzing; LDM, nurse centered)*

Stuart and Sundeen (1983), p. 500

285. C. Chlorpromazine (Thorazine) is used primarily for severe psychosis, anxiety, neurosis, and as an adjunct during alcohol withdrawal; it is not prescribed for antisocial personality disorders. Chlorpromazine does not depress the chemoreceptor trigger zone for emesis. There is no cure for antisocial personality disorder. *(NB, analyzing; LDM, nurse centered)*

Haber et al, pp. 397–398

286. D. Antipsychotic drugs such as chlorpromazine promote relaxation and clearer, less delusional thinking and reduce hallucinations. These medications do not alleviate depression or establish a more even mood. The medication should make the client feel better but this response is more vague than the correct option; it may also be perceived as false reassurance. *(NB, implementing; LDM, shared)*

Haber et al., pp. 397–398

287. C. Chlorpromazine possesses a relatively high degree of anticholinergic action and can induce urinary retention. Tachycardia is more likely to occur than bradycardia, and appetite may be increased to the point of weight becoming a problem. Libido is decreased with antipsychotics. *(NB, analyzing; LDM, shared)*

Haber et al., pp. 398–399

288. C. Benztropine mesylate (Cogentin) is a quick-acting antiparkinsonian drug used to treat extrapyramidal symptoms associated with antipsychotic drugs. Antianxiety agents such as barbiturates or benzodiazapines are used to relieve mild to moderate anxiety. Antipsychotic medications can produce sedation for the agitated patient and normalize unacceptable psychotic behaviors. *(NB, analyzing; LDM, nurse centered)*

Haber et al., pp. 400–404

289. B. During the intake interview it is important to document the client's medication history, including current prescribed drugs, dosage, reactions, etc. While trifluoperazine hydrochloride (Stelazine) generally produces minor sedative effects, it would be important to document the extent to which its sedative effect may be interfering with client functioning. Angina pectoris and tachycardia may occur with beta-adrenergic-blocking agents such as propanolol hydrochloride (Inderal). Antiemetic effect and muscle relaxation are nonspecific assessments and unrelated to the major medication for antipsychotic drugs. Blurred vision may occur with several medications, and craving for sweets can be a presenting symptom of depressive behavior. *(NB, assessing; LDM, shared)*

Haber et al., pp. 398–406

290. C. Clients should be taught to take missed doses of medication later in the day to ensure a therapeutic level of the medication. Medications must be taken regularly to avoid possible psychotic manifestations and they are not withheld during the menstrual period. Taking antacids within an hour of medication ingestion will interfere with absorption of the antipsychotic medication. *(NB, analyzing; LDM, client centered)*

   Wilson and Kneisl (1983), p. 676

291. D. Trifluoperazine comes in small dosages of 10-60 mg.; therefore the medication in this situation is mislabeled and should be returned to the pharmacy. Reading the label three times will not correct the basic problem of mislabeling; the medication should not be poured. Concentrated solutions of antipsychotic medications should be mixed with juices or milk because they are caustic to mucous membranes. The maximum therapeutic effect of this medication occurs 2-3 weeks after therapy is begun. *(NB, implementing; LDM, nurse centered)*

   Wilson and Kneisl (1983), p. 676

292. A. Most antipsychotic medications are ordered as a single dose at bedtime to maximize the drug's sedative properties and to decrease patients having to remember to take medication many times during the day. The patient should be encouraged to use a sunscreen when going to the beach while taking antipsychotic drugs since these drugs can cause photosensitivity. The medication should not be discontinued. While a dry mouth is annoying, it is a common side effect of antipsychotic medication; the medication should not be discontinued. Medication should not be increased without consulting with the physician. *(NB, evaluating; LDM, client centered)*

   Wilson and Kneisl (1983), p. 672

293. B. Tardive dyskinesia is characterized by bizarre facial and tongue movements, stiff neck, and difficulty swallowing; it is one of the extrapyramidal side effects of long-term antipsychotic medication therapy. Providing emotional support is an ongoing goal, not a priority at this time. Monitoring salt intake is important for clients taking lithium carbonate, and tyramine-rich foods are contraindicated for patients taking MAO inhibitors. *(NB, analyzing; LDM, shared)*

Stuart and Sundeen (1983), p. 502

294. C. Orthostatic hypotension is a side effect that can occur with antipsychotic medication; the client should be instructed to stand up slowly. Antidepressant medications act to increase perspiration, and excessive urination is a side effect of lithium carbonate. Alcohol is contraindicated with antipsychotic medication because it produces faster metabolism of the antipsychotic drug by the liver. *(NB, evaluating; LDM, client centered)*

Stuart and Sundeen (1983), p. 503

295. D. Severe muscle contractions, twisted neck, and eyes rolling upward are all symptoms of an acute dystonic reaction, a type of extrapyramidal side effect occurring after the first few days of treatment with an antipsychotic. Symptoms in option A are characteristic of autonomic blockade-type side effects, and those in option B are characteristic of cholinergic-type blockade effects. Option C indicates endocrine effects that can occur with thiothixene (Navane) therapy. *(NB, assessing; LDM, shared)*

Wilson and Kneisl (1983), p. 673

296. A. Dystonic reactions are usually controlled immediately by intramuscular injections of benztropine mesylate (Cogentin). Chewing gum and rinsing the mouth with water would relieve cholinergic blockade side effects. Charting rashes and bowel movements would document cholinergic blockade side effects. Liver function tests would be ordered if there was indication of cholestatic jaundice. *(NB, implementing; LDM, shared)*

Stuart and Sundeen (1983), p. 502

297. C. Long-term use of benztropine mesylate (Cogentin) predisposes clients to tardive dyskinesia. Antipsychotic medication should be slowly withdrawn. Drug "holidays" from antipsychotics are recommended to periodically assess for the existence of tardive dyskinesia, an indication to discontinue Cogentin. *(NB, planning; LDM, client centered)*

Stuart and Sundeen (1983), p. 502

298. B. Haloperidol (Haldol) is the drug of choice for managing highly agitated clients; it is quick acting and produces sedation in large doses. The medication dosage should be adjusted when the desired therapeutic effect is achieved, i.e., calm, less-agitated behavior. Hypoglycemia is unrelated to rapid tranquilization. There is no reason to restrict fluid intake or maintain the client on complete bed rest. *(NB, implementing; LDM, shared)*

Haber et al, pp. 398–399

299. D. Hypotension is a common side effect of antipsychotic drug administration, and haloperidol (Haldol) is associated with a high incidence of extrapyramidal side effects; therefore, monitoring vital signs and observing for development of these side effects is essential during rapid tranquilization. The CPK level is monitored following myocardial infarction. Group activities would be contraindicated during rapid tranquilization as would family visitation. *(NB, planning; LDM, shared)*

Haber et al., pp. 399–400

F. PERSONALITY DISORDERS

300. A. Of the 7% of Americans classified as having personality disorders, 2-5% are classified as antisocial personalities or sociopaths. *(NB, assessing; LDM, nurse centered)*

Burgess, p. 312

301. D. The antisocial person's history generally shows that early needs for satisfaction and security were met with delay, indifference, and rejection on the part of significant others. He has experienced rejection and had limited opportunities to trust as a child. None of the other options contain information pertinent to developing an antisocial personality. *(NB, assessing; LDM, shared)*

Haber et al., p. 511

302. B. The antisocial personality feels that any type of attachment to, or affection for, other people are traps. He fears loss of freedom if he becomes in any way dependent on others. Identifying his feelings about initiating a therapeutic relationship may decrease his fear of becoming dependent. Showing no emotion will not affect the client's behavior. Since this client's behavior is not admirable (i.e., he is impulsive, considers people as insignificant objects to be used) his behavior should not be supported. He has no guilt feelings, even though he understands guilt and can feign it readily. *(NB, implementing; LDM, shared)*

Burgess, pp. 312–313

303. C. Antisocial personalities use avoidance to withhold emotional involvement, escaping from feeling. It is important to provide interpersonal contact while respecting the client's need for distance. The nurse should convey an expectation that the client at some point will wish to relate in a different way and should not limit attention to the "bad" moments when the client is physically or emotionally withdrawn. Options A and B would perpetuate the client's pattern of avoidance. Since antisocial personalities often anger other clients, providing them with the opportunity to ventilate their feelings would serve to further alienate the antisocial personality from others. *(NB, planning; LDM, shared)*

Haber et al., pp. 517, 526

304. A. Observing the client's relational patterns with others will assist the nurse in dealing with the problematic themes documented. It is premature to think of this client in a leadership role since he has difficulty establishing and maintaining relationships. The client has no inclination toward depression, and assessing future goals is unrealistic because the client lives only in the present. *(NB, assessing; LDM, shared)*

Haber et al., pp. 510–511, 515

305. A. Committing a crime brings no remorse to the antisocial personality. Documenting the client's response can indicate the dynamic elements with which the nurse can begin to deal in a therapeutic relationship. Option B offers a means of excusing the client's behavior, thus preventing the client from learning the consequences of her behavior. Canceling the client's privileges will not provide a deterrent to recurrence, and bringing her family in will not deal with the underlying problematic behavior. *(NB, planning; LDM, shared)*

Burgess, pp. 312–313;
Haber et al., pp. 511–512

306. A. Automatically opposing all client behavior does not allow him to discriminate among various behaviors in self and others. By asking the client his intentions, the nurse conveys awareness of his manipulative behavior but also offers the possibility of meeting his needs within clearly defined limits. Options B, C, and D are responses that avoid the issue of the client's manipulative behavior. *(NB, implementing; LDM, shared)*

Haber et al., pp. 524–525

307. A. According to Freud, the drives of the primitive id are not under sufficient control by the ego and conflict with society's restrictions in the antisocial personality. A setting with appropriate limits would provide a reasonable outlet for the client's drives while controlling impulsive behavior. Punishment is ineffective because the superego is not adequately developed. The antisocial personality operates at a "pretrust" level, thus classes on trust would be ineffective. An overly sympathetic atmosphere provides greater opportunity for the antisocial personality to exploit and manipulate others. *(NB, analyzing; LDM, shared)*

Burgess, p. 314
Haber et al., pp. 510–511, 524

308. C. The antisocial personality has a very low tolerance for anxiety but has difficulty talking about feelings. By indicating she is available to talk about the situation, the nurse conveys concern for the client without acceptance of his behavior. Telling others to avoid confronting the client allows him to avoid responsibility for his actions. Leaving the client alone also helps him to avoid looking at his behavioral patterns. Telling the client that feelings are difficult to cope with is not useful in helping the client work through difficult situations. *(NB, planning; LDM, shared)*

Haber et al., pp. 510–511, 524

309. B. Observing client-family interaction can provide clues about the family's role in maintaining the client's dysfunctional behavior and provide dynamic themes for nurse-client interaction. Limiting family contact serves no useful purpose, especially when the family's relational pattern with the client is not documented. Sympathizing with the family is taking sides against the client, perpetuating his outsider position. The family cannot do much about the client's needs while he is hospitalized; some idea of their relational patterns with the client is needed so that they can contribute to helping the client. *(NB, planning; LDM, shared)*

Haber et al., p. 513

310. B. Anger constitutes the main affect the borderline personality experiences; this affect is directed at a variety of targets. Depression and feelings of loneliness are likely to be present, not joviality. Aggressiveness and arrogance are not affects associated with the borderline patient. *(NB, assessing; LDM, nurse centered)*

Burgess, p. 306

311. A. In guiding the borderline client to become an observer of her own behavior, it is necessary to identify those situations which provoke use of intellectualizing as an ego defense. The borderline client presents bland, nondescript, "as if" behavior with no sense of identity. Option C is an example of the nurse intellectualizing. The borderline client offers little spontaneity in response to situations, and intellectualizing promotes this type of withdrawal from social situations. *(NB, implementing; LDM, shared)*

Burgess, pp. 306–307

312. D. Verbal expression is a more mature way to express feelings than nonverbal ways which are inappropriate; the client is helped to gain insight into the reasons for such behaviors. Consistency is a necessary component for any individual who has difficulty controlling behavior. The staff needs to make group decisions about client care to decrease the possibility of being manipulated. Progress in borderline personality disorders is slow and the acting-out behaviors exist for a long time. *(NB, implementing; LDM, shared)*

Haber et al., pp. 471–480

313. A. Patients bordering on neurosis react with whining, crying, and sadness when dependent needs are not satisfied; thus fewer entries indicating these behaviors would indicate that the patient is effectively working through dependency. The borderline neurotic exhibits a childlike clinging depression not associated with anger or guilt feelings; he seems defeated, discouraged, and apathetically accepting of his state. *(NB, evaluating; LDM, client centered)*

Burgess, p. 306

314. A. Having the client keep a log of demands is a focused way of demonstrating to the client that he recognizes what he is doing and provides reinforcement when the behavior decreases in frequency. Several years of intensive therapy is required with the borderline client before he can function on his own, therefore it is unrealistic to expect evidence of this behavior in a short-term situation. Holding a staff meeting will promote consensus of approach but will not promote client insight into his behavior. Manipulation is to be expected from the borderline client and it needs to decrease in frequency with therapy. *(NB, implementing; LDM, shared)*

Burgess, pp. 308–309

315. B. Withdrawal is frequently used as a defense mechanism by the borderline client. This client is very acceptive, with both negative and positive affect missing. Having no sense of personal identity would make it virtually impossible for this client to act forcefully on her own behalf. Hallucinations would be associated with psychosis, not borderline personality. *(NB, analyzing; LDM, client centered)*

Burgess, pp. 306–307

316. D. The borderline client who is still hostile can act aggressively toward the staff. Her behavior can make the staff very defensive and unless their approach is consistent, the client can manipulate or split the staff to meet her needs. The borderline client has no established sense of identity. Increased staff efforts to help this client would indicate the patient is making some improvement. Denial, although used by the borderline client, is not related to the issue of hostility. *(NB, evaluating; LDM, shared)*

Burgess, pp. 308–309

317. D. Although their symptoms may vary, the underlying dynamics of dependent patients' behavior are similar. They are obsessed with their health and perceive themselves as worthless, accounting for their willingness to undergo painful procedures repeatedly. Their hostility is veiled by their helpless, passive appearance. Anxiety and isolation are not underlying dynamics, nor is passivity since they become resistant to becoming independent. *(NB, analyzing; LDM, client centered)*

Wilson and Kneisl (1979), p. 631

318. C. This conversation reflects the sense of omnipotence which characterizes narcissism. Loose association, obsession, and reaction formation are not characteristic of narcissistic personality disorder. *(NB, assessing; LDM, nurse centered)*

Haber et al., p. 539

319. C. When the needs of a passive-aggressive personality are not met, the client responds with feelings of helplessness, depression, and then anger and rage. This client uses intentional inefficiency, rather than helpfulness in relating with others. Procrastination, not punctuality, is characteristic of the passive-aggressive personality. Intellectualizing occurs in a variety of disorders but is not characteristic of the passive-aggressive personality. *(NB, analyzing; LDM, client centered)*

Burgess, p. 304

320. D. One characteristic of the person with pedophilia is lack of feelings of emotional security and self-confidence. Anger, sex role identity, and domination are not problems in pedophilia. *(NB, analyzing; LDM, shared)*

Haber et al., p. 660

321. B. A frank, warm, objective approach to clients whose sexual orientation is different from the nurse's will foster openness and encourage discussion of difficulties the client may be experiencing; in this situation acknowledging the client's loss of a partner and his feelings of alienation would provide support to the client. Telling the homosexual client to stay away from male patients is unrealistic, and avoiding him will only increase his sense of alienation. Placing this client in seclusion is unnecessary and inappropriate. *(NB, planning; LDM, shared)*

   Haber et al., pp. 657, 662–665

322. C. A staff meeting would be a useful way to help everyone consider his individual response toward a person with a different life-style; it would be an opportunity to clarify one's own feelings about sexuality and consider the sexual concerns of clients. Transferring the staff is a possibility but not an initial action, and assigning all male clients to female staff may not be a practical option. Confronting the male staff with their sexual biases is inappropriate; they may be experiencing a threat to their own sexual identity. *(NB, implementing; LDM, nurse centered)*

   Haber et al., pp. 659, 661, 665

323. C. This response indicates the client exhibits a realistic attitude toward his life situation. Options A and B indicate the client is still withdrawn and perhaps not ready for discharge. Option D indicates the client has not resolved conflicts about his homosexuality. *(NB, evaluating; LDM, client centered)*

   Wilson and Kneisl (1983), p. 587

324. D. Acceptance by the nurse is important for the client to accept his sexual identity and to begin counseling. Options A and D reflect inappropriate labeling by the nurse. Option B indicates that the nurses have not resolved their feelings toward the client's homosexuality. Option D also reflects lack of acceptance of the client's sexual preference. *(NB, evaluating; LDM, client centered)*

   Stuart and Sundeen (1983), p. 678

325. B. Assessing how much the client knows about possible sexual abuse is the first step in teaching him about sexual molestation or assault. Teaching the child to avoid males can interfere with subsequent relationships with men. After the child's knowledge is assessed, role playing can be used as a teaching strategy. Talking about dangerous situations can be introduced following the assessment. *(NB, implementing; LDM, shared)*

Burgess, p. 561

G. ORGANIC MENTAL DISORDERS

326. C. The label of "organic brain syndrome" is prejudicial in that it does not indicate degree of impairment while implying that little can be achieved therapeutically. Organic mental disorder can occur at any developmental stage. Not all neurologic illness in children can be diagnosed; general terms such as "hyperactivity" or "minimal brain dysfunction" are nonspecific. In some instances children may outgrow the symptomatic behavior, but not always. *(NB, analyzing; LDM, nurse centered)*

Pasquali et al., pp. 597–599

327. B. Lead produces fragility of the red blood cell membrane with subsequent destruction of nerve cells in the brain. Pica often involves chewing on items painted with older paint that is lead based. Not all nonfood substances would produce neuronal destruction; they do not furnish protein. Manganese is not found in paint. *(NB, analyzing; LDM, client centered)*

Pasquali et al., p. 583

328. D. The Mental Status Questionnaire consists of ten valid and reliable questions that are indicators of a person's mental status. Questions address orientation for time, place, and person; memory, recent and remote; and general information. The Minnesota Multiphasic Personality Inventory is an extensive test of responses forming a personality profile. The face-hand test is a series of double, simultaneous stimulations of the face and hand which can assess cortical neuronal loss. The Rorschach test is a complex test of inkblot interpretation. *(NB, assessing; LDM, shared)*

Haber et al., p. 833;
Wilson and Kneisl (1979), pp. 85–86

329. A. How a particular person responds to organic mental syndrome depends on personality type, interpersonal relationships, past experiences, the current environmental situation, etc. The client does not develop brand new personality traits. Physiologic changes account for the changes in brain functioning, and these changes can occur at any age. *(NB, analyzing; LDM, client centered)*

Wilson and Kneisl (1979), pp. 413–414

330. A. Elderly clients with organic mental disorders often generate frustration in their caregivers. Awareness that these feelings are developing is part of the resolution of potential problems, and examining individual feelings about aging will affect the nurse's responses to these clients. Nursing assistants may provide care to these clients, but the registered nurse needs to supervise their care provision. Making all patient decisions fosters client dependency, although it may be easier for the staff. Providing only physical care reduces the client to the status of an object and ignores client's emotional needs. *(NB, planning; LDM, nurse centered)*

Haber et al., pp. 843–845

331. A. Prominent symptoms of organic mental syndrome include disturbances in intellectual abilities, particularly memory, orientation, and judgment. Motor disturbance may be present in neurologic illnesses such as Parkinson's disease and Huntington's chorea but not in all organic mental disorders. Delusions are more often associated with schizophrenia but may occur in some acute states of delirium.

Disturbed mood is a prominent symptom of manic-depression but may occur in some organic mental disorders. *(NB, assessing; LDM, nurse centered)*

Pasquali et al., p. 567

332. C. Delirium refers to global impairments of acute onset that are usually transient in nature. Clinical features include clouded level of consciousness, cognitive impairment, disorientation, slowing electroencephalogram, hallucinations, and delusions. *(NB, assessing; LDM, shared)*

Wilson and Kneisl (1979), pp. 416–417

333. B. Chronic infections of the central nervous system have a gradual onset and may be detected only because of associated emotional or behavioral changes such as depression, insomnia, or psychosis. Acute infections produce classic neurologic signs that appear suddenly, as well as disorientation, confusion, or wild behavioral deviations. *(NB, analyzing; LDM, nurse centered)*

Wilson and Kneisl (1979), p. 419

334. B. Acute bacterial infections of the central nervous system in the form of meningitis, encephalitis, and brain abscess produce classic physical signs and acute mental changes characteristic of delirium. None of the other options are causes of delirium. *(NB, assessing; LDM, nurse centered)*

Wilson and Kneisl (1979), p. 419

335. D. When a client complains of insects that are not really there, the nurse should be alert to the possibility that the client is going into delirium tremens. Severe anxiety is accompanied by other subjective and objective symptoms. The client would probably remember having a nightmare. *(NB, analyzing; LDM, shared)*

Taylor, p. 434

336. A. The nurse who is calm and reassuring can better deal with her own feelings of anxiety that the patient's condition arouses, and thus will be able to provide a quiet environment for the patient. The nurse may not understand the patient's hallucinations and taking complete charge of the patient is unrealistic. When the patient is no longer confused, he may begin to identify with the nurse's mood. *(NB, planning; LDM, shared)*

Pasquali et al., pp. 593–594

337. C. In caring for the delirious patient speaking and moving slowly, softly, and deliberately helps convey to the patient that the nurse is there to help him. The nurse's voice provides contact with reality and her nonverbal behavior may not be understood by the patient. Opinion on the use of medication in controlling delirium is divided, particularly since there is a danger in giving too much on top of an unknown cause for delirium. Unless absolutely essential, exposure to stressful procedures such as x-rays and diagnostic tests is avoided because the procedures may precipitate panic. *(NB, planning; LDM, shared)*

Burgess, p. 336

338. A. Delirium refers to global impairments of acute onset which are usually transient in nature. Acute bacterial infections can produce acute mental changes characteristic of delirium. Dementia refers to irreversible impairments of either acute or gradual onset. Cerebral arteriosclerosis presents progressive mental impairment in the older patient. General paresis is the result of syphilitic infection. *(NB, analyzing; LDM, nurse centered)*

Wilson and Kneisl (1979), pp. 416–419

339. C. Delirium is characterized by bewilderment and disorientation. By providing short, simple answers the nurse will help the patient understand what is going on. A team of different nurses would tend to increase the patient's anxiety

because he needs a familiar environment. Darkness increases the patient's disorientation and increases unreality, and solitude adds to his anxiety because no one is there to clarify frightening stimuli. *(NB, implementing; LDM, shared)*

Pasquali et al ., p. 594

340. D. Confabulation is commonly seen in organic brain syndrome, occurring when the individual cannot recall specific events and supplements this loss with relevant but imaginary information. Circumstantiality is a disturbance in associative thought process; the person goes into unnecessary detail and inappropriate thought before expressing the main idea. Reminiscing is the process of recalling and expressing material or events from a previous time in life. Regression is the return to a previous developmental level. *(NB, assessing; LDM, shared)*

Pasquali et al., p. 571

341. C. Immediate recall and recent memory are the most seriously affected in irreversible brain damage; patients have difficulty shifting to the present. Confabulation is the tendency to fabricate a response to a question when one cannot remember the answer. Remote memory may remain intact. While disorientation can occur, it is not the most prominent characteristic. *(NB, assessing; LDM, client centered)*

Stuart and Sundeen (1979), p. 144

342. A. The cells of the central nervous system are very sensitive to even brief periods of decreased oxygen supply. Circulatory disturbances such as athersclerosis, infarction, and hypoxia decrease cerebral oxygenation and result in anxiety, headache, fatigue, and irritability. La belle indifference is the noticeable lack of affect in proportion to the apparent severity of symptoms in a conversion disorder. Flight-of-ideas and dissociative speech patterns are both seen primarily in psychopathology. *(NB, assessing; LDM, shared)*

Burgess, pp. 331–332

343. B. In the tonic phase of a grand mal seizure the patient loses consciousness, and if she falls in a rigid position, she is likely to hurt herself. Encouraging interaction with peers is of secondary importance in seizure control. Regulation of medication is the physician's responsibility, and checking the patient's gait would be one part of the assessment phase. *(NB, implementing; LDM, shared)*

Burgess, p. 330

344. D. Circumstantiality is a disturbance in associative thought processes in which the person digresses into unnecessary detail and inappropriate thoughts before communicating the main idea. Confabulation is the unconscious filling of gaps in memory with experiences that have no basis in fact. Blocking is the involuntary cessation of thought processes or speech because of unconscious emotional factors. Punning is a type of speech seen most often in schizophrenics. *(NB, assessing; LDM, client centered)*

Pasquali et al., p. 570

345. A. Attempts to intervene or complete a story can be frustrating to the client and arouse anger and anxiety. Isolating the patient fails to meet her need for socialization. Encouraging the patient not to talk can frustrate her and create dependency on others. Completing the patient's thought implies staff impatience and can create anger or other undesired patient reactions. *(NB, planning; LDM, shared)*

Pasquali et al., p. 570

346. B. Level of consciousness is not affected in persons with chronic irreversible brain syndrome, while memory and intellectual functioning are definitely impaired. The person also demonstrates labile affective behavior. *(NB, assessing; LDM, nurse centered)*

Stuart and Sundeen (1979), pp. 143–145

347. D. Dysmensia, impairment in the ability to retain and recall information, is the most prominent symptom of chronic irreversible brain syndrome. Immediate recall and recent memory are usually most seriously affected while remote memory may be intact. Attention-deficit is a neurologic condition producing motor-perceptual dysfunction and problematic behavior. Disorientation refers to dysfunction in one's orientation to time, place, or person. Dementia is the loss of intellectual abilities of sufficient severity to interfere with social or occupational functioning; it is another term for chronic organic mental disorder. *(NB, assessing; LDM, shared)*

Haber et al., p. 834;
Stuart and Sundeen (1979), pp. 144–145

348. D. The amount of brain involvement does not affect the patient's behavioral response to cognitive impairment, but responses are affected by personality characteristics, current affective state, and available support systems. Some patients with extensive brain involvement are able to compensate while others with little involvement demonstrate marked personality deterioration. *(NB, analyzing; LDM, shared)*

Wilson and Kneisl (1983), pp. 492–493

349. A. Providing challenge to the patient with irreversible organic mental disorder will serve as an additional stressor to her; she needs to be protected from awareness of her deficits. Maintaining a familiar environment, protecting the patient from harm, and reinforcing reality are all therapeutic nursing interventions. *(NB, planning; LDM, shared)*

Haber et al., p. 847

350. A. Chlorpromazine (Thorazine) or another member of the phenothiazide derivatives will reduce this client's agitation. Phenobarbital depresses cerebral functioning and is contraindicated. Lithium is used to treat manic-depressive illness, and methylphenidate (Ritalin) is a stimulant. *(NB, planning; LDM, nurse centered)*

Wilson and Kneisl (1983), p. 672
Burgess, pp. 366–367

351. B. Patients with irreversible brain syndrome may have a labile affective behavior if the limbic system is affected by the disease process. Impulsive sexual advances toward members of the opposite sex may occur, reflecting decreased inhibition and impaired judgment or a way of attempting to establish interpersonal contact. There are few social expectations of sexual behavior in a man of 80. Constantly watching this patient will not prevent recurrence of the behavior but will emphasize his loss of identity. *(NB, analyzing; LDM, shared)*

Stuart and Sundeen (1979), pp. 144–145

352. D. The administration of an anticoagulant greatly increases the patient's potential for bleeding complications. There are no data to support the need for seizure precautions, assaultive behavior, or if she does indeed have impaired ability to communicate. *(NB, planning; LDM, shared)*

Pasquali et al., p. 588

353. D. Patients with organic mental syndromes need contacts with others, especially family members or others known to the patients. Group activities would provide opportunity for self-expression and communication. Increasingly complex, lengthy tasks may only increase the patient's frustration. A reasonable balance of structure and freedom in activities is desirable. *(NB, planning; LDM, shared)*

Wilson and Kneisl, pp. 425–426

354. B. Unfamiliar surroundings increase confusion and raise the patient's anxiety level; to decrease further agitation she needs reassurance about being in a strange place. Promoting reality orientation and encouraging independent functioning are long-term concerns. When the brain is impaired organically equilibrium becomes precarious; too little or too much sensory input can precipitate further cognitive, perceptual, and affective deterioration. *(NB, implementing; LDM, shared)*

Pasquali et al., p. 600
Wilson and Kneisl (1979), p. 426

355. B. Attending occupational therapy provides stimulation from others and an opportunity for increasing self-worth. Options A, C, and D are all solitary activities that can inhibit social interaction. *(NB, implementing; LDM, client centered)*

Pasquali et al., pp. 600–601

356. C. Patients with chronic illnesses such as Parkinson's disease often experience grief and go through a psychobiologic process of mourning. The parkinsonian patient, particularly, experiences altered self-concept, and it is advisable to have this patient maintain his ordinary activities of daily living as much as possible to reduce depression. Options A, B, and D would all contribute to frustrating and isolating this patient. *(NB, planning; LDM, client centered)*

Haber et al, pp. 765-768

357. B. Special emphasis should be given to providing emotional and physical support to the client with organic brain dysfunction. Maintaining the client's physical capabilities, promoting reality orientation, and encouraging independent functioning are all relevant nursing approaches. *(NB, planning; LDM, shared)*

Pasquali et al., p. 600

358. C. Thiamine deficiency resulting from excessive alcohol use leads to lesions in the midbrain that produce classic neurologic signs and alterations in mental status such as confusion, disorientation, and memory loss. Deficiencies in ascorbic acid may show depression as an early symptom. Niacin deficiency can produce mental symptoms ranging from anxiety and depression to severe delirium. Iron deficiency is not related to mental status alterations. *(NB, assessing; LDM, client centered)*

Burgess, p. 326;
Wilson and Kneisl (1979), p. 424

359. C. A reduced alcohol intake and increased intake of thiamine is therapeutic for the patient with Wernicke's encephalopathy. *(NB, evaluating; LDM, client centered)*

Wilson and Kneisl (1979), p. 424

360. C. The delirious person should be placed in a quiet private room with a minimum of stimulation. Restraints should be avoided because they tend to confuse and excite the patient. Reality orientation should be done consistently to facilitate the patient's awareness and sense of security. Constant supervision is needed to prevent the patient from harming himself. *(NB, planning; LDM, nurse centered)*

Taylor, p. 432

361. D. Hallucinations occurring in delirium tremens are colorful, primarily visual, and frightening. Auditory hallucinations occur primarily in schizophrenia. *(NB, analyzing; LDM, client centered)*

Pasquali et al., p. 442

362. B. Huntington's chorea is a syndrome of progressive mental deterioration with a jerking movement of the face and limbs. Speech difficulties and an ataxic gait also may be problematic. *(NB, planning; LDM, client centered)*

Wilson and Kneisl (1979), p. 420

363. C. Diabetes may cause changes in mental functioning such as fatigability, irritability, and impotence. Polydipsia, polyuria, and polyphasia are all classic physiologic symptoms of diabetes. *(NB, analyzing; LDM, client centered)*

Wilson and Kneisl (1979), p. 420

364. A. The presence of a home health aide will assure proper food preparation and medication supervision and also provide social contact; she can also be an objective observer of the patient's status. Having the client's daughter assume responsibility for her father's meals may be difficult with her own family's needs. The client may be unable to retain all the details of a medication routine and subsequently mismanage medications. If this patient were adequately self-sufficient, he probably would not have required hospitalization. *(NB, planning; LDM, shared)*

Taylor, pp. 440–441

365. A. Sedatives could be one cause of organic mental disorders, and if diuretics are not properly monitored, fluid and electrolyte imbalance can result. There are no data to support evidence of alcohol abuse. Loneliness and poor socialization may contribute to disorientation over time, but again there are insufficient data to warrant this conclusion for this patient. *(NB, analyzing; LDM, shared)*

Haber et al., p. 830

366. B. There is no scientific evidence sufficiently supported to explain senile dementia, but metabolic, endocrine, vascular, and genetic factors are thought to strongly influence its development. Avitaminosis and intracranial tumors are not usually associated with senile dementia. Frontal lobe atrophy is associated with senile dementia. *(NB, assessing; LDM, nurse centered)*

Burgess, p. 332

367. D. Senile dementia is generally accompanied by other evidence of progressive aging affecting the entire body such as muscle wasting, speech disturbances, unsteady gait, and easy fatigability. Sensory and petit mal seizures are types of epilepsy. Retrograde amnesia and nausea can occur following head injury. Headaches and fainting may occur in cerebral-vascular episodes. *(NB, assessing; LDM, shared)*

Burgess, pp. 328–332

368. B. Cardinal symptoms of senile dementia include dysmnesia, disorientation, and difficulty in abstract reasoning. Dyspnea and anxiety may result from cerebral anoxia. Anorexia and insomnia may occur in delirium tremens, and irritability and sleep disturbance may occur in hyperthyroidism. *(NB, assessing; LDM, client centered)*

Burgess, pp. 327–328, 332–333

369. B Confabulation is the tendency of a confused person to fabricate a response to a question when he cannot remember the answer. To compensate, a person makes up for a deficiency in self-image by emphasizing another feature regarded as an asset. Depersonalization is a subjective experience involving feelings of unreality and alienation from the self. In dissociation, anxiety-laden experiences or thoughts are excluded from awareness. *(NB, assessing; LDM, client centered)*

Stuart and Sundeen (1983), pp. 436, 980–981

370. C. Alzheimer's disease is one of progressive mental deterioration beginning between ages 40 and 60. Emotional distress and agitation are common, and the person appears to be overactive. Loss of initiative, progressive memory decline, and extrapyramidal symptoms are associated with Pick's disease, another disease of mental deterioration. *(NB, assessing; LDM, nurse centered)*

Burgess, p. 334

371. C. Clients with Alzheimer's disease often save everything because they cannot distinguish between significant and insignificant items and they are fearful of discarding something of importance. Assisting the client to sort through items preserves the client's dignity and a sense of responsibility. Confrontation is not used because it increases anxiety and decreases functional ability and self-esteen. Exploration of feelings is counterproductive because it places the client in the position of having to face her deficits. Telling the client what she may keep assumes the ability to distinguish what must be discarded, an unrealistic expectation. *(NB, planning; LDM, shared)*

Haber et al, pp. 837, 847

372. A. Patients with Alzheimer's disease may not follow directions or requests because they do not know what to do. Repeating the information using clear, simple directions is the most appropriate initial intervention. Telling the patient the time assumes she can make the connection between the time and the event, highlighting one of the client's deficits. Grasping the client by the hand may instigate an impulsive assault and thus would be contraindicated. Commenting on the client's behavior forces her to examine her deficits, increasing her anxiety and maladaptive behavior. *(NB, implementing; LDM, shared)*

Haber et al., pp. 837, 848

373. C. The client should be kept mentally active within the parameters of her limitations, recognizing that if demands that are beyond her capabilities are placed on the client, disorganization may result. Watching television may stimulate social interaction without placing excessive demands upon the client. Activities in options A, B, and D require coordinated cognitive, psychomotor, and social functioning which can be overtaxing for the client. *(NB, planning; LDM, shared)*

Haber et al., pp. 836–837, 847

374. D. The client's agitation may be related to sensory overload in relation to the activity, thus removing her from the environment that may be precipitating the agitation is indicated. Exploration of feelings tends to increase anxiety and agitation. Medication may be used, but not initially, if agitation persists. Encouraging the client to join in the activity will increase the client's agitation. *(NB, implementing; LDM, shared)*

Haber et al., p. 848

H. CHILDHOOD DISORDERS

375. D. The autistic child may begin to manifest symptoms soon after birth or between the ages of 2 and 3 years; on the other hand symptoms of childhood schizophrenia develop gradually and occur later. Developmental histories of autistic children indicate that disturbed behavior patterns of feeding, elimination, and sleeping have existed from birth; motor development is usually normal. Withdrawal and inappropriate emotional behavior occur in both childhood schizophrenia and autism. *(NB, assessing; LDM, shared)*

Burgess, p. 615
Haber et al., pp. 1015–1016

376. C. Reflecting feelings consists of reverbalizing that which seems to be implied. The nurse attempts to identify latent and connotative meanings that may either clarify or distort the content. Option A closes off communication by offering reassurance without discussing the client's real feelings. Options B and D use the emotionally charged words, "guilty" and "bad" before the client has had an opportunity to clarify feelings. *(NB, implementing; LDM, shared)*

Haber et al., p. 244;
Wilson and Kneisl (1979), p. 114

377. D. The stage of initiative-vs-guilt occurs between the ages of 3–5, according to Erikson. The stage of trust-vs-mistrust occurs between birth and 18 months, while autonomy-vs-shame and doubt follows (18 months to 3 years). Identity-vs-role diffusion occurs between the ages of 12–20 years. *(NB, assessing; LDM, client centered)*

Wilson and Kneisl (1979), p. 181

378. C. The child's basic needs must be met before he can begin to deal with therapeutic intervention to reduce tension and anxiety. Options A, B, and C are long-term goals which cannot be met until basic needs are satisfied. *(NB, analyzing; LDM, nurse centered)*

Wilson and Kneisl (1979), pp. 489–491

379. C. A structured environment provides adult role models while peers are available for identification and acting out. In a therapeutic milieu the child feels accepted and may choose an adult who best meets his needs. Intervention may be necessary to keep the child in his treatment plan; you may need to plan interventions to promote his safety. Isolation will only reinforce the child's autistic behavior. *(NB, analyzing; LDM, shared)*

Wilson and Kneisl (1979), pp. 490–497, 514

380. B. The child will seek out the adult who best meets his needs in the milieu. Playing with a group of children would probably be the last evidence that milieu therapy was effective. Playing with one other child would be reasonable outcome of establishing a relationship with an adult. Hitting other children should stop after the child has established relationships with an adult and a child. *(NB, evaluating; LDM, nurse centered)*

Wilson and Kneisl (1979), pp. 499, 514

381. A. This option reflects the nurse's response to the child's nonverbal cues with verbal interpretations. Options B and C give directions to the child without giving him this opportunity to think through the situation. Option D threatens the child by challenging him. *(NB, implementing; LDM, shared)*

Wilson and Kneisl (1979), p. 497

382. C. Operant conditioning refers to conditioned responses of motor and cognitive behaviors versus autonomic behavior. The point of operant conditioning is to elicit adaptive motor and cognitive behaviors using techniques such as positive reinforcement, extinction, and negative reinforcement. Positive or negative reinforcement are techniques of conditioning. Demonstrating the desired response is called modeling. Shaping is the concept of reinforcing approximations of the desired behavior. *(NB, analyzing; LDM, nurse centered)*

Haber et al., p. 54–55

383. D. Praising the child for using the potty chair is an example of positive reinforcement, an operant conditioning technique used to increase the rate of response. If the child is anxious about sitting on the potty chair, desensitization could be used, but it is an unlikely solution with a child of this age; desensitization is not a component of operant conditioning. Demonstrating the use of the chair is a modeling technique. Punishing the child for not using the chair is unlikely to help since he must first learn what the desired response is. *(NB, implementing; LDM, shared)*

Haber et al., pp. 54–55

384. A. Going to the toilet by himself would be the long-term desired outcome. When the child indicates his need to go to the bathroom by gesturing, this is an early indication he has begun to achieve the goal of toilet training. Looking ashamed when he wets himself is not an indication that the child is achieving toilet training. Sitting on the potty chair without preparing to use it does not indicate goal achievement. *(NB, evaluating; LDM, client centered)*

Wilson and Kneisl, p. 498

385. C. Psychotropic drugs such as prochlorperazine (Compazine) can produce dry mouth and lips and constipation. Encouraging fluid intake will combat drying of mucous membranes and help prevent constipation. These drugs cause photosensitivity and the use of sunscreens is encouraged. Weight gain may occur in patients taking psychotropic drugs. Antiparkinsonian medication is not prescribed unless the patient experiences extrapyramidal side effects and large doses of antipsychotic drugs remain a necessity. *(NB, planning; LDM, shared)*

Haber et al., pp. 399–402

386. C. In some instances there is an apparent link between the hyperkinetic child and illness during infancy which has resulted in minimal injury of the central nervous system. A middle-class socioeconomic background is not a correlate of hyperkinesis. The mother's pregnancy, labor, and delivery were normal and resulted in no apparent birth injury. A moderate activity level during play or school is not unusual, and hyperkinesis occurs more frequently in boys. *(NB, assessing; LDM, shared)*

Haber et al., p. 1095

387. B. Learning to be effective parents involves them in a constructive task that helps them feel better about their parenting skills and their child's behavior. Reference books may be useful as an adjunct to active problem solving. Behavioral problems at school could be similar to, or different from, problems at home, and parental concerns are focused on home problems. Planning to get parents away from the problem only postpones the parents dealing with it. *(NB, analyzing; LDM, shared)*

Haber et al., pp. 1105–1106

388. A. This child has symptoms of minimal brain damage, and stimulants such as amphetamines or methylphenidate (Ritalin) have been demonstrated to be highly effective with such children. Placement in an activity therapy group may be useful after the child's response to medication is noted. Behavioral conditioning may also be a useful approach when response to medication is determined. Counseling about limit setting with this child implies the problem has no organic basis. *(NB, planning; LDM, shared)*

Haber et al., pp. 1100, 1110

389. B. If this child's problematic behavior continues while he is on a medication regimen the dosage may need to be increased to provide the desired results. The child with minimal brain damage (MBD) is hyperactive, and it is unlikely that he will fall asleep in class, even when taking medication. The child with MBD develops a "bad child, dumb child" self-image when the nature of his problem is undiagnosed. Easy distractability is one cognitive symptom of MBD. *(NB, evaluating; LDM, client centered)*

Haber et al., pp. 1096–1097, 1110

390. A. An organic disturbance of uncertain origin is thought to be the basis of hyperkinesis; the primary symptom, difficulty with attention span, is the same as that presented by the hyperactive child. The electroencephalogram for a hyperkenetic child may contain borderline changes, but there is no evidence of mental retardation and no specific central nervous system pathology. *(NB, assessing; LDM, nurse centered)*

Wilson and Kneisl (1979), p. 494

391. A. Side effects such as anorexia and insomnia occur frequently during initial treatment with stimulants but do not usually persist. The administration schedule and drug dosage may need adjustment. Chances of addiction to stimulants, including Ritalin, are minimal when taken as prescribed. Therapeutic effectiveness is usually seen within 2-3 weeks after medication is initiated. This stimulant works by increasing levels of norepinephrine in the brain, promoting attention to tasks and limiting impulsivity. *(NB, evaluating; LDM, shared)*

Haber et al., p. 1110

392. C. Some families become isolated from the extended family and support systems because they feel guilty and overwhelmed by the child's behavior. This isolation deprives the family of support which might be available to them. Options A, B, and D all reflect progress toward stated goals by limit setting, incorporating the child into family activities, and positive reinforcement of the child's progress. *(NB, evaluating; LDM, client centered)*

Haber et al., pp. 1105–1107, 1109, 1100–1102

393. C. Children who are distractible and have limited attention spans will be better able to concentrate in a quiet, low-stimulus environment. Complex tasks such as constructing a model airplane would only frustrate this child and because of his restlessness, fine motor games such as jacks will not provide an adequate discharge of his energy. With difficulty in concentrating, making a long list of tasks will be impossible to master. *(NB, planning; LDM, client centered)*

Haber et al., pp. 1096, 1106–1107

394. D. Childrens' self-esteem is enhanced by consistent expectations in accordance with their capacities. Therefore, the schedule and supervision for completing household chores needs to be known and consistently followed, and the child not allowed to choose when chores are to be done. All other options describe desirable aspects of a behavior modification program for control of hyperkinetic behavior. *(NB, implementing; LDM, shared)*

Haber et al., p. 1107

395. A. School-related learning tasks geared to meet most students' abilities may be inappropriate for the hyperkinetic child who is experiencing development lags in cognitive areas and becomes frustrated by complex tasks. All other options describe desirable, supportive school environments for the hyperkinetic child—predictable, clearly set limits, and supplementary help. *(NB, analyzing; LDM, shared)*

Haber et al., pp. 1096–1097; 1102, 1107

396. B. By not acknowledging the child's undesired behavior and thus reinforcing it, the undesirable behavior should be extinguished, according to behavior theory. Reinforcing desired behavior at regular intervals serves as positive reinforcement technique. The behavioral therapy approach is not punitive in nature and would preserve the child's self-esteem. Direct confrontation serves to reinforce the undesired behavior and to threaten the child's self-esteem. Promising not to repeat the undesired behavior is unrealistic for a child who is impulsive, distractible, and restless. "Time out" is a form of punishment which perpetuates the child's low self-esteem. *(NB, planning; LDM, shared)*

Haber et al., pp. 54–55, 1107

397. D. Distractibility is one cognitive sign of hyperkinesis, along with limited attention span. Several short, focused sessions are more effective for this child than one long session. Perceptual deficits such as accurate perception of time, space, and form may affect the project but not the spacing of time to spend on the project. The hyperkinetic child often has difficulty grasping cause-and-effect relationships, which may affect the type of project to develop. Emotional immaturity would not be a factor in limiting the time spent on the project. *(NB, planning; LDM, shared)*

Haber et al., pp. 1096–1097

398. B. Masturbation is a normal sexual activity for people of all ages, and many boys have experienced nocturnal emissions before the age of 15 years. Masturbation is a frequent mode of discharging tension and is unrelated to sexual preference. Nocturnal emissions are a normal part of development. *(NB, planning; LDM, shared)*

Wilson and Kneisl (1983), pp. 586–587;
Stuart and Sundeen (1983), p. 777

399. C. For an adolescent girl with a weight problem, professional counseling to help her understand the dynamics of her overeating (i. e., feelings and possible physical causes) not simply the eating itself is likely to be most useful. It is very likely that this girl already knows about the four basic food groups, and lack of information is not her problem. Eating whatever she wants has contributed to her present weight problem. Diets themselves do not explore the cause or meaning of excessive weight gain. *(NB, analyzing; LDM, shared)*

Wilson and Kneisl (1983), p. 589;
Stuart and Sundeen (1983), p. 785

400. C. By late adolescence the person usually has fewer intimate friends but a broader social circle. A girl of 17 who has no close friends is a person who is isolated, and this may make her angry, depressed, or anxious in dealing with teachers and peers. The IQ, chronologic age, and maturity level are not synchronized in the adolescent and may create additional anxiety. Superior academic standing indicates ability, not maturity. Uncertainty about the future is not uncommon in late adolescence. *(NB, analyzing; LDM, shared)*

Haber et al., p. 1042–1044
Stuart and Sundeen (1983), pp. 783–785

401. B. Adolescents seek to create a language all their own. Word meanings vary from group to group, so even applying common street meanings may indicate the nurse is an outsider. The nurse needs to identify the meaning of the words, then communicate with the adolescent in this language. Use of profanity and obscene words are often part of the adolescent's identity, anger, and fears; helping the adolescent express these feelings is desirable, not prohibiting communication because it is profane. If restricted language is used for the nurse's comfort, this can be nontherapeutic. *(NB, planning; LDM, shared)*

Wilson and Kneisl (1983), p. 580

402. D. The double-bind of making good grades which results in personal rejection leads to feelings of worthlessness and helplessness. Scapegoating involves blaming and projecting on others. This girl did not intend to set up the situation described and cannot balance her performance and her peers response; therefore she is more angry than anxious. Her response to the situation more than tests the limits of diet and academic regime. *(NB, analyzing; LDM, client centered)*

Stuart and Sundeen (1983), p. 781;
Wilson and Kneisl (1983), pp. 580–585

403. C. Adolescents are curious about death; it is a major theme of adolescent intellectualization. The intellectualization acts as a defense against the impulses by distancing them. When anxiety is high, emotional processes dominate cognitive processes, and the ability to rationalize and problem solve are lost. When this occurs, curiosity about death has no safe, self-protective way of expression. Triggering events for suicide include loss of a significant person or breakup of a love relationship, parental conflict, emotional and sexual problems. Suicide attempts are a nonverbalized cry for help. *(NB, analyzing; LDM, client centered)*

Haber et al., pp. 1045–1046, 1059

404. D. An objective, nonjudgmental validation of the pregnancy is the most appropriate course of action. Sexual activity in teenagers and teenage pregnancy are not uncommon. In option B, the nurse seeks information but does not act to confirm or deny the pregnancy, while in option C, the nurse is passing judgment on the girl. *(NB, implementing; LDM, shared)*

Stuart and Sundeen (1983), p. 779;
Wilson and Kneisl (1983), pp. 587–588

405. D. The unwed adolescent should be aware of options such as adoption or foster placement, special school programs, work potential, parental support, etc. The adolescent's ambivalence about the baby is part of her problem, not an option or solution. *(NB, planning; LDM, client centered)*

Haber et al., p. 1047;
Stuart and Sundeen (1983), p. 779;
Wilson and Kneisl (1983), p. 331

406. C. Therapeutic groups are oriented toward providing information and help. Option A is unlikely to be true as "everyone" does not want anything. Hearing other people's problems may not help the client solve her problems. Groups do not provide direction in terms of what to do. *(NB, analyzing; LDM, client centered)*

Stuart and Sundeen (1983), pp. 702, 709;
Wilson and Kneisl (1983), pp. 220–221

407. C. This option reflects the client's wishes and choice; it does not imply correctness of that decision. Option A reflects parental pressure, not the client's decision. Option B reflects the boyfriend's position, not the client's desire. Option D reflects a perceived message from the group, not the client's wishes. *(NB, evaluating; LDM, client centered)*

Stuart and Sundeen (1983), p. 779

I. DEVELOPMENTAL DISABILITIES

408. C. Mental retardation is defined as significantly sub-average general intellectual functioning existing concurrently with deficits in adaptive behavior and manifested during the developmental period. Options A, B, and D are characteristics of developmental disability. *(NB, assessing; LDM, nurse centered)*

Haber et al., pp. 1093, 1017

409. C. This child's abilities reflect a level of moderate retardation. It is appropriate for her to learn self-care and acceptable social behavior. Option A describes an appropriate goal for a profoundly retarded client. Option D reflects an appropriate goal for a client with borderline retardation. *(NB, analyzing; LDM, shared)*

Haber et al., p. 1095

410. C. Helping the child develop a sense of value or self-worth is essential and can be established through a one-to-one nurse-patient relationship. Complex relationships would be beyond the client's intellectual capabilities, and a detailed history would be better obtained from the parents. Reinforcing feelings of rejection and worthlessness would not be therapeutic. *(NB, planning; LDM, shared)*

Wilson and Kneisl (1979), p. 411

411. D. The retarded child has problems with forming and maintaining relationships because of reduced cognitive capacities, in addition to constitutional deficiencies such as irritability, restlessness, and short attention span. Thus impaired adaptive ability will mean the child will have problems with independence and responsibility. The IQ level is not particularly helpful in understanding mental retardation. This child's disabilities exceed those of a learning disability, but they are not so profound as to require permanent institutionalization. *(NB, evaluating; LDM, shared)*

Wilson and Kneisl (1979), pp. 409–410

412. D. Down's syndrome results from a nondisjunction of chromosomal material, leading to an extra chromosome. This extra genetic material is known to cause several enzymatic defects. Option A describes the basis of phenylketonuria (PKU), and option B, Tay-Sachs disease. Option C describes hemophilia. *(NB, analyzing; LDM, nurse centered)*

Wilson and Kneisl (1979), pp. 404–406

413. C. Behavior modification therapy is based on the principle that behavior is determined by its consequences. Option A describes play therapy and option B, psychodrama. Psychoanalysis uses techniques of free association. *(NB, analyzing; LDM, nurse centered)*

Wilson and Kneisl (1979), pp. 507–509, 512–513

414. B. What is rewarding to the child helps to positively reinforce appropriate behavior. Depriving the child of things that she enjoys is punishment, not necessarily related to her behavior modification plan; punishment places more emphasis on undesirable behavior. Rewarding undesirable behaviors will only reinforce these behaviors. *(NB, planning; LDM, shared)*

Wilson and Kneisl (1979), pp. 512–513

415. B. A major goal in working with retarded children is developing the client's sense of self-worth and counteracting feelings of worthlessness. This father's statement is demeaning to his child and will contribute to her maintaining low self-esteem. His statement alone will not prevent his daughter from becoming independent, and his lack of patience with her behavior leads to his labeling her as a "dummy." *(NB, analyzing; LDM, client centered)*

Wilson and Kneisl (1979), p. 411

416. D. The father's statement reflects his cooperation in achieving the stated goal. Most retarded children can learn to dress themselves if enough time is spent in this activity. Helping the child will not enable her to become independent in dressing herself. Helping the child, even one time, contributes to continued dependence. *(NB, evaluating; LDM, client centered)*

Haber et al., pp. 1104–1106

417. A. Since their child has a genetically linked form of mental retardation, these parents would find genetic counseling helpful. Mental retardation can occur as the result of factors occurring prenatally, or postnatally. Errors in metabolism are only one known cause of mental retardation. The decision to have or not to have other children should be made by the parents, after considering accurate information about the genetic prognosis. *(NB, planning; LDM, client centered)*

Wilson and Kneisl (1979), pp. 404–406

418. A. A realistic care plan for a retarded adult living in a supportive-living home should be based upon assessment of socioadaptive capacity, maturity, and self-help skills. This client would not be in a supportive-living home with psychotic behavior. Organic factors, motor abilities, and neurologic causes will not help determine the client's plan of care. Aspects in option D are unrelated to this client's assessment. *(NB, assessing; LDM, shared)*

Wilson and Kneisl (1983), p. 477

419. B. Making simple decisions without help is an appropriate short-term goal for the client. It is unrealistic to expect this client to go shopping without assistance or to control all angry outbursts within 1 week. Leading a residential meeting would be appropriate as a long-term goal. *(NB, analyzing; LDM, shared)*

Wilson and Kneisl (1983), pp. 476–477

420. C. Benztropine mesylate (Cogentin) is an antiparkinsonian agent prescribed to control extrapyramidal symptoms. Thiothixene is a major tranquilizer, diazepam is a minor tranquilizer, and imipramine is an antidepressant. None of these drugs would be used to control extrapyramidal symptoms. *(NB, analyzing; LDM, shared)*

Stuart and Sundeen (1983), p. 502

421. D. A sore throat can be a symptom of agranulocytosis. Liver complications would include fever, jaundice, and flulike syndrome. Extrapyramidal symptoms are neurologic, not upper respiratory. A sore throat is unrelated to postural hypotension which can occur with chlorpromazine. *(NB, analyzing; LDM, shared)*

Stuart and Sundeen (1983), p. 503

422. D. Dressing without assistance, improvement in decision-making skills, and control of emotional outbursts all indicate the client is ready for more advanced goals. Behaviors in option A indicate the client needs more structure and supervision. Behaviors in option B are indications for increased nursing support and intervention. Dependency, ambivalence, and worthlessness are all indications that the present approach is ineffective. *(NB, evaluating; LDM, client centered)*

Wilson and Kneisl (1983), p. 476

J. PERSON ABUSE

423. B. The school-aged stage begins when the firstborn child is 6 years old and ends when the child enters adolescence, 13 years. Marriage marks the beginning stage of a new family. The launching center stage is characterized by the first child leaving the parental home and ends when the parents are alone again. The empty nest stage begins when the last child leaves home and ends with retirement or the death of one spouse. *(NB, assessing; LDM, client centered)*

Friedman, pp. 49–71

424. D. Alcoholism, as well as divorce, drug addiction, unemployment, etc., play major roles in leading the potential abuser to strike out at a child or spouse. Effective coping with stress would not contribute to abusive behavior nor would realistic expectations about marriage. *(NB, analyzing; LDM, nurse centered)*

Friedman, p. 255

425. C. Because of feelings of guilt and shame, battered women do not always seek treatment for their assault and emotional pain. Victims usually have evidence of physical aggression, although the signs may be well hidden by protective clothing. This client's mannerisms may provide a clue to her battering but not as obvious one as the appearance of bruises. Her relationship to her parents is not pertinent to her battering, and her loyalty to her husband should be considered but is a secondary concern at this point. *(NB, planning; LDM, shared)*

Stuart and Sundeen (1979), pp. 550–551

426. A. Any plan of action is based on the client's own decision. The client should be helped to describe her situation and critically examine her alternatives, to be made aware of community resources, and to be supported in her decision making. Decisions about seeking employment and leaving her husband are the client's, not the nurse's. Reporting her abuse to the police is also the client's decision. *(NB, planning; LDM, client centered)*

Stuart and Sundeen (1979), pp. 550–551

427. B. The husband who abuses his wife tends to have been abused as a child and to have observed wife beating in his family. He feels insecure in his marital relationship and roles outside the home, with a fragile male self-image. *(NB, analyzing; LDM, nurse centered)*

Haber et al., pp. 980-981;
Stuart and Sundeen (1979), p. 549

428. B. If child abuse is strongly suspected, hospitalization is often recommended to protect the child from further injury and to allow additional time for assessment of the family. Assessment may reveal recent or old fractures that are unexplained. Separating mother and child may be necessary but only when abuse is confirmed. The physician can be informed of the family history following the nursing assessment. The parents already feel guilty and frightened by what has happened to their child, and confronting them (or the mother, in this situation) will produce denial and hostility. *(NB, implementing; LDM, shared)*

Haber et al., p. 990

429. A. The abusing parent typically expects her child to perform as an adult and severely punishes her when she fails to meet parental expectations. In this situation, it would also be important to document the father's expectation of his daughter. There are insufficient data to determine whether the mother's use of defense mechanisms is ineffective or if there is a significant age difference between these parents. Child abuse occurs in all socioeconomic and educational levels. *(NB, analyzing; LDM, nurse centered)*

Stuart and Sundeen (1979), pp. 548-549

430. A. Ethnicity is not related to violent behavior as violence cuts across all cultural groups. Violence is frequently associated with psychosis, drug use, and delirium, among other factors. *(NB, assessing; LDM, nurse centered)*

Burgess, pp. 476-477

431. C. Children are immature in their biopsychosocial development and sexual abusers can capitalize in self-serving ways on the naivete of the child, exploiting the child physically, socially, psychologically, and emotionally. *(NB, analyzing; LDM, nurse centered)*

Burgess, p. 551

432. C. Primary prevention emphasizes promotion of healthy personality development, healthy families, and healthy communities through reduction of factors considered harmful to these systems. Courses in parenting would be a primary prevention modality. Hospitalizing the abused child is a means of secondary prevention. Criminal punishment is probably a form of tertiary prevention. Separating parents and child is a form of secondary prevention. *(NB, planning; LDM, shared)*

Haber et al., pp. 22, 988

433. A. Before the nurse can effectively assist the rape victim, it is essential to be aware of any bias held and the extent to which it affects one's belief system about rape and one's nursing care with victims. Calling for assistance may be traumatic at this time; the client may need privacy. Taping the conversation without the client's consent or knowledge is illegal. The person working in a rape crisis clinic should already be familiar with the myths of rape. *(NB, planning; LDM, nurse centered)*

Stuart and Sundeen (1979), p. 428

434. C. Assessment of the signs and symptoms of physical and emotional trauma assume priority in the care of a rape victim. Identification of the client's support systems is an important part of the plan of care and would follow the assessment. Knowledge of legal responsibilities is a secondary concern. The victim should not be left alone at this point. *(NB, assessing; LDM, shared)*

Stuart and Sundeen (1979), p. 439

435. D. The nurse can provide the victim with adequate information about what her rights are and what she can expect from the staff to reduce her sense of anxiety and helplessness. The woman will resolve the crisis better if she finds the nurse supports her beliefs and her own value system. The examination is important, but the client needs to make this decision herself. The client's parents should be involved only if she wishes them to be notified. The police will be notified if this is the client's decision. *(NB, implementing; LDM, shared)*

Stuart and Sundeen (1979), pp. 442–445

436. A. The nurse needs to ask the client what she wants to know during the physician's examination, then provide this information; this provides the woman with a sense of control. Written explanations of the procedure are not useful when the client's concentration is probably limited, nor is it appropriate to ask her for a written description of the incident at this time. Assurance of the type in option D is probably unwarranted. *(NB, implementing; LDM, shared)*

Stuart and Sundeen (1979), p. 446

437. D. Evidentiary material should be gathered and held for release to the police. Laboratory specimens should be gathered by a physician in the presence of a witness and personally handed to a technician or pathologist. It is not necessary for the physician to personally conduct the laboratory analysis, and the laboratory technician or pathologist must sign the laboratory results. Findings and evidentiary material should not be released without the client's consent. *(NB, implementing; LDM, nurse centered)*

Stuart and Sundeen (1979), p. 444

438. B. Half of all rapes occur in a private residence, and a third to a half are committed in the victim's residence. Rapes also can occur in parks and cars and are unlikely in the rapist's residence. *(NB, assessing; LDM, nurse centered)*

Stuart and Sundeen (1979), p. 429

439. C. Rape is a violent attack using sex as the weapon. About 68% of rapes are planned in advance by the rapist. *(NB, analyzing; LDM, nurse centered)*

Stuart and Sundeen (1979), p. 429

440. B. One myth of rape is that rape is provoked by the victim when in fact, a woman does not ask for rape by acting in normal socially defined ways. Any woman can be a rape victim, regardless of socioeconomic class, appearance, age, or place of residence. Rape is the fastest rising violent crime in the United States and most rapes are intraracial. *(NB, analyzing; LDM, nurse centered)*

Stuart and Sundeen (1979), pp. 429–431

441. D. In taking responsibility for herself, the battered woman acknowledges her husband will not, or cannot, stop his violent behavior. In making decisions for herself, she begins to build self-esteem. *(NB, analyzing; LDM, client centered)*

Stuart and Sundeen (1979), p. 551

442. B. Physical and emotional abuse and neglect appear to have intergenerational influences. The characteristic dominance of emotionality and minimal use of cognitive processes contribute to members' impulsivity when stress occurs within the family. Abusive families tend to be socially isolated and distrustful of others. Some members of fundamentalist religious groups abuse their children. *(NB, analyzing; LDM, nurse centered)*

Haber et al., pp. 983–984

K. SUBSTANCE ABUSE

443. B. High-risk factors for development of alcoholism include coming from an Irish or Scandanavian cultural background, coming from a broken home or a home with an absent or rejecting father, and a family history of alcoholism or teetotalism. Sibling position or husband's job are not related to development of alcoholism. *(NB, analyzing: LDM, client centered)*

Burgess, p. 504

444. C. Alcohol is a central nervous system depressant with slight excitatory effects on respiratory centers. The stimulating qualities of alcohol are felt to be the release of inhibition. Hallucinogens and phenothiazines are different classifications of drugs. *(NB, assessing; LDM, nurse centered)*

Burgess, pp. 500–501

445. B. Defense mechanisms most commonly identified with alcoholism are rationalization, denial, projection, and dissociation. Knowledge of these mechanisms is helpful in determining the accuracy of the data received. The defense mechanisms in the other options are not usually associated with alcoholism. *(NB, analyzing; LDM, client centered)*

Burgess, pp. 504–505

446. C. The alcoholic has feelings of guilt, inadequacy, and low self-esteem which may be projected on the nurse. The client then feels that the nurse regards her as unworthy and responds to the nurse with anger and hostility. Strategies for improving the client's self-concept would be an important part of her plan of care. There are insufficient data to warrant confronting her about parenting, encouraging her to seek a divorce, or the need to learn breast self-examination. *(NB, planning; LDM, shared)*

Burgess, p. 504

447. A. The nurse needs to be aware of her own attitudes and not allow her own values to prevent her from being therapeutic. She also needs to help the alcoholic connect his painful feelings with his need to drink. Giving the alcoholic advice keeps him dependent and prevents him from being responsible for his own decisions. The alcoholic needs help sorting out his feelings and pamphlets primarily address cognitive needs. Stressing unfairness may further increase guilt and decrease self-worth. *(NB, implementing; LDM, shared)*

Burgess, pp. 508–509

448. B. Because the nurse's attitude toward drinking and alcoholism have a direct relationship to the response made to the patient with a drinking problem, the nurse needs to be aware of his personal attitudes, the reasons for them, and how they can be modified. All other options describe positive attitudes and behaviors regarding the alcoholic and alcoholism. *(NB, analyzing; LDM, nurse centered)*

Burgess, pp. 508–512

449. C. A blood level concentration of 0.15 or more is the legal test for inebriation in many states. There are insufficient data to conclude this client has developed tolerance to alcohol, a serious alcohol problem, or is feeling depressed. *(NB, analyzing; LDM, nurse centered)*

Wilson and Kneisl (1979), p. 34

450. A. Alcoholic intoxication is classified as an acute reversible brain syndrome in which neurochemical and electrical responses are altered as a result of the stressor, alcohol. Metabolic disturbances can alter cerebral demands for oxygen and metabolites. *(NB, analyzing; LDM, nurse centered)*

Stuart and Sundeen (1979), pp. 141–142

451. A. Alcohol addiction develops when there is a physiologic dependence on alcohol. Dependence is demonstrated by appearance of withdrawal symptoms when the alcohol is stopped. Alcohol withdrawal syndrome includes symptoms of diaphoresis, tachycardia, elevated blood pressure, tremors, nausea and vomiting, anorexia, and restlessness. As this syndrome progresses, hallucinations, convulsions, and delirium tremens occur. *(NB, assessing; LDM, shared)*

Haber et al., pp. 505–506

452. D. Since convulsions can occur during alcohol withdrawal, it is important to determine if the client has previously experienced withdrawal seizures. Regardless of whether or not seizures have occurred previously, seizures should be prevented. Ability to tolerate job-related stress or to express emotions are better assessed when the effects of alcohol have subsided. Tranquilizers are used only when the client's agitation interferes with his sleep or physical safety. *(NB, assessing; LDM, shared)*

Haber et al., pp. 519–521

453. C. During detoxification the client must be protected from injury and allowed to rest as comfortably as possible. The nurse observes the client for any signs of a psychologic or physiologic instability which suggests the development of alcohol withdrawal syndrome. Teaching relaxation techniques and about liver disease is more appropriate after detoxification, as is exploring maladaptive defenses. *(NB, implementing; LDM shared)*

Haber et al., p. 520

454. B. Delirium tremens is a medical and nursing emergency, an acute pathologic state of consciousness resulting from interference with brain metabolism. Symptoms include increased psychomotor activity, confusion and disorientation, fearfulness, signs of vasomotor lability, tachycardia, fever, and hallucinations. Oversedation would control symptoms of alcohol withdrawal. Other data would be needed to establish a diagnosis of renal failure. *(NB, evaluating; LDM, nurse centered)*

Haber et al., p. 506

455. B. According to Maslow's hierarchy of needs, this patient is seeking love and belonging. Assisting him to be self-directing, to establish meaningful relationships, and to develop positive ways of dealing with behavior are all important interventions. While attempting to kiss a nurse may be inappropriate, it is not out of control, nor are sufficient data provided to determine if he has fallen in love with her. There are also insufficient data to determine if the patient has a deep-seated sexual problem; as Maslow stresses, love is not synonymous with sex. *(NB, analyzing; LDM, shared)*

Haber et al., pp. 8–9

456. A. One of the stabilizing functions of alcohol abuse in families is facilitating maintenance of emotional distance in relationships. If emotional demands in a relationship are too steep, the person can distance from the demands with excess alcohol, relieving his anxiety. There is no particular insight reflected in this client's comment, but it may be his rationalization. The client is not being harsh on his family, simply expressing his perception of them. There are insufficient data to determine if this client is suicidal. *(NB, analyzing; LDM, shared)*

Haber et al., pp. 507–508

457. A. Frequent automobile accidents, outbursts of rage, suicidal gestures when drinking, and decreased tolerance to alcohol are all characteristic of the late stage of alcoholism. There are some similarities between the antisocial personality and the alcoholic, but the history of drinking behavior would be a significant differentiating factor. *(NB, analyzing; LDM, shared)*

Burgess, p. 312
Estes, Smith-Dijulio, and Heinemann, p. 17

458. B. Alcoholics can be confused and may deny their disease because they do not experience negative effects each time they drink. Constant confrontation is ineffective unless the client is ready to accept his diagnosis. Teaching this client the consequences of alcohol abuse before he accepts this diagnosis is ineffective, as is ignoring his denial. *(NB, planning; LDM, nurse centered)*

Estes, Smith-Dijulio, and Heinemann, p. 39

459. D. Delirium tremens (DTs) is an acute complication of alcoholism. Signs preceding DTs include increasing tremors, restlessness, irritability, headache, nausea, insomnia, and nightmares. Tremulousness is an early sign. Coma is a late complication. Hypoglycemia is more often found in alcoholics than hyperglycemia. *(NB, assessing; LDM, nurse centered)*

Haber et al., p. 506

460. D. Individual, group, and family treatment modalities are used to repattern behavior in alcohol abuse. The nurse acts as a role model in a therapeutic relationship to facilitate trust and socialization. Giving the client time alone reinforces his isolation, but having him rejoin his "drinking buddies" will interfere with developing abstinence from alcohol. This client may not be ready for the complex relationships involved in being unit president. *(NB, planning; LDM, shared)*

Haber et al., pp. 521, 525

461. D. This response indicates that the client has achieved the goal of socialization and also some degree of insight into his problems. Drinking alone is a continuation of the client's isolation. Option B reflects the client's reluctance to establish social relationships, and option C indicates that drinking is an escape from loneliness for this client. *(NB, evaluating; LDM, client centered)*

Estes, Smith-Dijulio, and Heinemann, p. 42

462. A. Alcoholics Anonymous (AA) is the original self-help program in which sober alcoholics, by their support and example, help the active drinker achieve sobriety. There are also group support programs for other family members. Alcoholics Anonymous does not provide job referral or referral to community physicians. *(NB, analyzing; LDM, nurse centered)*

Burgess, p. 507

463. C. Sober alcoholics are assigned to work with active drinkers; thus the fact that this client has been assigned another client indicates his recovery. *(NB, evaluating; LDM, client centered)*

Burgess, p. 507

464. D. During the first group session the group is in the orientation phase and the leader's role is to provide information and structure. It is too soon to begin functioning as a therapist, but being nondirective is equally inappropriate at this time. Leaving the group when members begin to talk will remove the direction needed during group orientation. *(NB, analyzing; LDM, nurse centered)*

Stuart and Sundeen (1979), p. 330

465. B. A rap session is an informal group session where the nurse's role is primarily that of listener and clarifier. Such sessions can often improve and expedite information and communication, and the nurse should limit offering her opinions and should not be manipulated by clients. Controlling the group is counterproductive to expressing feelings. *(NB, analyzing; LDM, shared)*

Stuart and Sundeen (1979), pp. 322–323

466. B. The initial client assessment during detoxification should focus on respiratory or cardiac function and evidence of bleeding because these are potentially life threatening. Options A and D are less significant factors. Assessments in option C are more significant but still less important than cardiac and respiratory function. *(NB, assessing; LDM, nurse centered)*

Estes, Smith-DiJulio, and Heinemann, p. 187

467. D. Stabilizing the client's overall physical condition is the most appropriate acute care goal for this client. Option A suggests a goal appropriate to the continuing treatment phase, and options B and C, goals that would be appropriate following stabilization of the client's conditioning. *(NB, analyzing; LDM, shared)*

Haber et al., pp. 518–519

468. C. A temperature of 102°F indicates the need to force fluids to reduce fever, which should also assist in reducing pulse rate. A calm environment will not reduce the client's fever, nor will giving a prescribed hypnotic. The client does not feel well enough to socialize with others at this point. *(NB, implementing; LDM, shared)*

Haber et al., pp. 520–521

469. C. Normal vital signs and no signs of agitation would indicate this client is safely out of the acute withdrawal phase. Drinking beer continues to provide alcohol intake, which is to be avoided for full recovery. If the client is semiobtunded and is having seizures, demonstrates petechie and scleral icterus, he is still in the acute phase of alcoholism. *(NB, evaluating; LDM, shared)*

Estes, Smith-DiJulio, and Heinemann, p. 186

470. D. The benzodiazepines such as chlordiazepoxide (Librium) are believed to have a depressant effect on the central nervous system and would be used to prevent DTs. Librium has no effect on nutritional status nor does it interfere with alcohol consumption. Librium is not an adversive agent. *(NB, analyzing; LDM, nurse centered)*

Haber et al., pp. 402, 520–521

471. B. Disulfiram (Antabuse) blocks the metabolism of alcohol with the result that the client becomes very ill. Unless the gourmet dinner involves no use of wine in food preparation, he will become ill after eating. Antabuse is a long-acting drug which does not cure alcoholism but aids in preventing the client from drinking impulsively. Reactions can be produced for days after the medication has been stopped. *(NB, evaluating; LDM, client centered)*

Estes, Smith-DiJulio, and Heinemann, p. 203

472. D. Disulfiram produces elevated blood levels of acetaldehyde when alcohol is consumed, precipitating an unpleasant reaction marked by nausea, vomiting, sweating, and flushing. A severe reaction can produce hypotension, shock, and death. Symptoms in the other options are unrelated to disulfiram reactions. *(NB, planning; LDM, shared)*

Burgess, p. 506

473. B. Assessing the client's psychomotor activity would assume priority since this can be indicative of impending delirium tremens (DTs). Perceptual ability is not directly pertinent, and assessment of self-esteem and hygiene would better be made at a later time. *(NB, assessing; LDM, nurse centered)*

Haber et al., pp. 506, 520-521

474. D. Since this client is agitated, she needs to be protected from impulsive, self-destructive behavior. Hygiene is not a priority factor, and vital signs would better be assessed when the client is calmer. Motivating the client for treatment is inappropriate during this acute phase of alcohol withdrawal. *(NB, analyzing; LDM, shared)*

Haber et al., pp. 520-521

475. D. While the client is intoxicated and belligerent, she may be prone to falling or hurting herself so safety factors must be provided. Giving the client a backrub at this time may increase her agitation, and evaluation of her work situation and family responsibilities would be better postponed until the acute withdrawal phase has passed. Discussing alcoholism is also inappropriate at this time. *(NB, planning; LDM, shared)*

Haber et al., p. 521

476. B. A blood alcohol level of 0.10% is considered indicative of intoxication. Options C and D are unrelated to blood alcohol concentration levels. *(NB, analyzing; LDM, nurse centered)*

Estes, Smith-DiJulio, and Heinemann, p. 27

477. A. Alcoholism cannot be cured, only controlled; this option indicates client insight into the nature of her problem. Abstinence is the only effective control measure. Option C reflects the client's use of projection onto her mother, and option D indicates unresolved feelings about discharge. *(NB, evaluating; LDM, client centered)*

Estes, Smith-DiJulio, and Heinemann, p. 200

478. A. Malnutrition is a common chronic health problem associated with alcohol abuse. Follow-up of initial nutritional teaching should be arranged. Fear and anxiety are problems associated with acute alcohol withdrawal syndrome. Insomnia and susceptibility to intercurrent respiratory infections are health problems associated with initial alcohol withdrawal. *(NB, implementing; LDM, shared)*

Haber et al., pp. 521–522

479. D. Communicating both positive and negative feelings to family members increases client self-esteem through interpersonal relationships rather than alcohol. The alcoholic should allow appropriate dependence and interdependence with others because it is not possible to be totally independent nor to avoid all contact with people who drink. Confronting the grief he has caused others focuses primarily on negative feelings. *(NB, evaluating; LDM, client centered)*

Haber et al., pp. 507–508, 528–529

480. B. This client's symptoms may result from physiologic or psychologic sources, or both. It would be most important to obtain his nursing history to identify what these sources are. No medication should be prescribed without identifying the client's underlying problem. The client's symptoms do not indicate that he is a source of problems to other client's. Fluid intake would not need to be restricted unless the nursing history identified a reason for so doing. *(NB, implementing; LDM, nurse centered)*

Haber et al., pp. 835–836, 838

481. A. Seizures can result from a variety of physiologic problems such as hyperpyrexia, central nervous system infections, metabolic disorders, and drug withdrawal. Therefore it is most essential to determine any known history of seizures from a previously identified cause. Medication history is also important as it may reveal that the patient has stopped taking a drug preventing seizures or that he is experiencing withdrawal symptoms. Nutritional status and psychologic history are of secondary importance here. *(NB, analyzing; LDM, shared)*

   Haber et al., pp. 832, 838–839

482. B. Antipsychotic drugs such as chlorpromazine are used in alcohol withdrawal syndrome but would be contraindicated for the client with a history of liver disease. Insomnia may be helped by chlorpromazine. A history of excessive caffeine intake and multivitamin therapy are unrelated to alcohol withdrawal syndrome or to chlorpromazine. *(NB, analyzing; LDM, nurse centered)*

   Haber et al., pp. 400, 520–521

483. A. Hallucinogens produce unusual sensations and changes in self-perception. They do not produce physical dependence but can produce psychologic dependence and mild tolerance. Hallucinogens do not alter respirations, nor do they produce both stimulation and depression. *(NB, analyzing; LDM, client centered)*

   Burgess, pp. 525–526;
   Wilson and Kneisl (1979), p. 552

484. A. The common need demonstrated in the personality of the drug abuser is dependency. Many patients initially assume a defensive, hostile veneer because they expect their requests will be denied and that they will be dealt with in a prejudicial manner. Regression is the return to a previous developmental level, and displacement is the severing of an emotion from its original connection and attaching it to substitute persons or objects. These defense mechanisms are not usually associated with the drug abuser. *(NB, planning; LDM, shared)*

Burgess, p. 27, 529

485. C. In drug tolerance the dosage required to obtain the desired effect gradually increases. There are no data presented that support the other options of blackouts, physical illness, or withdrawal symptoms. *(NB, analyzing; LDM, client centered)*

Burgess, p. 522

486. C. Psychologic dependence implies emotional dependence, desire, or compulsion to continue taking the drug. Withdrawal symptoms are characteristic of physical dependence on the drug, and the continual need for larger drug dosage is drug tolerance. Use of several drugs is common but some addicts use only one type. *(NB, assessing; LDM, nurse centered)*

Burgess, p. 522

487. D. The manipulative tactics of the substance abuser are exacerbated by excessive rigidity or permissiveness, inconsistencies, or ambiguities in environmental expectations. Nursing actions should include limit setting, which is appropriate in this situation. Calling the security guard defers responsibility for setting and maintaining expectations, an important part of the therapeutic relationship. Ignoring or accepting the client's behavior serves to condone it. *(NB, implementing; LDM, shared)*

Haber et al., p. 524

488. A. In withdrawal from amphetamine it is important to stay with the person and watch for indications of suicidal intent. Muscle cramping and pain are symptoms of narcotic withdrawal. Amphetamines do not produce respiratory distress as part of withdrawal. Euphoria is one of the major reasons for taking amphetamines. *(NB, assessing; LDM, shared)*

Wilson and Kneisl (1979), p. 550

489. B. Mild narcotic withdrawal symptoms resemble a common cold and include sore throat, rhinorrhea, lacrimation, sweating, and slightly elevated temperature. Lack of coordination, slurred speech, and confusion are associated with depressant withdrawal. Combativeness and dizziness are among the symptoms of amphetamine overdosage. *(NB, assessing; LDM, shared)*

Burgess, p. 524
Wilson and Kneisl (1979), p. 550

490. B. An overdose of sedatives can result in progressive respiratory depression and coma; therefore maintaining a patent airway and adequate respiratory function assumes priority. There is no known antagonist for a sedative overdose. Intravenous therapy can be initiated later if needed, and an accurate drug history can also be obtained when basic physiologic needs have been met. *(NB, implementing; LDM, nurse centered)*

Wilson and Kneisl (1979), p. 551

491. A. Acute withdrawal from barbiturates can produce seizures, therefore nursing actions should be directed toward preventing seizure activity. Psychiatric complications would be of secondary importance. Developing client identity and insight would be components of treatment following detoxification. *(NB, implementing; LDM, nurse centered)*

Burgess, p. 523;
Wilson and Kneisl (1979), p. 551

492. D. Symptoms of heroin overdosage include a depressed level of consciousness and a depressed respiratory rate. Maintaining support of all vital functions is imperative. Contact with reality is not a problem with heroin overdosage, and adequate fluid is not a priority. A safe environment is also unrelated to heroin overdosage. *(NB, planning; LDM, nurse centered)*

Wilson and Kneisl (1979), p. 551

493. D. For the person who overdoses with hallucinogens and has a "bad trip," a nonthreatening environment with subdued and pleasant stimuli is important because this person experiences perceptual distortion. Goal-directed activity is beyond the capability of the person with perceptual distortion. Preventing flashbacks is not a possibility. Physiologic dependence does not occur with hallucinogens, and the cardiovascular system is unaffected. *(NB, implementing; LDM, shared)*

Wilson and Kneisl (1979), pp. 331, 552

494. A. Symptoms of cocaine overdosage are essentially the same as for amphetamines, including cardiac arrhythmias, shock, and death. Gangrene, septicemia, and vascular rupture are not associated with cocaine overdosage. *(NB, assessing; LDM, nurse centered)*

Wilson and Kneisl (1979), p. 551

495. D. Drug dependence may result from taking prescribed drugs for a physiologic problem such as low-back pain. It would be important to obtain a medication history from this patient to determine if he has been taking any drugs that could result in withdrawal symptoms. Assessing financial status and family support are secondary concerns. There is insufficient information to indicate that this person is anything but fully conscious. *(NB, assessing; LDM, shared)*

Burgess, pp. 522–523

496. D. Benzodiazepines such as diazepam (Valium) potentiate the central nervous system depressive action of alcohol, making this a potentially lethal combination. Tranquilizers have been associated with birth defects and would not be safe during pregnancy. Prescription drugs taken as directed can produce physical dependency. Nutritional status and dependency on antianxiety agents are not related. *(NB, planning; LDM, client centered)*

Haber et al., pp. 402–403

497. C. Addicts frequently seek help only when external pressures from courts, family, or job, force them to do so. These addicts may represent excellent candidates for successful treatment, since research indicates such patients do almost as well as individuals entering programs on a purely voluntary basis. In most cases psychologic dependence rather than physical dependence poses the greatest obstacle to recovery. Withdrawal states from narcotics are uncomfortable but not dangerous. Addicts use drugs because of unconscious psychologic conflicts and use defense mechanisms to avoid reality. *(NB, analyzing; LDM, shared)*

Burgess, pp. 525–529

498. C. Long-range treatment of the addicted client is based upon helping the person learn better mechanisms for coping with stress and problems. Positive reinforcement of problem solving that is not drug oriented would help the client improve his low self-esteem. Demanding abstinence from drugs without providing knowledge of alternative resources or opportunity to practice skills necessary for lifestyle changes is an unrealistic, self-defeating approach. Imposing restrictions does not support positive behavioral changes; a more appropriate method of limit setting is preferred. Using street language may be perceived as accepting use of drugs. *(NB, planning; LDM, shared)*

Haber et al., pp. 524–525, 530;
Wilson and Kneisl (1979), p. 332

499. B. Recreational use of caffeine is not considered problematic. Use of alcohol daily may accelerate, particularly in a vulnerable person. Smoking a pack of cigarettes daily maintains physical dependence upon nicotine and can be harmful to the person's general health. Use of marijuana would be discouraged in a person who is being rehabilitated in a drug abuse program. *(NB, evaluating; LDM, client centered)*

Burgess, pp. 525–527

500. A. Opiates and amphetamines have strong reinforcement capacity as pleasure-producing agents and escapes from internal and external psychic stress. Hallucinogens produce psychologic dependence and mild tolerance, and users gain secondary reinforcement from belonging to a user group. Marijuana produces psychologic dependence but its effects are less potent than those of other drugs. Sedatives produce physical and psychologic dependence and can be used to escape from interpersonal difficulties; their use produces secondary reinforcement. *(NB, evaluating; LDM, client centered)*

Burgess, pp. 523–526

501. C. Assuming that this client's old friends are still using drugs, it would be easy to slip back into previous drug habits since they would support his reentry into their special group. This client does need the support of others, but his support would be better obtained through the clinic staff. Social stigma does not appear to be an issue for this client. Methadone maintenance is a useful treatment modality for heroin addicts, and there is no evidence this approach would be ineffective for this client. *(NB, evaluating; LDM, shared)*

Haber et al., p. 510;
Burgess, pp. 533–534

502. B. Specially developed day-care programs are useful for individuals unwilling to enter residential facilities because they provide structure and concentrated group experience. Reinforcing a decision that is not in the patient's best interests would not be appropriate. The client's family may ultimately need to become involved in the outpatient treatment plan. There are no data to support the conclusion the client is being manipulative. *(NB, analyzing; LDM, shared)*

Burgess, pp. 532–533

References

Aguilera, D. and Messick, J.: *Crisis Intervention: Theory and Methodology,* 4th Ed. St. Louis: C.V. Mosby, 1982.

Blattner, B.: *Holistic Nursing.* Englewood Cliffs, N.J.: Prentice-Hall, 1981.

Burgess, A.: *Psychiatric Nursing in the Hospital and the Community,* 3rd Ed. Englewood Cliffs, N.J.: Prentice-Hall, 1981.

Clunn, P.A. and Payne, D.B.: *Psychiatric-Mental Health Nursing: Nursing Outline Series,* 3rd Ed. Garden City, N.Y.: Medical Examination Publishing Co., 1982.

Diagnostic and Statistical Manual of Mental Disorders, 3rd Ed. (DSM III) Washington, D.C.: American Psychiatric Association, 1980.

Estes, N., Smith-DiJulio, K., and Heinemann, M.: *Nursing Diagnosis of the Alcoholic Person.* St. Louis: C.V. Mosby, 1980.

Fields, S. and Sherman, J.: *Guide to Patient Evaluation,* 4th Ed. Garden City, N.Y.: Medical Examination Publishing Co., 1982.

Freidman, M.: *Family Nursing: Theory and Assessment.* New York: Appleton-Century-Crofts, 1980.

Grace, H. and Camilleri, D.: *Mental Health Nursing,* 2nd Ed. Dubuque, IA: William C. Brown, 1981.

Haber, J., Leach, A., Schudy, A., and Sideleau, B.: *Comprehensive Psychiatric Nursing,* 2nd Ed. New York: McGraw-Hill, 1982.

Hahn, A. et al.: *Pharmacology in Nursing,* 15th Ed. St. Louis: C.V. Mosby, 1982.

Kolb, L.C., *Modern Clinical Psychiatry,* 10th Ed. Philadelphia: W.B. Saunders, 1977.

Lancaster, J.: *Adult Psychiatric Nursing.* Garden City, N.Y.: Medical Examination Publishing Co., 1980.

Luckmann, J. and Sorensen, K.: *Medical-Surgical Nursing,* 2nd Ed. Philadelphia: W.B. Saunders, 1980.

Morgan, C.T., King, R.A., and Robinson, N.M.: *Introduction to Psychology,* 6th Ed. New York: McGraw-Hill, 1979.

Pasquali, E., Alesi, E., Arnold, H., and De Basio, N.: *Mental Health Nursing.* St. Louis: C.V. Mosby, 1981.

Patterson, C.H.: *Theories of Counseling and Psychotherapy.* New York: Harper and Row, 1966.

Robinson, L.: *Psychiatric Nursing as a Human Experience,* 3rd Ed. Philadelphia: W.B. Saunders, 1983.

Schultz, D.: *Theories of Personality.* Monterey, CA: Brooks-Cole Publishers, 1976.

Stuart, G. and Sundeen, S.: *Principles and Practice of Psychiatric Nursing.* St. Louis: C.V. Mosby, (1st Ed., 1979; 2nd Ed., 1983).

Taylor, C.: *Mereness' Essentials of Psychiatric Nursing,* 11th Ed. St. Louis: C.V. Mosby, 1982.

Wilson, H. and Kneisl, C.: *Psychiatric Nursing.* Menlo Park, CA: Addison-Wesley, (1st Ed., 1979; 2nd Ed., 1983).